# PRAISE FOR *EAT MORE, WEIGH LESS*

"If you were to read only one book on diet and nutrition, this should be it. Dr. Ornish raises this subject to a new level. This book will change your body, mind and health."

Larry Dossey, M.D.,
author of *Meaning and Medicine*

"A fabulous book. The whole concept is brilliant. This book presents a compelling philosophy of life that will revolutionize your relationships— to yourself, to your loved ones, and to the universe."

Joan Borysenko, Ph.D.,
author of *Minding the Body, Mending the Soul*

"Thanks to Ornish's ultra-low-fat program, you can eat more, eat more frequently and still lose weight simply, safely and easily. . . . The highlight of the book is the lineup of creative low-fat recipes. . . . These are innovative meals with many layers of magnificent flavor. Ornish proves beyond a doubt that there is flavor after fat."

*Houston Post*

"Dr. Ornish has done it again! His program is sound science, is very practical, and is very personal. It makes sense in every way. This book is must reading."

T. Colin Campbell, Ph.D.,
Jacob Gould Shurman Professor of
Nutritional Biochemistry and Director,
China Diet Health Project, Cornell University

"The noted doctor and bestselling author strikes gold again. . . . Ornish explains how and why foods we eat make us not only fat but also weak and susceptible to disease. You'll learn the latest on why yo-yo dieting ultimately fails; why moderate exercise is more effective than heart-pumping aerobics for weight loss; and some different ways to nourish your soul without a visit to the refrigerator."

*Longevity*

"*Eat More, Weigh Less* is compelling, whether you follow the program religiously for medical or weight-loss reasons or simply sprinkle the healthful and creative recipes into your own cooking repertoire."

*Food & Wine*

"Startling as it sounds, 'Eat more, weigh less' can make sense. . . . His diet is easy to grasp: As long as you eat until you're full, not stuffed, you can have as much as you want of fruits, vegetables, grains and legumes. You can consume other fat-free and very low-fat foods in moderation. . . . Despite several lapses over the course of the month, our dieters lost from three to six pounds. . . . The dieter who stuck with it most faithfully was hoping to lower her high cholesterol count. In one month her cholesterol plummeted from 270 to 160. . . . At the two-week point, several of the women said they felt more energetic. . . . Cravings aside, all participants found the diet relatively easy to follow at home."

*Glamour*

## Books by Dean Ornish, M.D.

LOVE AND SURVIVAL

EVERYDAY COOKING WITH DR. DEAN ORNISH

EAT MORE, WEIGH LESS

DR. DEAN ORNISH'S PROGRAM FOR REVERSING HEART DISEASE

STRESS, DIET, AND YOUR HEART

# *Eat More,* WEIGH LESS

## Dr. Dean Ornish's Program for Losing Weight Safely While Eating Abundantly

DEAN ORNISH, M.D.

HarperTorch
*An Imprint of* HarperCollins*Publishers*

Grateful acknowledgment is made for permission to reprint a *Cathy* cartoon. *Cathy* copyright © 1987 by Cathy Guisewite. Distributed by Universal Press Syndicate. Reprinted with permission. All rights reserved.

The height and weight tables on pages 52–53 are reprinted courtesy of Metropolitan Life Insurance Company.

The recipes for Spicy Cinnamon-Chili Paste, Tomato Ketchup, and Persimmon Relish are from *Adventures in the Kitchen* by Wolfgang Puck. Copyright © 1991 by Wolfgang Puck. Reprinted by permission of Random House, Inc.

HARPERTORCH
*An Imprint of* HarperCollins*Publishers*
10 East 53rd Street
New York, New York 10022-5299


ISBN: 0-06-109627-X



First HarperTorch paperback printing: January 2002
First HarperCollins mass market printing: April 1997
First HarperCollins trade paperback printing: August 1994
First HarperCollins hardcover printing: June 1993

HarperCollins®, HarperTorch™, and ™ are trademarks of HarperCollins Publishers Inc.

Printed in the United States of America

Visit HarperTorch on the World Wide Web at www.harpercollins.com

20 19 18 17

*For Molly*

# *Contents*

## PART THREE

# *Eat More,* WEIGH LESS

# *Foreword*

I wrote *Eat More, Weigh Less* in 1993 in hopes that it would help people lose weight, feel better, and become healthier. Since then, I have received thousands of letters every year from people who have lost weight and kept it off.

Recently, for example, a man named Mark Nichols came to my office and showed me a photograph of how he looked two years earlier. I hardly recognized him—because he weighed 335 pounds then and only 165 pounds now. He lost 170 pounds by following the program outlined in *Eat More, Weigh Less* and has not regained it.

I find it gratifying to know that when people make the diet and lifestyle changes I recommend, they not only lose weight but also improve their health and well-being. That's why I wrote *Eat More, Weigh Less*, to provide a doorway to better health as well as the easiest and most optimal way to lose weight and to keep it off. Safely. Simply. Easily. Without hunger, and with feelings of abundance rather than deprivation.

It is true that one can lose weight on just about any diet if calories are restricted and/or energy expenditure is increased (i.e., exercise). There are three major ways of eating fewer calories:

1. *Eat fewer calories by eating less food.* Count calories, restrict portion sizes, etc. Sooner or later, most people get tired of feeling hungry and deprived, get off the diet, gain the weight back, and blame themselves for not having enough discipline or motivation or willpower, which is why most diets work in the short run but not in the long run. Also, when you restrict the amount of food, then metabolic rate decreases as well since your body thinks you are starving. If you really are in a famine, then you want to burn calories more slowly, as this gives you a survival advantage. But if you are trying to lose weight, then this can be frustrating.
2. *Eat foods that are less dense in calories (i.e., lower fat) and higher in fiber (i.e., avoid sugar and other simple carbohydrates).* When you eat less fat, you eat fewer calories without having to eat less food. As you know, fat has over twice as many calories/serving as protein or carbohydrates. So, when you go from a high fat to a low fat diet, even if you eat the same amount of food, you consume fewer calories without feeling hungry and deprived. Also, because the food is high in fiber, you get full before you consume too many calories. You can eat whenever you're hungry and still lose weight. And since you are not restricting the amount of food, metabolic rate does not decrease.
3. *Eat less sugar.* When you eat a lot of sugar and other simple carbohydrates, you consume a lot of calories without feeling full. Also, you provoke an insulin response which helps convert those calories into fat. However, a diet high in fiber and complex carbohydrates doesn't cause a spike in blood glucose because the fiber slows the rate of absorption. And the fiber fills you up before you get too many calories. You can only eat so many apples or pears before you get full, but you can consume virtually unlimited amounts of sugar without feeling full.

To me, the real issue is not only losing weight but also enhancing health. When you go from a meat-based diet to a plant-based diet, there is a double benefit: reducing the intake of disease-promoting substances (cholesterol, saturated fat, oxidants) and increasing the intake of disease-protecting substances (phytochemicals, bioflavinoids, retinols, isoflavones, etc.).

Also, it is not all or nothing. People often confuse the reversing heart disease diet, which is strict (because that's what it takes to reverse heart disease) with the weight loss diet, which can be more moderate. To the degree you move in that direction, there is a corresponding decrease in weight. How much change someone wants to make is a personal decision.

In 1998, my colleagues and I at the non-profit Preventive Medicine Research Institute published our research findings in the *Journal of the American Medical Association.*[1,2] We found that most of the study participants were able to maintain comprehensive diet and lifestyle changes for at least five years.

You can lose weight on just about any diet. Keeping it off is a lot harder. A few years ago, the government reviewed all the different weight loss plans. They found that two-thirds of people gained back all the weight they lost within a year, and 97 percent gained it all back within five years.

However, we found in our research that the average person lost twenty-four pounds in the first year and kept off more than half that weight five years later, even though they were eating more food, and more frequently, than before. Without hunger or deprivation. Simply. Safely. Easily.

And they weren't even trying to lose weight.

They not only *felt* better, they *were* better. We also found that they had even more reversal of heart disease after five years than after one year, and two-and-a-half times fewer cardiac events, including heart attack, stroke, bypass surgery, and angioplasty. The more closely people followed the program, the better they were. Clearly, if you can reverse heart disease by eating this way, then you can help prevent it as well.

In contrast, the randomized comparison group (who were making more moderate changes in diet and lifestyle with a 30 percent fat diet) showed progression (worsening) of their heart disease after one year and became even worse after five years. They also gained weight during the study.

A few months earlier, my colleagues and I published the results of the Multicenter Lifestyle Demonstration Project in the *American Journal of Cardiology*.[3] In the past, lifestyle changes have been viewed only as *prevention*, increasing costs in the short run for a possible savings years later. Now, our program is offered as a scientifically-proven alternative *treatment* to many patients who otherwise were eligible for coronary artery bypass surgery or angioplasty, resulting in an immediate and substantial cost savings.

In brief, we found that almost 80 percent of people who were eligible for bypass surgery or angioplasty were safely able to avoid it by making comprehensive lifestyle changes in the hospitals we trained. Mutual of Omaha calculated an immediate savings of almost $30,000 per patient. These patients reported reductions in angina (chest pain) comparable to what can be achieved with bypass surgery or angioplasty without the costs or risks of surgery.

More recently, Highmark Blue Cross Blue Shield has been providing as well as covering this diet and lifestyle program. Their results have been spectacular: of their first 300 patients, 299 avoided bypass surgery or angioplasty.

By now, you might be saying, "Hey, I don't have heart disease, I'm just trying to lose weight." But if it works this well to reverse heart disease, imagine how well it can work to help keep you healthy in other ways.

Increasing evidence shows that the *Eat More, Weigh Less* diet may help to prevent a wide variety of other illnesses in addition to enabling you to lose weight and to keep it off. These include breast cancer in women, prostate cancer in men, colon cancer, lung cancer, lymphoma, osteoporosis, diabetes, hypertension, and so on.

Also, heart disease is, by far, the leading cause of death in women as well as in men. Women don't undergo bypass surgery or angioplasty as often as men; when they do, they don't do as well.

Here's the good news: women seem to be able to reverse heart disease more easily than men. Many women are prescribed estrogen to lower their risk of heart disease or osteoporosis even though it increases the risk of breast cancer—not a good trade-off. When you go on the *Eat More, Weigh Less* diet, you may lower your risk of heart disease, osteoporosis, *and* breast cancer—without having to make these painful choices.

We tend to think of advances in medicine as a new drug, a new laser or surgical technique, something high-tech and expensive. We may have a hard time believing that the simple choices we make in our lives each day—like what we eat, how we respond to stress, exercise, smoking, and psychosocial support—can make such a powerful difference in our health and well-being, but they do. In our research, we used the latest high-tech, state-of-the-art measures to prove the power of these very ancient, low-tech, and low-cost interventions.

One of the interesting findings in our earlier studies was that older people showed just as much improvement as younger ones. No matter how old they were, on average, the more people changed their diet and lifestyle, the more they improved. This is a very hopeful message for Medicare patients, since the risks of bypass surgery and angioplasty increase with age, but the benefits of comprehensive lifestyle changes may occur at any age.

Because of these findings, Medicare began the first project to demonstrate if our program of comprehensive changes in diet and lifestyle may be a safe and cost effective alternative to conventional medical treatments for selected Medicare patients. This is exciting, because most other insurance companies follow Medicare's lead, thereby making the program available to the people who most need it.

My colleagues and I are trying to create a new model of medicine that is more caring and compassionate as well as more cost effective by addressing the causes of such chronic diseases as obesity and coronary heart disease rather than just bypassing them literally or figuratively . The program is a new model for lowering health care costs without compromising the quality of care or access to care.

Given so much success with our program, I am distressed that people are fatter than ever. A recent study by the Centers for Disease Control and Prevention found that the number of Americans considered obese—defined as being more than 30 percent over their ideal body weight—soared from about one in eight in 1991 to nearly one in five last year.[4]

It's not hard to figure out why. Americans are eating more fat than ever. For example, there was a 13 percent increase in fat consumption among men nineteen to fifty years old between 1990 and 1995, and a 21 percent increase in their total caloric intake over the same period, according to the USDA. In 1990 the average man ate 2,215 calories a day; in 1995, he was consuming 2,672 calories.[5]

The theme of all of my work is simple yet radical: if you don't address the underlying causes of a problem—any problem, including heart disease or obesity—then the same problem often comes back again, or you may get a new set of problems or side effects, or you may have painful choices. Whenever I lecture, I often begin by showing a cartoon of doctors busily mopping up the floor around a sink that's overflowing without also turning off the faucet.

One of my favorite movie scenes was in *Raiders of the Lost Ark* in which Harrison Ford, playing Indiana Jones, is confronted by a man whirling a sword doing his best kung fu routine. Bemused, Indiana Jones just pulls out a gun and shoots him.

A lot of people take the same approach to health and to losing weight. "Why bother to fool around with all this touchy-feely stuff like diet and exercise and meditation when you can just take a pill like fen-phen or Xenical or go on a high protein diet or have liposuction? Why change your diet and lifestyle when you can just fix it with a bypass operation or an angioplasty?"

Many people are finding that the quick fix doesn't last. Just as bypass surgery and angioplasty operations tend to clog up again within a few months or a few years, people who lose weight using the quick-fix approaches usually gain it all back or suffer side-effects ranging from annoying to disastrous.

For example, fenfluramine, sold as Pondimin, and dexfenfluramine, sold as Redux—taken together as "fen-phen"—were taken off the market, because they caused serious damage to heart valves. Some people dream about a drug that allows you to eat all the fat you want and not to absorb it. In real life, though, it remains just a dream.

The drug, orlistat, marketed under the brand name Xenical is not a quick fix. Xenical works by blocking absorption of one-third of the fat you eat each day. That means a patient taking the drug who eats 60 grams of fat a day may absorb only 40 grams of fat, and the other 20 grams will be excreted through the digestive tract. This drug will block about one-third of the fat you eat, but it is such a backwards approach. It makes so much more sense just to eat one-third less fat.

Like all drugs, Xenical has side effects. It acts in the intestines to block fat absorption. The drug prevents enzymes in the gastrointestinal track from breaking down the fat you eat into smaller molecules that can be absorbed by the body. Since it blocks the absorption of fat, it also blocks the absorption of some important fat-soluble vitamins, carotenoids, and other essential nutrients. One of the more disturbing side-effects for many people is anal leakage, two words that should never go together.

Confusion reigns. With the rise of the Internet, people have access to more information than ever, yet there is even less knowledge and wisdom to make sense of it. When the experts don't agree, many people are beginning to throw up their hands in exasperation and say, "These damn doctors, they can't make up their minds, to hell with 'em, I'll eat whatever I want and forget about it!"

For example, a recent story on the front page of *The New York Times* proclaimed, "Hormone that Slimmed Fat Mice Disappoints as Panacea in People." Yet the front page of the *San Francisco Chronicle* on the same day said, "Americans Getting Fatter Fast—Hormone Study Offers Hope." A cover story in *Time* magazine described the controversy over diets low in carbohydrates, but the lead article the same week in the *Journal of the American Medical Association* talked about the benefits of diets high in fiber and complex carbohydrates.

I am a scientist because the whole point of science is to say, "Prove it!" Just as Tom Cruise as Jerry Maguire said, "Show me the money!" a scientist says, "Show me the data!" To have something published in a peer-reviewed journal, you have to convince a "jury of your peers"—other well-regarded scientists—that what you say has facts to back it up.

Part of the value of science is to help you sort out conflicting claims, to distinguish fact from fancy, what sounds good from what is real. I'm not trying to tell you what to eat; just to provide you with scientifically-based information so that you can make more informed and intelligent choices. To the best of my knowledge, none of the high-protein diet authors has ever published any studies in any peer-reviewed journals documenting that their approach can help people lose weight safely, keep it off, and improve their health. In contrast, my colleagues and I at the non-profit Preventive Medicine Research Institute have published our findings in the leading peer-reviewed medical journals.

I wrote *Eat More, Weigh Less* as a doorway for helping people make changes in the name of losing weight that also will help improve health in many other ways. Unfortunately, there has been a resurgence of interest in diets high in protein and low in carbohydrates in the past few years that have the opposite effect.

When people follow a high-fat, high-protein diet to lose weight, they may mortgage their health in the process. Having seen what a powerful difference changes in diet and lifestyle can make, I want to pull out what's left of my hair to see the renewed interest in diets that may be harmful to your health. These diets are hazardous to your health. They were first popularized by an undertaker in the 1800s—maybe he needed more business.

For example, a recent study by Richard Fleming, M.D., published in the peer-reviewed journal *Angiology*, examined blood flow to the heart in those who followed a high protein diet or who followed a low-fat, whole foods diet.[6] After a year, blood flow to the heart became measurably worse in those on a high protein diet but improved significantly in those on a low-fat, whole foods diet. (For a picture of these scans, as well as a list of recommended vitamins and supplements and lots of recipes, please go to my web site at WebMD by going to www.Ornish.com.) This is not surprising, since studies have shown that even a single high-fat meal can impair blood flow.[7]

To the best of my knowledge, none of the high-protein diet authors has ever published any studies in any peer-reviewed journals documenting that their approach can help people lose weight safely and keep it off. In contrast, my colleagues and I at the non-profit Preventive Medicine Research Institute have.

Telling people that pork rinds and sausage are good for you is a great way to sell books, but it is irresponsible and dangerous for those who follow their advice. I would like to be able to tell you that these are health foods, but they're not.

Fortunately, there is a way to safely lose even more weight while eating great foods in abundance. Here's the real skinny on fat:

There is a large body of scientific evidence from epidemiological studies, animal research, and randomized controlled trials in humans showing that high protein foods, particularly excessive animal protein, dramatically increase the risk of breast cancer, prostate cancer, heart disease, and many other illnesses. In the short run, they may also cause kidney problems, loss of calcium in the bones, and an unhealthy metabolic state called ketosis in many people. The American Dietetic Association recently condemned high-protein diets as being dangerous, "a nightmare of a diet."

In contrast, whole foods such as fruits, vegetables, grains, and beans contain literally thousands of other substances that are protective, having anti-aging, anti-cancer, and anti-heart disease properties. These include fiber, isoflavones, carotenoids, bioflavinoids, retinols, lycopene, geninstein, on and on.

Most people don't really think anything bad will ever happen to them. They think prevention is *borrrrr-ing*: "I don't care if I die sooner, I want to *enjoy* my life."

So do I. But how much fun are you having if you're feeling tired, lethargic, and impotent? Or dead?

When you go on a high protein diet, you may get less blood flow to your most important organs. When you get less blood flow to your brain, you may feel more tired and you think less clearly. (Think about a time when you had a rich Thanksgiving feast, and how you felt afterwards.) When you get less blood flow to your heart, you increase your risk of chest pain or a heart attack. And when you get less blood flow to your sexual organs, your sexual potency decreases.

When I was in medical school, we were taught that most impotence began in your brain—psychological. We now know it usually begins in your arteries—physiological. The reason that Viagra is one of the best-selling drugs of all time is that so many people need it. Impotence, also called "erectile dysfunction," is a silent epidemic, present in at least one-half of men over the age of forty. Did you know you're much more likely to be impotent if your cholesterol level is elevated?[8, 9, 10] Knowing this is a lot more motivating for many men than telling them they're going to live to be eighty-six instead of eighty-five—even when they're eighty-five.

Not to mention bad breath and body odor. Your body excretes toxic substances like excessive amounts of meat in your breath, perspiration, and bowels. When you eat a lot of meat, it takes a long time for it to make its way through your digestive tract. As it putrefies and decays, your breath smells bad, your sweat smells bad, and your bowels smell bad. Not very attractive. You may want to lose weight to attract people to you, but when they get too close, it becomes counterproductive.

A study commissioned by Dr. Atkins of his diet plan, conducted by Dr. Eric Westman of Duke, was presented by him at a debate that I had with Dr. Atkins earlier this year that was sponsored by the United States Department of Agriculture.[11] In this study, not yet published, 65 percent of the participants had halitosis, 70 percent were constipated, 10 percent reported hair loss, and 54 percent reported headaches.

Yet many people do lose weight on high-protein diets, and cholesterol levels may even decrease. How can this be?

*The important distinction to make is between simple carbohydrates and whole foods,* also called complex carbohydrates. The dangerous half truth is this: simple carbohydrates may cause you to gain weight, but complex carbohydrates help you lose weight. This is not a new idea, and I wrote about this in *Eat More, Weigh Less* when it was first published in 1993 (please refer to the section in chapter 4 entitled, *"How Sweet it Isn't"*). The goal is not to switch from simple carbohydrates to a diet consisting mainly of high-protein foods like meat but from simple carbohydrates to whole foods, while reducing your intake of high-protein animal foods. As I wrote in that section, you can actually gain weight on a low-fat diet if it's high in sugar and other simple carbohydrates.

Simple carbohydrates—sugar and other concentrated sweeteners, and alcohol, which your body converts to sugar—are absorbed quickly, causing your blood sugar to increase rapidly. White flour (including foods like white flour pasta) and white rice are also absorbed quickly, because the fiber and bran have been removed. In response, your body secretes insulin to lower your blood sugar levels to normal.

However, chronically elevated insulin levels also accelerate the conversion of calories into fat, raise your cholesterol level, and have other harmful effects. Over time, like the boy who cried wolf, the insulin receptors say, "Oh, not more insulin!" and become less sensitive to its effects, causing your body to secrete even more insulin in a vicious cycle.

The high-protein authors advise us to avoid all carbohydrates and eat high-protein foods, because these are less likely to provoke an insulin response. Instead of going from simple carbohydrates to pork rinds, a better choice is to go from simple carbohydrates to complex carbohydrates, or whole foods.

Whole foods (complex carbohydrates)—including whole

wheat, brown rice, and fruits, vegetables, grains, beans, and soy products in their natural form—are rich in fiber, which slows their absorption. Since they are absorbed slowly, your blood sugar does not spike, and so your body does not need to produce elevated levels of insulin.

Instead of the rapid swings in blood sugar, you experience a more constant feeling of energy throughout the day. You become more sensitive to insulin rather than resistant to it; diabetics often are able to reduce or discontinue insulin under their doctor's supervision when they eat a low-fat, whole foods diet.

Even white flour pasta is OK in moderation if you eat it with lots of veggies or legumes on top, as the fiber from these foods will slow their absorption. A recent article in the *Journal of the American Medical Association* clearly documented that high fiber diets lower insulin levels.[12] In contrast, meat has virtually no dietary fiber.

Why do some people lose weight on the high protein diets? Most people in this country eat a lot of simple carbohydrates, so there is a lot of room for improvement when they switch to a high protein diet. A recent study showed that one-third of the vegetables eaten in the United States are either French fries or potato chips. And consumption of sugar, white flour, and processed foods has increased significantly in the past two decades, along with obesity.

Eating a lot of meat instead of all those simple carbohydrates will help lower their insulin response, causing them to lose weight. But they may be mortgaging their health in the process.

There is a better way. If you switch from simple carbohydrates to a whole foods, low-fat plant-based diet, then you don't provoke an exaggerated insulin response—so you get the insulin benefit similar to being on a diet high in animal protein without the many harmful effects. Also, you are eating whole foods that are much lower in fat and cholesterol, so you lose even more weight than on a high-protein diet and your cholesterol levels come down even further.

In our studies, for example, we found a 40 percent *average* reduction in LDL cholesterol without using drugs. And you're getting thousands of substances that are protective rather than harmful.

Most weight loss plans are based on deprivation: counting calories, restricting portion sizes, and eating less food. Sooner or later, people get tired of feeling hungry, so they get off the diet, regain the weight, and usually blame themselves for not having enough discipline, willpower, or motivation, when the real problem is that they were going about it in the wrong way.

Here's a better way: if you change the *type* of food, you don't have to reduce the *amount* of food. To lose weight, you have to reduce intake of calories. The laws of physics and thermodynamics still apply.

One way is to eat less food, which is difficult. The other is to change the type of food, to eat foods that are less dense in calories.

Fat has nine calories per grams whereas protein and carbohydrates have only four calories per gram. So, when you eat less fat, you eat fewer calories even if you eat the same amount of food—because low-fat foods are less dense in calories. You feel better and you become healthier. You really can eat more and weigh less if you know what to eat.

For example, if you go from a 40 percent fat diet to a 10 percent fat diet, even if you eat the same amount of food, you consume almost one-third fewer calories. Excess calories of any kind—whether they come from carbohydrates, fat or protein—will eventually be converted by insulin into body fat. The easiest way to reduce your intake of calories is to reduce your intake of fat and simple carbohydrates.

It's not all or nothing. Many people think that the only diet I recommend is 10 percent fat because this is the diet that we found could reverse heart disease. But if you're only trying to lose weight, you don't have to eat such a restrictive diet. To the degree you move in that direction, you will get a corresponding benefit. You have a spectrum of choices.

In short, when you switch from a diet based on animal protein and simple carbohydrates to a whole foods, plant-based diet, you get a quadruple benefit:

- the high fiber content of fruits, vegetables, grains, and beans reduces insulin levels, so you lose weight and lower cholesterol levels;
- when you eat less fat, you eat fewer calories without eating less food;
- you avoid the animal-based products rich in substances that cause illnesses; and
- you get thousands of other substances that are protective.

If you eat a low fat diet based on whole foods, you are likely to lose even more weight than on a high protein diet, your cholesterol levels may come down even more, and you may feel better, look better, and love better. The more you move in this direction, the more benefits you receive. And you may significantly reduce the risk of heart disease, cancer, and other illnesses rather than increasing it. You can lose weight and gain health.

—Dean Ornish, M.D.
Founder and President,
Preventive Medicine Research Institute
Clinical Professor of Medicine,
University of California, San Francisco
Sausalito, California
September 21, 2001

**REFERENCES:**

1 Ornish D, Scherwitz L, Billings J, et al. Can intensive lifestyle changes reverse coronary heart disease? Five-year follow-up of the Lifestyle Heart Trial. JAMA. 1998; 280:2001-2007.

2 Ornish D. Concise Review: Intensive lifestyle changes in the management of coronary heart disease. *Harrison's Principles of Internal Medicine* (online), edited by Eugene Braunwald et al., 1999.

3 Ornish D. Avoiding Revascularization with Lifestyle Changes: The Multicenter Lifestyle Demonstration Project. *American Journal of Cardiology.* 1998; 82:72T-76T.

4 Mokdad AH, Serdula MK, Dietz WH, et al. The Spread of the Obesity Epidemic in the United States, 1991-1998. JAMA. 1999; 282:1519-1522.

5 Sugarman C. Eat fat, get thin? *The Washington Post.* Tuesday, November 23, 1999, page H12.

6 Fleming RM, Boyd LB. The Effect of High-Protein Diets on coronary blood flow. Angiology. 200:51(10), 817-26.

7 Vogel RA, Corretti MC, Plotnick GD. Effect of a Single High-Fat Meal on Endothelial Function in Healthy Subjects. *Am J Cardiol.* 1997; 79:350-354.

8 Azadzoi KM, Saenz de Tejada I. Hypercholesterolemia Impairs Endothelium-Dependent Relaxation of Rabbit Corpus Cavernosum Smooth Muscle. *Journal of Urology.* 1991; 146(1):238-40.

9 Butler RN, Lewis MI, Hoffman E, Whitehead ED. Love and sex After 60. *Geriatrics.* 1994; 49(10):27-32.

10 Kim JH, Klyachkin ML, Svendsen E, et al. Experimental Hypercholesterolemia in Rabbits Induces cavernosal Atherosclerosis with Endothelial and Smooth Muscle Cell Dysfunction. *Journal of Urology.* 1994; 151(1):198-205.

11 A complete transcript of this debate is available at www.USDA.gov/cnpp.

12 Ludwig DS, Pereira MA, Kroenke CH, et al. Dietary Fiber, Weight Gain, and Cardiovascular Disease Risk factors in Young Adults. *JAMA.* 1999; 282:1539-1546.

# *Author's Note*

Dr. Ornish's Program is an adjunct to, not a substitute for, conventional medical therapy. If you have coronary heart disease, obesity, or other health problems, please consult your physician before beginning this program. Each person is different, and decisions affecting your health are personal, ones that you should make only after consulting with your physician and other health professionals. If you are taking medications, your physician may wish to decrease or discontinue some or all of these if your clinical status improves. Do *not* make any changes in your medications without first consulting your doctor; it can be very dangerous to suddenly stop taking some drugs.

No treatment program, including drugs, surgery, or lifestyle changes, is effective for everyone. Some people may not lose weight or may become worse despite any treatments or lifestyle changes.

This book is based on the latest in scientific information. Since science is always evolving, further understanding of human nutrition may lead to changes in the recommendations contained here.

One of my goals in writing this book is to help increase your understanding of how powerful lifestyle choices can be in affecting your health and well-being. Another goal is to strengthen the communication between you and your doctor.

In this context, you may wish to share this book with him or her. Discuss it with your doctor so that the two of you can work together more effectively to help you achieve greater health and happiness.

# *Acknowledgments: "You're Writing What?"*

Whenever I told my research colleagues that I was writing a new book, they usually asked me, "So, what are you going to call it?" When I replied, "*Eat More, Weigh Less,*" they would usually blink a few times and, trying to be diplomatic, reply, "Oh, *that's* nice. . . ." The more forthright said, "You're writing *what*? Don't you think you might lose some of your credibility as a researcher if you write a weight-loss book? Some people might start thinking of you as a diet doctor!"

But this is really much more than just a weight-loss book. And I am a research scientist and a specialist in internal medicine, not a diet doctor.

This is a book about improving your health and well-being. It's a book about learning how to begin healing emotional pain, loneliness, and isolation in your life. And, yes, this is a book that describes a new program that can really help you to lose weight without deprivation or hunger.

Besides helping you to lose weight and keep it off, this program has other benefits that mean even more to me, as a physician, than weight loss. But if I wrote a book entitled *How to Prevent Heart Disease, Obesity, Stroke, Breast Cancer, Prostate Cancer, Colon Cancer, Osteoporosis, Diabetes, Hypertension, and Lots of Other Illnesses,* you might not read it. The same might be true for a book on emotional and spiritual transformation. I hope that the attraction of really being able to eat more and weigh less also opens the door for you to better health and well-being in many other ways.

A rather large number of people have made this book possible, either directly by contributing to it or indirectly by helping to make possible the research upon which it is based. It gives me great pleasure to write this section and to remember how grateful I am for each person's contribution. Of course, the fact that I have acknowledged them here does not necessarily mean that they agree with everything in this book.

I especially appreciate the gifted chefs who have created recipes for this book. These are chefs' chefs, the crème de la crème (probably not the most appropriate metaphor), the best of the best. We have learned that the optimal way to make low-fat foods taste great is not necessarily to work with vegetarian chefs or health food chefs; instead, we found the best well-trained chefs and asked them to work within these dietary guidelines. In this book, I am honored and grateful to include recipes from Paul Bertolli (Chez Panisse, Berkeley), Daniel Boulud (Le Cirque, New York), Judith Ets-Hokin, Susan Feniger (City Restaurant, Los Angeles), Jean-Marc Fullsack (California Culinary Academy, San Francisco), Joyce Goldstein (Square One, San Francisco), Hubert Keller (Fleur de Lys, San Francisco), Michael Lomonaco ("21," New York City), Deborah Madison (*The Greens Cookbook*), Michael McDermott (*The Healthful Gourmet*), Mary Sue Milliken (City Restaurant, Los Angeles), Donna Nicoletti (Undici, San Francisco), Bradley Ogden (Lark Creek Inn, Larkspur, California), Catherine Pantsios (Zola's, San Francisco), Alfred Portale (Gotham Bar & Grill, New York City), Wolfgang Puck (Spago, Los Angeles, and Postrio, San Francisco), Tracy Pikhart Ritter (Golden Door Health Spa, Escondido, California) assisted by Jill O'Conner, Alain Rondelli (Ernie's, San Francisco), Martha Rose Shulman (*Mediterranean Light*), and Barbara Trapp (China Moon, San Francisco). Also included are recipes from John and Phyllis Cardozo, Joe and Anita

Cecena, Hank and Phyllis Ginsberg, Victor and Lydia Karpenko, Conrad and Marsha Knudsen, Sharon Luce, Dennis and Margaret Malone, Myrna Melling, Natalie Ornish, Paul Paulsen and Don Vaupel. Recipes were tested and, in some cases, modified by Tina Salter and Christina Swett.

This book is based on three research studies that my colleagues and I have conducted during the past seventeen years.

Principal research collaborators included William T. Armstrong, M.D., Paul Baum, Ph.D., James H. Billings, Ph.D., M.P.H., Richard J. Brand, Ph.D., Shirley Brown, M.D. (co-principal investigator), Amy Gage, K. Lance Gould, M.D., Richard Kirkeeide, Ph.D., LaVeta Luce, R.N., Marjorie McClain, Pat McKenna, M.D., Sandra McLanahan, M.D., Myrna Melling, Terri Merritt, M.S. (who, along with George Leonard and Michael Murphy, also provided background research on exercise for chapter 5), Barbara Musser, M.B.A., Carol Naber, Thomas Ports, M.D., Mary Dale Scheller, M.S.W., Larry Scherwitz, Ph.D. (co-principal investigator), Lawrence Spann, P.A.C., and Stephen Sparler, M.A.

Other collaborators included Celeste Burwell, Pamela Lea Byrne, Ph.D., R.N., M.S., M.F.C.C., Mary Carroll, Carol Connell, Jean-Marc Fullsack, Richard Goldstein, M.D., Mark Hall, Mary Haynie, R.N., Mary Jane Hess, R.N., Georgie Hesse, R.N., Dale Jones, R.T., David Liff, Ana Regalia, Yvonne Stuart, R.T., and Mary Tiberi, R.N.

Referring physicians and angiographers included William T. Armstrong, M.D., Damian Augustin, M.D., G. James Avery, M.D., Richard Axelrod, M.D., Wayne Bayless, M.D., Robert Bernstein, M.D., Robert Blau, M.D., Craig Brandman, M.D., Bruce Brent, M.D., Roger Budge, M.D., Michael Bunim, M.D., Michael Chase, M.D., James A. Clever, M.D., Keith E. Cohn, M.D., James Cullen, M.D., Daniel Elliott, M.D., Richard Francoz, M.D., Gordon Fung, M.D., Kent Gershengorn, M.D., Gabriel Gregoratos, M.D., Lloyd W. Gross, M.D., Robert Hulworth, M.D., Timothy Hurley, M.D., Gerson Jacobs, M.D., Herbert Jacobs, M.D., Lester Jacobson, M.D., Thomas J. Kaiser, M.D., William Kapla, M.D., Hilliard Katz, M.D., John Kelly, Jr., M.D.,

Jonathan Keroes, M.D., Edward Kersh, M.D., Frederick London, M.D., Randall Low, M.D., Myron Marx, M.D., Roy Meyer, M.D., Felix Millhouse, M.D., Frederick Mintz, M.D., Gene Nakamoto, M.D., Gerald Needleman, M.D., Morris Noble, M.D., Paul Ogden, M.D., Philip O'Keefe, M.D., Thomas Olwin, M.D., James Reid, M.D., J. Patrick Robertson, M.D., John Sarconi, M.D., H.C. Segars, M.D., Arthur Selzer, M.D., Gene Shafton, M.D., Joel Sklar, M.D., Richard Strauss, M.D., Brian Strunk, M.D., Martin Terplan, M.D., William Thomas, M.D., Anne Thorson, M.D., Michael Volen, M.D., Jon Wack, M.D., and Mark Wexman, M.D.

William T. Armstrong, M.D. (Chief of Cardiology, California Pacific Medical Center), Keith Marton, M.D. (Chief of Medicine, California Pacific Medical Center), and Floyd C. Rector, M.D. (Chief of Medicine, School of Medicine, University of California, San Francisco) provided ongoing support for our clinical research, and I am grateful.

Our research was conducted under the auspices of the Preventive Medicine Research Institute (PMRI), a nonprofit, independent research institute. Board members Martin Bucksbaum, Jenard Gross, Frank Lorenzo, Stuart Moldaw, Jay Pritzker, and Fenton R. Talbott. They provided encouragement, guidance, and financial support at a time when this project was only a dream, and they have provided ongoing vision and leadership, for which I remain deeply grateful. I feel blessed by their friendship.

The major hospitals collaborating on our study have been Presbyterian Hospital of California Pacific Medical Center, Moffitt Hospital of the University of California, San Francisco, University of California, Berkeley, and the University of Texas Medical School, Houston.

Generous support was also provided by the John E. Fetzer Institute (with special appreciation to the late John Fetzer, Robert Lehman, Judith Skutch Whitson, Bruce Fetzer, and others), the National Heart, Lung, and Blood Institute of the National Institutes of Health (RO1 HL42554, with appreciation to Stephen Weiss, Ph.D., Peter Kaufmann, Ph.D., Fred Heydrick, Ph.D., Antonio M. Gotto, Jr., M.D., and Claude Lenfant, M.D.), the Department of Health Services of the

State of California (#1256SC-01, with special appreciation to Assemblyman John Vasconcellos, Senators Art Torres and Nicholas Petris, Kenneth Kizer, M.D., Neal Kohatsu, M.D., the late Senator Bill Filante, and former governor George Duekmejian), Houston Endowment Inc. (J. Howard Creekmore and Jack Blanton), Gerald and Barbara Hines, the Henry J. Kaiser Family Foundation (Alvin R. Tarlov, M.D.), The Enron Corporation Foundation (Kenneth Lay), Continental Airlines/Texas Air Corporation (Frank Lorenzo), ConAgra, Inc. (Charles M. Harper, Philip Fletcher, and others), The First Boston Corporation (Fenton Talbott and others), Texas Commerce Bank (Ben Love), The Quaker Oats Company, The Emde Company, Corrine and David R. Gould, Dick and Kathy Dawson, General Growth Companies (Martin and Melva Bucksbaum), the Phyllis & Stuart Moldaw Philanthropic Fund, Gross Investments (Jenard and Gail Gross), Pritzker & Pritzker (Jay and Cindy Pritzker), Henry and Carol Groppe, Transco Energy Co., Pacific Presbyterian Medical Center Foundation (Dr. Bruce Spivey and Aubrey Serfling), Arthur Andersen & Co., Marvin and Marie Bomer, The Ziegler Corporation (Jack and Vyola Ziegler), Corporate Property Investors (Hans Mautner), The Ray C. Fish Foundation (James L. Daniel, Jr., Robert J. Cruikshank, CPA, and others), The Weatherhead Foundation (Albert and Celia Weatherhead), and the Nathan Cummings Foundation (Charles Halpern, Andrea Kydd, and others).

Additional support was provided by The Glenn Foundation (Paul Glenn and Mark Collins), Johnson & Johnson (Frank Barker), the M.B. Seretean Foundation, The Jewish Community Endowment Fund, United Savings Association of Texas, The Margoes Foundation (John Blum), Drexel Burnham Lambert (Michael Milken and Harry Horowitz), Hugh R. Goodrich, Edward O. Gaylord, Fayez Sarofim & Co., Eileen Rockefeller Growald, Lucy Rockefeller Waletzky, M.D., Biopsychosocial Research Fund of the Medical Illness Counseling Center, United Energy Resources, The Duncan Foundation (John Duncan), Mesa Petroleum (T. Boone Pickens), The Communities Foundation of Texas, Brown & Root, Inc. (T. Louis Austin, The Sackman Foundation, Physis Health Center (John Bagshaw, M.D.), Fenton and Judith Talbott, Leo Fields Family Philanthropic Fund, Bill and Uta Bone, Richard and Rhoda Goldman, Dr. and Mrs. James Langdon, Charles and Louise Gartner Philanthropic Fund, Frank A. Liddell, William and Lucero Meyer, Marianne Pallotti, Robert Finnell, T.B. Hudson, the Bob Hope International Heart Research Institute, Jeffrey Rhodes, Arnold and Carol Ablon, The William and Flora Hewlett Foundation, the Institute of Noetic Sciences (the late O'Regan), Pat McKenna, M.D., Werner and Eva Hebenstreit, Mel and Lenore Lefer, Amos and Dorian Krausz, Robert McAleese, Thomas Russell Potts, Victor and Lydia Karpenko, Edwin and Natalie Ornish, Simon and Paula Young, Doug Hawley, Van Gordon Sauter, PPG Industries, Burton Kaufman, James and Margaret Keith, Howard B. Wolf & Co., Joseph Frelinghuysen, Edward F. Kunin, David Harrison, Dr. Kit Peterson, Joseph Forgione, the Institute for the Advancement of Health, and others.

Jim Billings, Ph.D., has been like the big brother I never had, teaching me by his example. Alexander Leaf, M.D., has been both a mentor and a role model. Henry and Carol Groppe, Jenard and Gail Gross, and Gerald and Barbara Hines have been guardian angels. I feel grateful for our friendships.

For the past several years, I have been consulting with ConAgra, makers of Healthy Choice foods, to develop the "Advantage\10" line of frozen low-fat dinners in order to make it easy, convenient, and inexpensive to follow the program described in this book. I am particularly indebted to Brue Rhode, Tim McMahon, Jack McKeon, Frank Lynch, Steve Bakke, and John Mieckma.

David and Nora Plant contributed office space to the Preventive Medicine Research Institute, thereby making our work possible, and for which I am deeply grateful. Henry Feldman of the Claremont Hotel and Resort gave us rooms for our retreats at a discount, as did Manu Mobedshahi at the Sherman House, Ed Cohen at the Sherith Israel kitchen, and Marc Kaski at the Fort Mason Center.

Perhaps the person most directly responsible for this book

is Susan Moldow, who was editor-in-chief and vice-president of HarperCollins, the publisher of this book. Working with Susan has been an unmitigated pleasure, and I have grown to respect and admire her greatly. Others at HarperCollins who made important contributions to this book include: C. Linda Dingler, Carole Lalli, Kim Lewis, Joseph Montebello, Nancy K. Peske, David Rakoff, and Bill Shinker. More recently, I have been indebted to Diane Reverand and Jane Friedman at HarperCollins.

I wrote this book myself, so please do not hold the editors responsible for any lapses in grammar or style. Occasionally, I will violate standard usage (like starting a sentence with an adverb . . . ) if it makes the tone more relaxed and friendly. Some sentences are incomplete, and others are intentionally redundant to emphasize a point.

My appreciation and respect for Michael Rudell and Esther Newberg only increases over time. They embody a rare combination of intelligence, competence, and compassion.

I will always be indebted to my parents, Edwin and Natalie Ornish, for giving me the love, support, and education that enabled me to do this work, and to Louvada Reeves, who helped raise me. I am fortunate to be close with my siblings—Laurel, Steven (and his wife, Marty), and Kathy. Laurel also read the manuscript and provided helpful comments. Ronald Moskowitz has been my local family.

Much of what is in this book is a direct outgrowth of twenty years of study with Swami Satchidananda, the renowned spiritual teacher, for whom I have the deepest respect and appreciation.

The research upon which this book is based would not have been possible if the study participants had not had the courage, faith, and dedication to volunteer for our research. They demonstrated with their own lives that many people really can make and maintain comprehensive lifestyle changes for several years while living in the real world. No one else has ever demonstrated this. Their example gives us new hope, new possibilities, and new choices.

In the final analysis, this is really a book about transformation, not just a book on losing weight. Being overweight is not just a physical problem, so it needs to be addressed in a broader context. If you are overweight, then you know what it means to be in emotional pain. When you're suffering, though, your distress can be a catalyst, your wound an open doorway, to real healing.

# *Eat More,* WEIGH LESS

# PART ONE

# 1

# *Fed Up with Diets?*

Eat more, weigh less?

This book challenges the conventional wisdom. In it, I will present new scientific evidence that you really can eat more and weigh less—if you know what to eat. And that it's easier to make big changes in diet than moderate ones—if you know what changes to make.

When the conventional wisdom isn't working, an unconventional approach is worth considering. And the conventional wisdom about weight loss isn't working. A recent panel of weight-loss experts convened by the National Institutes of Health Nutrition Coordinating Committee concluded that none of the conventional approaches to losing weight is effective—in other words, most diets don't work.

"Evidence suggests that weight-loss regimes do more harm than good," said the panelists. "There is a strong tendency to regain weight, with as much as two-thirds of the weight lost regained within one year of completing the program and almost all by five years." Only 3 percent of those who take off weight keep it off for at least five years. Worse, the "yo-yo" pattern of going on a diet, losing some weight, and then gaining it back may be more harmful to your health than not going on a diet in the first place.

This pattern is familiar to just about anyone who has gone on a diet. And each time you go on another diet of deprivation, the weight becomes more difficult to lose, so you may become even more discouraged. This discouragement often leads to eating even more, causing more depression and overeating in a vicious cycle. You may blame yourself for being "destined to be fat" or for having "insufficient willpower," when what is really needed is clear, scientifically based information to help you make more successful choices.

The panelists went on: "Very-low-calorie diets and fasting are associated with a variety of short-term adverse effects. Patients frequently report fatigue, hair loss, dizziness, and other symptoms, but these appear to be transitory. More serious is the increased risk for gallstones and acute gallbladder disease during severe calorie restriction. . . ."

When I systematically reviewed the medical literature on diet, lifestyle, and weight loss, I was dismayed to learn how unsuccessful most weight-loss programs have been. In November 1992, for example, *The New York Times* ran a three-part series of front-page articles with titles like "For Most Trying to Lose Weight, Dieting Only Makes Things Worse" and "Commercial Diets Lack Proof of Their Long-Term Success." Here is a not-unusual example from *The New England Journal of Medicine* and *The New York Times* quoting a prominent weight-loss researcher:

> Over the years, he has been the leading proponent of the view that obesity is innate, or that some people are born to be fat . . . . "They will feel miserable," he said. "But if they can diet, they will be better off . . . . I don't want to discourage people about losing weight, but they will have to pay for it."

Here's a leading obesity specialist from Harvard Medical School:

> At least half of obese people—those who are more than 30% overweight—who try to diet down to "desirable" weights listed in the height-weight tables suffer medically, physically, and psychologically as a result, and would be better off fat.

According to a leading weight-loss researcher from the University of Pennsylvania:

> There is not one single commercial weight loss program that makes available any data on its results or even wants to know what they are . . . . It isn't happenstance that there's not a single bit of scientific evidence that they are effective. The studies are actively opposed by the weight reducing industry.

And in perhaps the most gloomy assessment, the editor of the *Harvard Medical School Health Letter* wrote:

> I can see no ethical basis for continuing research or treatment on weight loss.

In the face of this, is it any wonder that a growing number of people are asking, "Why bother? What's the use?" According to a recent front-page story in *The New York Times:*

> A growing number of women are joining in an anti-diet movement . . . which encourages people to stop weight-loss regimes, to eat in accord with their natural appetites and to make peace with their body size. They are forming support groups and ceasing to diet . . . . Others have smashed their bathroom scales . . . .

I understand this frustration. According to the conventional wisdom, you lose weight by counting calories, carefully keeping track of everything you consume, and depriving yourself by limiting the amount of food you eat. And "diet food" usually doesn't taste very good. Eventually you grow tired of the complexity, the hunger, the lack of flavor, and the feelings of deprivation. You abandon the diet and gain back the weight you lost—sometimes even more.

Despite the frustration with conventional diets, about one-half of women and one-fourth of men are currently trying to lose weight, with an additional one-quarter trying to maintain their weight. Even children are heavier than ever. Over one-third of children were overweight in 1991, compared with less than one-fourth only seven years earlier. One out of three girls ages eleven to eighteen is on a diet to lose weight.

## WEIGH MORE, EARN LESS

If it's so hard to lose weight, why do people keep trying? Because they know they'll look better. They'll feel better. And they know that being overweight may lead to serious health problems.

For example, in a recent study of more than 115,000 American women thirty to fifty-five years of age who were followed for eight years, those who were as little as 5 percent overweight were 30 percent more likely to develop heart disease. Those who were mildly to moderately overweight had a risk of coronary disease 80 percent higher than their lean counterparts. And those who were 30 percent or more overweight were over *300 percent* more likely to get it. Put in a more positive way, losing even a little weight may significantly improve your health and well-being. So even if you're only interested in losing ten or twenty pounds to look better, you'll also benefit in many other ways.

Overweight people are less likely to be hired for a job. They make less money for a given job than someone who is not overweight. For example, one study found that people are paid an average of $1,000 less in salary for each pound that they are overweight. Also, they are less likely to be promoted to higher paying jobs.

I'm sure you have many reasons of your own for wanting to lose some weight.

## WHY IS THIS PROGRAM SO DIFFERENT FROM CONVENTIONAL DIETS?

The program that I describe in this book is not just a diet to get on and then fall off—it's a more healthful way of eating and a happier way of living. It takes a new approach, one scientifically based on the *type* of food rather than the amount of food. Within the guidelines of the program, you have an exciting array of foods from which to choose, creating a sense of abundance rather than deprivation.

The average American consumes almost 40 percent of calories as fat. Diets such as Weight Watchers, Lean Cuisine, Jenny Craig, Nutri/System, Diet Center, the American Heart Association diet, and others reduce fat consumption to approximately 30 percent, so they must rely on small portion sizes to reduce calories sufficiently. Because the portion sizes are small, people often feel hungry and deprived.

On this program, in contrast, you'll consume less than 10 percent fat and almost no cholesterol. Because the meals are so low in fat, you'll get full before you consume too many calories. You can eat more frequently, eat a greater quantity of food—and still lose weight. Simply. Safely. Easily.

And the food is delicious, nutritious, and beautifully presented. In our research, we learned that the best way to make low-fat food taste good is to work with the best chefs and have them work within these guidelines.

In Part Three of this book, you'll find more than two hundred fifty recipes from some of the country's most celebrated chefs—like Joyce Goldstein of Square One in San Francisco, Paul Bertolli of Chez Panisse in Berkeley, Hubert Keller of Fleur de Lys in San Francisco, Susan Feniger and Mary Sue Milliken of City Restaurant in Los Angeles, Bradley Ogden of The Lark Creek Inn in Larkspur, California, Deborah Madison, author of *The Greens Cookbook,* now at Cafe Escalera in Santa Fe, Jean-Marc Fullsack, formerly of Lutèce in New York and an instructor at the California Culinary Academy, Michael Lomonaco of the "21" restaurant in New York City, and others.

CATHY / Cathy Guisewite
THIS IS MY LUNCH ??
THAT'S YOUR 300-CALORIE LUNCH.
THIS IS A 300-CALORIE LUNCH ??
THAT'S A 300-CALORIE LUNCH.
STAFF
WHEN I MAKE A 300-CALORIE LUNCH, IT'S 25 TIMES MORE FOOD THAN THIS.

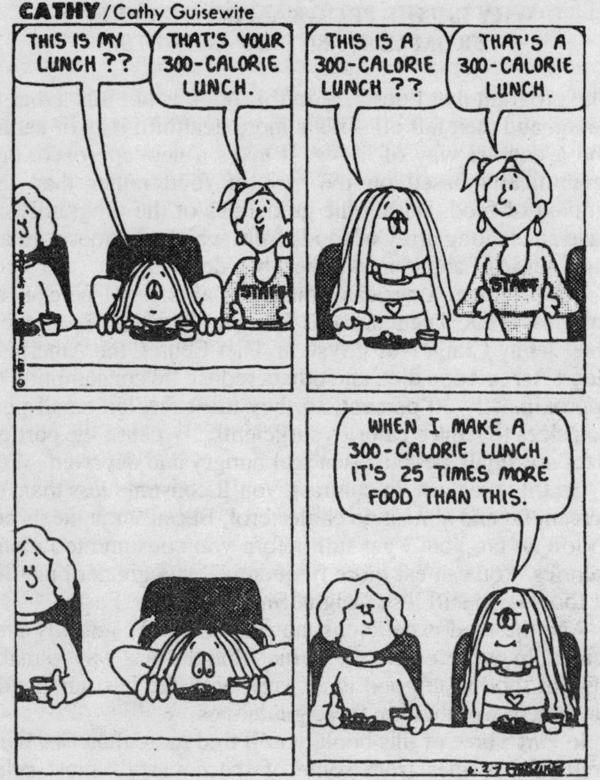

## HOW THIS PROGRAM WAS DEVELOPED

I did not start out to study weight loss. And as I mentioned in the introduction, I am not a "diet doctor." The major focus of the medical research that my colleagues and I have been conducting during the past sixteen years has been on preventing and reversing heart disease. Along the way, we learned that our program also has dramatic effects on weight.

Our research, called the "Lifestyle Heart Trial," was the first randomized, controlled clinical study scientifically demonstrating that the progress of even severe coronary heart disease can often be reversed by making lifestyle changes alone (including diet, stress management training, smoking cessation, moderate exercise, and emotional support), without cholesterol-lowering drugs or surgery. Also, we learned what really motivates people to make and maintain comprehensive lifestyle changes over many years while living in the real world.

In 1977, when I first began conducting research in this area, most scientists did not believe that heart disease could be reversed. "At best, maybe the relentless progression of heart disease can be slowed," they said, "but not reversed. Impossible." However, we found that the "natural history of heart disease"—to worsen over time—is really unnatural and can often be changed. Instead of becoming worse and worse over time, we learned that many people can become better and better. This gives many people new hope, new possibilities, and new choices.

My colleagues and I presented the results of our research at numerous international medical conferences, including the annual scientific meetings of the American Heart Association, the American College of Cardiology, the International Society of Behavioral Medicine, the American Dietetic Association, and many others. Our research findings were published in a number of professional medical journals, including *The Lancet, The American Journal of Cardiology, The Journal of the American Medical Association, The Journal of the American Dietetic Association, Hospital Practice, Circulation,* and several others.

Now, as other scientists are beginning to confirm our research findings, most of the medical community believe that heart disease is reversible for many people. And so is being overweight. Like heart disease, obesity can be reversed—if we address the more fundamental *causes* of gaining weight, not just the behaviors that lead to it.

An unexpected—but very important—discovery in our research was that people who followed this program improved not only their hearts but also their waistlines. During the first year, patients in our study lost an *average* of twenty-two pounds, even though they were eating more food, and more frequently, than before entering our study. Without counting calories. Without measuring portion sizes. Without hunger. Most of the patients reported feeling a sense of abundance rather than deprivation. These findings have powerful implications for anyone who wishes to control his or her weight.

When I lecture at scientific meetings, the major question remains, "OK, *your* patients changed their lifestyles, but *my* patients never would. I can't even get them to make small changes in diet and lifestyle—how do you expect them to make the big changes you propose?"

But it's not just our research participants who are able to make these comprehensive lifestyle changes. My colleagues and I are training other physicians in our program, and they are reporting similar successes with their patients. To make our research findings and program more widely available, I wrote a book for the general public, *Dr. Dean Ornish's Program for Reversing Heart Disease.* Since then, I have received more than fifteen thousand letters and calls from people from all over the world. Many of them, just by reading my book, were able to change their lifestyles. (One of my favorites was a letter from China addressed, "Dear Dr. Onions. . . .") Most talked about their improvements in cholesterol, blood pressure, chest pain, and heart disease, but many also described how much weight they lost. Here are two illustrative examples. The first is one that I received from Mrs. Joy Muñoz in South Carolina, whom I have never met:

> I barely know how to begin this letter—you have changed my life in such a profound way that "thank you" is so inadequate.
>
> I first became aware of your book when I read about your work in a magazine article. I was impressed by the simple common sense that you espoused. It coincided with a crossroads I was at, when I knew I had to start doing something to take control of my life. I don't have any heart problems that

I'm aware of, but my father and all of his brothers and sisters have died of or survived heart attacks, and one of my cousins survived a coronary at the age of 35.

I'm a 44-year-old woman and have been obese since I gained 75 pounds with my first pregnancy and never lost it and, in fact, added some more. I'm 5'3" and for the last 24 years of my life have weighed in the 190- to 220-pound range. I'd tried many times to diet and only once had a little success (on an all-liquid diet—of course, you know what happened when I started eating food again!). I counted calories the other times, but could never lose unless I ate 500 calories a day or less. After a week or two, I was so hungry that I could eat anything I could get my hands on.

I purchased your book and read it over Christmas vacation. It was so easy to read, and you made it seem like such a simple, logical thing to do that I chose to jump in with both feet on January 3, 1991. That day I weighed 205 pounds. My blood pressure for the last few years hovered around 140/90. Yesterday [June 11, 1991], I weighed in at 158 pounds. My blood pressure was 111/63. I had a fasting blood chemistry done and all other factors were normal.

I've never felt healthier, or happier. My husband, who thought I was going to drop dead from lack of meat, has become very supportive of my efforts. I cook for me and add a chicken, turkey, or seafood portion for him. I'm a phenomenon at work and I have to say the praise and compliments from coworkers have been such a morale booster.

I've had wonderful side effects I never expected. Incredibly, from the very first month on your program, I had no extra breast pain of a cyclical nature. In fact, I no longer have the terrible menstrual cramps or the uncomfortableness in the days before the onset. I'm just in awe of the wonderful, unexpected benefits I've received. I thank God every day for the incredible changes in my life.

She wrote me again to let me know how she was doing:

It has been nearly a year since I last wrote to you, and what an exciting and wonderful year!

In eight months' time last year, I lost 65 pounds, and since last August, have lost only 2 more. But with no effort at all, I stay within 2 or 3 pounds of the same. I'm so delighted—I thought it could never happen for me. But your concern is not weight loss alone. So for the other good news. . . .

In January 1991, my total cholesterol was 238, and this March it measured at 160! I danced for days over that! My blood pressure, which used to be around 140/90, is consistently around 105/55 now. But best of all, I feel so GREAT all of the time. I must add that my husband is delighted with my looks and new attitude. He says I'm a lot more self-confident and assertive.

I still want you to know how grateful I am. I'm sure the changes I can see and measure on the outside are mirrored on the inside. God bless you and your work.

The following is from Debbie Voltura, a well-known singer who lives in northern California:

I began following your program in November 1992, after my father-in-law began reading your book. I'm a professional singer, so how I look is important to me in my work.

In the past four months, I've lost 52 pounds! And the fat is melting off in the places where I needed it to the most. Before, I thought the less you ate, the more you lost, so I never ate anything before noon. I felt deprived and hungry all the time.

Not anymore! Now, I'm never hungry, because I'm eating even more than before, and I'm eating more frequently. I'm on the road 50 weeks a year, performing concerts and singing for thousands of people. But it hasn't been hard following your program even when I travel.

I just love the energy. People who see me say I look terrific, not just that I look thinner. My skin is smoother and my eyes are clearer. I used to get headaches all the time, and I'd go through a bottle of aspirin or other painkillers every week. I haven't had a headache since I went on your program. Before, I slept poorly and needed at least eight or nine hours of sleep. Now, I sleep great and wake up feeling refreshed after only six or seven hours.

I've been on so many different diets, lost weight, and always gained it back—and then some. But this is not a diet that I'm going to follow for a few months and then get off. This is a lifestyle change, a new way of eating and living.

## THE POWER OF ADDRESSING THE REAL *CAUSES* OF OUR PROBLEMS

•

How is it possible for people like these to make and maintain such major changes in lifestyle just from reading a book? If we try to change our behaviors without addressing the underlying causes, then the same problem tends to come back again, or we may find ourselves with a new set of problems. Instead, if we address the underlying causes, then improvements can occur more quickly than we had once thought possible.

Our lifestyle choices are the major cause of heart disease: what we eat, how we respond to stress, smoking, lack of exercise, and so on. In my last book, I described why conventional approaches to treating coronary heart disease—drugs, angioplasty (blowing up a balloon inside a blocked coronary artery), and coronary bypass surgery—cause only *temporary* improvements because they literally or figuratively *bypass* the underlying causes of the problem. As a result, the same heart problem often recurs or new problems and side effects may develop.

Despite the tremendous expense of bypass surgery and angioplasty (billions of dollars each year), these procedures are not always successful. Up to one-half of bypass grafts become clogged again after only five years, and one-third of angioplastied arteries become clogged after only four to six months. When this occurs, then coronary bypass surgery or coronary angioplasty is often repeated, thereby incurring additional costs.

In contrast, because they are addressing the *causes* of the problem, most of the patients in the Lifestyle Heart Trial who are following this program are showing even more improvement after five years than after one year. Sadly, patients in the comparison group of our study who have followed the conventional dietary and lifestyle recommendations are much worse after five years than after one year.

Similarly, conventional approaches to losing weight usually don't last because these, too, do not address the underlying causes of the problem. So, more often than not, even when people temporarily lose weight they soon gain it back again.

## THE PROGRAM

You may have tried different diets. You may have lost and regained weight many times, and you may feel terribly discouraged. If so, this book may give you hope.

Most diets that require you to deprive yourself of food by restricting calories (for example, Nutri/System, Jenny Craig, Diet Center, and Weight Watchers) may make you feel hungry and may cause your metabolism to slow down, but this is not true of this program. (Your metabolism determines how quickly or slowly you burn calories.) Some diets may even cause medical problems. This is especially true of high-protein diets that recommend increasing consumption of meats and eggs and reducing dietary carbohydrates. These can increase the risk of heart disease, stroke, kidney disease, and many other health problems. They cause rapid weight loss primarily by causing you to lose water, but the water and the weight are just as rapidly regained.

In the pages that follow, I share with you information that may give you renewed hope and help you to regain control of your life. In chapters 3 through 7, I describe the real causes of being overweight, and why these are not dealt with on most other diets. I explain how addressing these causes can help to transform your life for the better.

Chapter 4 of the book describes the nutritional guidelines of the *Eat More, Weigh Less* diet. Also, I discuss how to exercise and manage stress more effectively in chapters 5, 6, and 7.

Section Two is an introduction to nonfat cooking, various methods and techniques, advice on stocking a low-fat pantry and equipment, and a sample week's menus.

Section Three is a "cookbook-within-a-book," with more than two hundred gourmet recipes designed to show you that even food so low in fat can taste great.

For the past several years I have been consulting with ConAgra, makers of Healthy Choice foods, to develop the "*Advantage\10*" line of frozen low fat dinners in order to make it easy, convenient, and inexpensive to follow the program described in this book.

This is not to suggest that everyone can be very skinny. Your weight is partially determined by your genes, but only to some degree. According to Dr. Albert Stunkard, a leading weight-loss researcher, even though a tendency to be obese is inherited, "you have to have the environment to bring it out." For example, while it is true that overweight parents tend to have overweight children, they also tend to have overweight pets.

On this program, you really *can* lose weight and keep it off. Even more important, though, you can be happier and healthier. The rest of this book shows you how.

I have also written a cookbook, *Everyday Cooking with Dr. Dean Ornish,* that includes simple recipes that are quick and easy to prepare with ingredients you can find easily.

# 2

# *Fat Accompli*

*"It's not over until the fat lady sings."*

One day, the telephone rang and the very resonant voice on the line said, "Dr. Ornish? I'm Paul Plishka, and I want to thank you for making me feel and look so good."

Paul Plishka is a leading singer with the world-renowned Metropolitan Opera. One night, he and his wife, Judy, invited me to dinner, and the following conversation ensued. I found their story to be so interesting and heartening that it helped inspire me to write this book. So I am including almost our entire conversation from that dinner here in hopes that it may also help to motivate you.

**Paul:** Well, about a year ago, I was doing a role in the New York Metropolitan Opera production of *Don Giovanni.* I played Leporello, who is Don Giovanni's sidekick. This was a production by Franco Zeffirelli, the well-known film director and opera designer, and it required me to carry a lot of bags and books and papers and all sorts of paraphernalia while I'm singing this aria. It's a very long aria with a lot of physical activity. I've been singing this role for over twenty-five years.

When I came off the stage at the end of the play, I just leaned against the wall, breathing heavy, and I felt like I was dying. I said to myself, "I'm in trouble." I just turned fifty this summer, and I've always been big and strong, as you can see. I can get away with murder, but I guess it catches up with you. My past history of eating, being of Ukrainian background and Slavic and all the cooking—

**Judy:** Not *my* cooking . . .

**Paul:** Not Judy's—my mother made the Ukrainian food, the potatoes and the pirogi, and all those things. Also, we spent a lot of time in Europe, and I got really hooked on pâté de foie gras [goose liver paste]. I *loved* it. In fact, at one point we even bought our own geese, and I was going to force feed them to be able to get my own foie gras! So, I was eating a lot of fat, I was getting very fat, and I knew that I was probably well on my way to clogging up my arteries with fat.

**Judy:** I've never liked to eat meat. So, we would go out to a restaurant, and we would order some meat, and I'd eat—

**Paul:** She likes corned beef or pastrami sandwiches, but—

**Judy:** Reuben sandwiches.

**Paul:** But when she got the sandwich, she would take off every piece of meat in it. Then, like a surgeon, she would take her knife and cut off all the fat and make her sandwich out of part of what was left. And sometimes in New York the sandwiches are really thick! I'd eat my pastrami sandwich, and then I'd ask the waiter for two more slices of rye bread. I'd take all the stuff that she'd cut off, make it into another sandwich and I'd eat it, too. It was even better than the first one. Because the fat was the thing. It's like an addiction. I think that you can really get addicted to fat.

And once in a while, although I haven't really discussed this too much with Judy, I would get this very strange sensation in my chest. It could have been indigestion, but that, along with the weight and the huffing and puffing, began to scare me.

One day, after a rehearsal, I was watching the *Today* show in the morning, and you were being interviewed about your book on reversing heart disease. And I said, "Wow, that's fascinating! To begin opening arteries with just diet and lifestyle alone—I mean, that's impressive." I was moved by the interview. Several days later, I got your book, went home, and started reading it.

I'm very lucky to be at the top of the hill in the opera business. It's a high-stress occupation, and with my past history of eating, I said to myself, "I'm probably well on my way to a heart attack. Let me give this a try." Judy liked the recipes in the book, so we started doing it.

**Judy:** Also, we began walking a lot. You got him into walking fast. He used to just amble.

**Paul:** Five or six days a week, for forty minutes to an hour, we walked from 71st Street up to 106th Street, thirty-five blocks there and then thirty-five blocks back as fast as we could go to keep me huffing and puffing. When we first started walking up Broadway in the Lincoln Center area, I know probably half the people who live there, or they know me, so the problem was that we were stopping every two or three blocks to say hello. Eventually, we learned to walk over to Riverside Drive or West End Avenue.

Anyway, I started following your program, and I was really very strict with it—because I was inspired by how much better I began to feel. And how quickly! Between September 21 and December 21, I lost fifty pounds in that three-month period!

I would make my own pizzas. Judy makes a pasta sauce, like a red sauce. She'll get a can of Progresso crushed tomatoes, and she'll put it in a big microwaveable measuring cup. And we'll cut up vegetables, any kind of vegetables, whatever is there, and put them in with a little garlic and onion. I would make pizza dough for a *big* pizza, add Judy's red sauce and then the vegetables. There was no oil in it at all, no fat. The other trick I learned—I would buy the best Parmesan cheese I could find, because then you only need a little bit of it.

We didn't worry about counting calories. We just left out most of the fat. We ate a lot of different pastas. And I was eating a lot of fruit during that time.

A lot of people eat just to survive. They have no idea what they're eating, and there's no real pleasure in it for them. They just eat, and it doesn't matter what they eat. But a lot of people find a great deal of pleasure in eating, and I do, too. However, if you eat something that's terrible, you have to eat ten more of those things to be satisfied, and even then you're not really happy. So, I would go to the best Korean markets in New York, and I would buy the best produce—the best peaches, nectarines, grapefruit, and so on. I'd eat any kind of fruits and vegetables and grains and tabouli I could get my hands on.

I never counted calories. But even though I was eating the same amount of food or more, I began losing weight. I could still eat something whenever I felt an impulse, just as long as there was *no meat, no fish, no whole-milk dairy, no oil.* Those words were my Bible. As long as I left those out, I was all right.

So then, when I went back to the opera house after losing the weight, people were just in shock. Because I'd been there for twenty-five years and I've always been very big. They asked, "What did you do, how did you do it?" And I said, "Well, I followed Dr. Ornish's program. It's wonderful."

When we were first married, I worked in an ice cream factory. It was very rich, high-quality ice cream, and I ate ice cream and milk shakes all the time. Lately, I've become very addicted to salsa, which is not bad because you can make it without oil or fat, but the chips are deadly because they're fried in oil.

Because of the pressure I'm under, to eat and chew on something is very important to me. I really have to control myself, because I really love to eat chips. It gets the anxiety out of my body—to chew into things, you see—and they were very good for that. But I can go through a bag of those without even thinking. One of the reasons people eat is to chew, to get out their frustrations by grinding their teeth, you know. And that's the good thing about eating greens and vegetables, because they give you that chewy kind of thing. I *love* them! And I can't get enough of the beans and grains.

I lost fifty pounds between September and December. By the end of January, I had lost a total of sixty-five pounds.

Well, some people in my business got worried. Opera is famous for big, fat, opera singers. They come on the scene, and the manager tells them that they have to lose weight. They go on a diet, they lose weight, and 99.9 percent of the time the voice goes with the weight. Almost always. But I have been singing this way for over thirty years. I've had one teacher, one technique for that time. It's the only way I know. I don't know if my voice could go anywhere else if it wanted to.

So, when I came back to New York weighing 215, my teacher and everyone else were hysterical. They said, "What are you doing? How do you sound? Oh, my God!"

**Judy:** His teacher said, "You *can't* lose any more weight!"

**Paul:** And I said, "Well, this is going to be up to the public, the listeners. They're the ones who are going to tell me whether or not the voice is gone." I spent from January to April in New York. I did some of the most difficult repertoire in the business, and I got some of the best reviews in New York that I've ever had!

The other thing I noticed was something that I never saw in a diet book, but it's something that I think is very important but is never mentioned. The word is *resentment.*

**Judy:** From other people for the weight loss.

**Paul:** It's a major factor. I've sensed resentment from people who have not been able to lose weight, or who lost and regained it. Sometimes, they're people in very powerful positions, people who are capable of moving my career in one direction or another.

For example, recently I was doing a job with a company that I have worked with in the past. One of the people in the company was a person I have known very well. When his wife saw how much weight I had lost—and he's gained quite a bit—she just nagged him the entire time I was there.

**Judy:** She said, "Look at that nice jacket Paul has on, why can't *you* wear that?"

**Paul:** I think it's one of the reasons that people say things in a very funny way to you, like, "Don't lose any more weight."

But it's worth putting up with the resentment, because I feel so good! And, of course, feeling good about yourself is really the best part of it. I have had no more chest discomfort. And I have a lot more energy. I mean, a hundred times more. I feel terrific, just really great.

**Judy:** I can't leave him in a clothing store alone.

**Paul:** I just buy everything in sight. I threw out all my old clothes. I was wearing a size 48 waist, and even then my pants were very tight on me. And now I'm in a size 40.

It has made a major improvement in my career. It's made me much more marketable. I mean, before, a 280-pound man is not a very romantic figure—unless you're Pavarotti, and then you make some allowances. And I've been working with him several times since then, and he keeps asking me, "How did you do it? How?" and I keep referring him to your books. And in New York, when I'm on television programs, they always ask me how I did it, and I tell them about your program. It has caused a big fuss in my business.

When you eat this way, your sense of taste improves. You taste things that you didn't experience before. Have you ever been to Venice? A few years ago, we went to a wonderful place there for lunch one day with some friends of ours from the States who came to visit us. There was a huge buffet. And, of course, we filled our plates with all these appetizers that the Italians have a wonderful way of making.

We were just shoveling this stuff down. There was one item on the plate, and Judy asked, "What is that? How does it taste? Is it fish?" And none of us could tell her what it was. We liked the taste of it, but our taste was not discriminating enough to be able to say, "It has a little bit of this in it and some of that." Everything becomes sort of bland, so you need to eat a lot of it.

But now, my palate has become much more discriminating. For lunch today, we made a little risotto. I bought some canned chick-peas, green beans, and red kidney beans, drained them, put some salad on a plate, and sprinkled some of the beans on top of the salad. Judy made a delicious dressing with balsamic vinegar, but I started eating the salad with just the beans and the greens and I didn't want anything on it. I just wanted the individual tastes. In the past, it would not have tasted like anything, it would have been so bland. It would have been uninteresting to me. Now it was delicious. And I felt so good afterwards!

When I occasionally eat a fatty meal, I suffer the next day. I have unbelievable bloatedness, like I just want to die. I just want to crawl up in a corner and be left alone. I really do notice a huge difference.

I mean, I like this feeling of being able to walk away from the table feeling comfortable. Not stuffed. Before, I could never before go away from the table without having that bulging, bloating kind of Thanksgiving Day feeling. And now, I really like how I feel after I eat. I've become more refined. Like a high-performance sports car.

This September, I'll be playing the lead role in *Falstaff,* which will be broadcast on PBS. The lead character is supposed to be about 300 pounds, and I was cast for the part three years ago when I weighed so much more. When they saw me now, they said, "Oh, no, what have you done!" So now I'll be wearing padding. But it's a lot easier to take off the padding after the performance than to carry all of that extra weight around.

Paul and Judy showed how it really is possible to eat and to *enjoy* a variety of foods that meet the guidelines of this program, even while living very busy, productive, interesting lives. They adapted many of their favorite foods to meet these guidelines, and they discovered how tasty and satisfying these foods can be. And they shared how these changes improved the *quality* of their lives and their careers. You may find that it can do the same for you.

# 3

# *Amazing Graze*

## WHAT CAUSES YOU TO GAIN WEIGHT?

The conventional wisdom is that you gain weight when there is an imbalance between energy intake (calories) and expenditure (exercise and metabolism). This is true, but it is only part of the story. The more fundamental questions are:

- Are all calories alike?
- What affects the rate at which you burn calories?
- What really motivates us to make and maintain *lasting* changes in our behaviors?

Let's examine the first two questions in this chapter. I will address the third one in more depth in the following chapters.

## ALL CALORIES ARE NOT THE SAME

What makes this diet so effective? Researchers have demonstrated that not all calories are alike. A fat calorie is not the same as a calorie from protein or carbohydrate, either in the number of calories it contains or in the way it is metabolized by the body.

Fat has over twice as many calories as either protein or carbohydrate. (Fat has nine calories per gram, whereas protein and carbohydrate only have four calories per gram.) So, when you reduce fat consumption from the typical American intake of 40 percent of calories down to the 10 percent fat levels in this diet, you can eat almost one-third more food yet take in the same amount of calories. Put in a more healthful way, you can consume the same amount of food yet take in far fewer calories.

Your body easily converts dietary fat calories into body fat. One hundred fat calories can be stored as body fat by expending only 2.5 calories, whereas your body must spend twenty-three calories—almost ten times as much—to convert one hundred calories of dietary protein or carbohydrate into body fat. Only about 1 percent of dietary protein and carbohydrate end up as body fat, because your body would rather use them up right away than waste energy to store them. So, by keeping fat consumption low, as you do on this diet, not only do you tend to consume fewer calories, but also those calories are less likely to be converted into body fat.

The reason your body converts dietary fat into body fat so easily is that fat is how your body stores energy. Calories are stored energy, like batteries. Since fat stores nine calories per gram, whereas protein and carbohydrate store only four calories per gram, then your body can store over twice as much energy in the form of fat. Until a few hundred years ago or so, most people ate foods similar to the diet I recommend. Even now, the majority of people on earth still do. They just happen to live in less affluent and less industrialized countries.

Your body only needs about 4 to 6 percent of calories as fat to synthesize what are known as essential fatty acids. The diet I recommend for many people is about 10 percent fat, so it provides more than enough fat without giving you more than you need. It's the excessive amounts of fat and cholesterol in your diet that lead to excess weight, heart disease, and other illnesses. As I describe more fully in chapter 4, you don't have to have a minor in mathematics to calculate a 10 percent fat diet. When you eat primarily fruits, vegetables, grains, and beans, that's what you end up with. And that's what your body has evolved to handle. It's not all or nothing, but less fat equals fewer calories.

## WHAT'S EVOLVED TO PROTECT YOU MAY HARM YOU

A central theme of this book is that you are living in a world to which your mind and body have not yet had time to adapt. The human body evolved a number of exquisitely complex mechanisms that were designed to help the species survive. But evolution of the body is a gradual process, one that occurs over very long periods of time—thousands of years. Yet there has been more change in the American diet and lifestyle during the past hundred years than in the past ten thousand years. You are eating a diet that the human body has not had time to adapt to.

It's not that you're designed wrong—but that these very mechanisms that evolved to protect the species can prove harmful or even lethal in a modern society. Heart disease, for example, is the result of a number of adaptive responses gone awry. Blockages in your coronary arteries are formed when the lining of the artery is injured. The body attempts to heal that damage with an inflammatory response, like putting on a Band-Aid. And that's good.

But when your arteries are repetitively injured, then it's like piling one Band-Aid on top of another. Over time, the result is blocked arteries. It's only relatively recently that people have had to deal with the causes of repetitive injuries to their arteries: too much fat, smoking, high blood pressure, and so on.

To complicate matters even more, during times of emotional stress, your body activates what is called the fight-or-flight response: Your adrenaline, heart rate, and blood pressure increase, your blood clots faster, and your arteries constrict. If a saber-tooth tiger jumps out in front of you, then these changes help you survive: You have more energy to fight or to run. If the tiger should bite your arm or leg, then your blood clots faster and your arteries constrict, so this helps keep you from bleeding to death.

However, in modern times, there are "tigers" everywhere, and these mechanisms are often chronically activated. Because of this overstimulation, the blood may clot and the arteries may constrict not only in your arms and legs but also in your heart. This can lead to a heart attack. (I discussed these mechanisms more fully in my last book, *Dr. Dean Ornish's Program for Reversing Heart Disease.*)

## SURVIVAL OF THE FATTEST

Weighing too much is a relatively modern problem. For the prior ten thousand years or so, the major concern for humans had been finding *enough* food, not having to deal with too much of it. (Food abundance is *still* a problem only in certain parts of the globe. Africa, as we have seen so dramatically in recent reports, is still trying to feed, not diet.) Consequently, because fat is a very efficient way for your body to store energy, your body's physiology evolved to conserve body fat. In a world of scarcity, those who gained weight easily had an evolutionary advantage—survival of the fattest, you might say.

We have already learned that the body converts dietary fat into body fat very easily. Now we know that this was so the body could store energy for a time when food might be scarce. To further complicate matters for those trying to lose weight today, it also evolved that during times of scarcity, the body's metabolic rate slowed down to help conserve energy.

These two mechanisms were designed to help you survive when the food supply was unreliable. But in the modern world, these same mechanisms can become harmful to you because your diet is so different from what people used to eat.

Until this century, the typical American diet was low in

animal products, fat, cholesterol, salt, and sugar, and high in carbohydrates, vegetables, and fiber. Vigorous physical activity was common. Early in this century, with the advent of refrigerators, freezers, good transportation, mechanized agriculture, and a prosperous economy, the American diet and lifestyle began to change radically. Now most people in the United States eat a diet high in animal products, fat, cholesterol, salt, and sugar, and low in carbohydrates, vegetables, and fiber. Being sedentary is common. Your body—your genes—have not had enough time to adapt to such a fundamental change in your diet and lifestyle from the way your ancestors ate and lived both in the recent past and during the previous ten thousand years.

## HOMEOSTASIS: YOUR FAT THERMOSTAT

Homeostasis, another word for equilibrium, is another evolutionary adaptation that makes dieting by traditional methods difficult. Your body resists change—both for better and for worse. It's good, for example, that if your body temperature begins to rise, you start to sweat to cool it down. It's not helpful today, however, that when you lose weight your body tries to regain it. But that's exactly what happens on a physiological level.

When you overeat, your fat cells grow larger. If you keep overeating, you begin forming new fat cells. You also gain weight. The size of your fat cells may decrease if you restrict food intake for a while, but the number does not. This helps to explain why it becomes harder to lose weight each time you go through the yo-yo cycle of gaining and losing weight. When you first lose weight by restricting the amount of food you eat, you lose both muscle and fat tissue. But when you gain weight back, you regain proportionately more fat than you lost.

When you deprive yourself of food, as with conventional diets, the size of your fat cells shrinks although the number does not decrease. As a result, in addition to feeling hungry, your body thinks you're starving (because you are), and it tries to compensate for the reduced intake of food by slowing down how fast you burn it. If you reduce your food intake by 25 percent, then your metabolic rate may slow down by as much as 20 to 25 percent. Like a thermostat that's been readjusted, your metabolic "set point" may change, causing your metabolism to remain at a lower rate. When your metabolism is lower, then you burn calories more slowly.

Homeostasis also affects your emotions and motivations—what you might call "psychological homeostasis." In chapter 6, I discuss why it's so hard to change your lifestyle if you focus only on your behaviors without also addressing what underlies your actions.

According to the set point theory, because of homeostasis your body tries to maintain your weight, even when you go on a calorie-restricted diet. As you start to lose weight, your body tries to compensate on the supply side by increasing your appetite to make you eat more calories, and on the demand side by causing your metabolic rate to drop.

When your metabolism is lowered, you burn calories more slowly, just as a car driven at a slower speed burns less gasoline. Because of this, even if you stay on a calorie-restricted diet, you may stop losing weight. This is the dread "plateau" phenomenon familiar to just about everyone who has tried to lose weight, and it really dampens your motivation. Eventually, you continue to eat less, yet weigh the same. Worse still, because repeated dieting leads to greater and greater lowering of your metabolic rate, when you get tired of feeling hungry and go off the diet, you may gain back even more than you lost—even if you only eat the same amount of food as you did before starting to diet.

Dr. Kelly Brownell and others at the University of Pennsylvania School of Medicine studied rats who lost and regained weight. Each time they lost and regained weight, their metabolism slowed down even more. In the second cycle, it took twice as long to lose the weight as it did the first time, and they regained the weight three times faster.

Dr. Brownell observed similar changes in metabolism in

wrestlers who went on crash diets before matches and then regained the weight afterwards. In another study, he also found that the more your weight fluctuates—the more you yo-yo—the higher your risk of heart disease.

## BYE-BYE TO YO-YO

Something different—and wonderful—happens on this diet. Your metabolism stays the same or even increases, so you burn off calories more quickly. You have more energy. And you can eat the same amount of food, or even more, yet consume fewer calories.

The whole grains, legumes, fruits, and complex carbohydrates that form the basis of the diet I recommend are bulky, high in fiber, and low in calorie-rich fat and sugar, so in addition to having an increased metabolic rate, you feel full before you eat too many calories. This diet is high in fiber, which slows down the absorption of food, so you feel full longer than when you're eating small portions on a calorie-restricted diet. And since these foods are high both in fiber and in complex carbohydrates, your blood sugar remains more stable, helping to give you a greater sense of equanimity and well-being.

Dr. Olaf Mickelsen of Michigan State University found that slightly overweight men lost weight when they included twelve slices of low-fat bread each day with their meals. One group ate low-fiber bread and one group ate high-fiber bread. Both groups lost weight, but those eating the high-fiber bread lost even more.

In contrast, you can eat large quantities of fat without feeling full. For example, 1.5 ounces of potato chips have the same number of calories as a twelve-ounce baked potato. You'd still be hungry after eating the potato chips, but you'd feel full after eating the potato. Eating carbohydrates takes care of your hunger and makes you feel full in about twenty minutes.

Recently, nutrition researchers at Cornell University published a study in the *American Journal of Clinical Nutrition* designed to disprove the set point theory, yet the results ended up confirming it. In the study, active and slightly overweight women ages twenty-two to fifty-six were randomly assigned to either a low-fat diet or a calorie-restricted typical American diet. Both groups were allowed to eat whenever they wanted, including snacks.

After eleven weeks, the women on the low-fat diet consumed about 15 percent fewer calories than those on the typical American regimen, even though both groups reported liking the food about the same. Women on the low-fat diet had lost twice as much weight as the women on the calorie-restricted typical American diet—about one-half pound per week. The researchers wrote, "These results demonstrate that body weight can be lost merely by reducing the fat content of the diet without the need to voluntarily restrict food intake." They went on to conclude:

> First, it seems that some degree of weight loss can be achieved without the necessity of dieting, i.e., voluntarily limiting the amount of food consumed. There is a great deal of evidence that conscious reduction in the amount of food consumed results in rapid losses of body weight; but almost invariably this lost weight is regained. Reductions in the fat content of the diet with no limitation on the amount of food consumed may lead to a more permanent weight loss than can be achieved through dieting. Second, the realization that reducing fat intake may lead to weight loss may help motivate the public to make dietary changes that will also reduce the incidence of heart disease and cancer.

According to the principal investigator, Dr. David Levitsky, your metabolic rate is related to the amount of carbohydrates you consume. "Maybe the body can't detect a reduction in the amount of fat coming in [if carbohydrates stay the same or increase], so the metabolism doesn't change. The results of this study confirm this hypothesis."

When you increase consumption of complex carbohydrates, your metabolic rate may increase. On this diet, you eat more carbohydrates and much less fat, so your metabolic rate stays the same or even increases.

Why? Your thyroid gland is a key regulator of your metabolism. Thyroid hormone increases your metabolic rate. Your thyroid gland makes a thyroid hormone called thyroxin, which can be converted to either an active or an inactive form. When you eat a diet high in carbohydrates and low in fat, then more thyroid hormone is converted to the active form.

## AMAZING GRAZE

It is very difficult to "graze" on a typical American diet, yet researchers have found that eating frequent, small portions often has many benefits, both physiological and psychological. On most diets, you probably would not want to divide your meals into smaller, more frequent snacks because there would not be enough food to go around. On the diet I recommend, though, you may find that you develop a natural tendency to graze, because (a) you get hungry sooner, (b) you feel full faster, and (c) you are able to eat more food without increasing the number of calories.

A study in the *New England Journal of Medicine* by Dr. David Jenkins and his colleagues at the University of Toronto reported that grazing is good for you in a remarkable variety of ways. The researchers randomly divided people into two groups. Both groups ate the same type and amount of food. However, one group ate the food divided into three meals a day, whereas the other group ate it divided into seventeen meals a day (what the researchers called "the nibbling diet").

After only two weeks, they found that the nibbling diet:

- reduced blood cholesterol levels by over 15 percent. Lower cholesterol, of course, reduces your risk for heart disease and stroke.

- reduced cortisol levels by over 17 percent. Since your body makes cortisol during times of stress, lower cortisol levels indicate less stress on your body.
- reduced blood insulin levels by almost 28 percent. Your pancreas produces insulin as a way of regulating your blood sugar. When you eat a typical American diet high in fat and sugar, then your blood sugar goes up and your pancreas releases more insulin in order to bring your blood sugar back down. Sometimes your pancreas may produce too much insulin, causing your blood sugar to fall even lower than it was before you started eating, causing you to feel tired. By nibbling throughout the day, your blood sugar stays more constant, so you don't need to make as much insulin. When your blood sugar stays constant, your energy level remains more even, without the ups and downs.

Besides regulating your blood sugar level, insulin plays an important role in fat metabolism. Because insulin increases the secretion of lipoprotein lipase, an enzyme that increases the uptake of fat from your bloodstream into fat in your body's cells, when your body produces more insulin, you are more likely to convert dietary calories into body fat.

When you try to lose weight by reducing the *amount* of food you eat instead of changing the *type* of food, your body responds not only by increasing the amount of insulin and lipoprotein lipase, but also by increasing your body's sensitivity to the effects of these. A double-whammy. As a result, your body increases the uptake of fat from your bloodstream and you tend to regain the lost weight.

Reducing insulin levels has other benefits. Insulin also plays a key role in increasing cholesterol synthesis. When your insulin levels rise, your liver makes more of an enzyme called HMG-CoA reductase which, in turn, causes your body to make more cholesterol. (Incidentally, this enzyme is the major target of the newest cholesterol-lowering drugs.)

Besides increasing your cholesterol level, insulin enhances the growth and proliferation of arterial smooth muscle cells.

These smooth muscle cells help to clog up your arteries and can lead to heart attacks. Other studies have shown that people with high insulin levels have higher rates of heart attacks. And people with high blood pressure secrete even more insulin than those with normal blood pressure; it is less clear if high levels of insulin may elevate your blood pressure.

Insulin also affects your stress level. When insulin levels increase, your sympathetic nervous system gets stimulated, just as it is stimulated during times of emotional stress. More on this later.

## ARE YOU AN APPLE OR A PEAR?

But insulin's final role in this story is even more critical, because insulin affects the *distribution* of your body's fat as well. Insulin tends to distribute weight in your upper body, making you apple-shaped instead of pear-shaped. If you are an "apple" (more common in men), your excess weight is carried in your upper body, above your hips and around your belly. Your waist may be bigger than your hips. If you are a "pear" (more often seen in women), your extra weight is carried around your hips, buttocks, and thighs. Your waist may be smaller than your hips.

Upper-body fat—being an apple—is much more harmful to your health than being a pear. For reasons that are not entirely understood, most of the health risks of being overweight are due to fat in your abdomen. Unfortunately, when you lose weight and regain it, you are more likely to regain it in your waist and upper body—one more reason why yo-yo dieting can be harmful.

Besides weight gain, in several studies upper-body fat distribution was found to be associated with:

- fifteen times greater risk for uterine cancer
- increased risk of breast cancer
- increased risk of heart disease, including smoking, low exercise levels, high LDL ("bad") cholesterol, low HDL ("good") cholesterol, and high blood pressure

- higher levels of anger, anxiety, and depression and lower levels of social support
- higher risk of diabetes

Losing weight can help much more than your appearance.

Are you apple-shaped or pear-shaped? Measure your hips, then your waist. Divide your waist measurement by your hip measurement. If the result is 0.75 or less, then you're pear-shaped; 0.75–.080 is mildly apple-shaped; greater then 0.80 is very apple-shaped. For example, if your waist is 33 inches and your hips are 40 inches, then your result is 0.825, meaning that you are apple-shaped.

Your body will tend to first burn up the fat you most recently stored. So if your waist has been growing recently, it may be the first to shrink on this program, helping you to turn an apple into a pear.

## LIVING LEANER MAY HELP YOU LIVE LONGER

As we've seen, increasing scientific evidence links diets high in animal fat not only with obesity but also with coronary heart disease, stroke, breast cancer in women, prostate cancer in men, colon cancer in both, osteoporosis, diabetes, hypertension, gallbladder disease—many of the most prevalent diseases. And these are the illnesses for which medicine does not have very effective treatments.

Breast cancer, for example, afflicts one in nine American women. If you ask American physicians what women can do to prevent breast cancer, they usually reply, "Get a mammogram every year after age forty." Yet mammograms do not *prevent* cancer, they *detect* cancer.

In Japan and other countries where the consumption of animal fat is much lower, breast cancer is rare. It's not because their genes are different. When Japanese women move to the United States and begin consuming a high-fat diet, they develop breast cancer at about the same rate as Americans—more than 400 percent higher than in Japan.

In part, this may be because a diet high in animal fats

increases both the production and the biological activity of estrogens. Nonvegetarian women have about 50 percent higher blood estrogen levels than vegetarians. High levels of estrogens, in turn, promote the growth of many breast tumors.

On the diet I recommend, most people will consume fewer calories than before, even though they are not eating less food. A diet lower in calories has been shown to retard aging and dramatically prolong the life span of many animals. The same is probably true in humans, but studies in people would be much more difficult to conduct.

In some of these studies, prolonging life depended not only on reducing the *number* of calories but also the *type* of calories. In one study, for example, mice that were given a calorie-restricted, high-fat diet lived twice as long as mice allowed to eat all they wanted. Yet when mice were placed on a low-fat, calorie-restricted diet, they lived *three times longer* than mice allowed to eat all they wanted. The authors concluded, "Clearly, although energy intake restriction provides significant influence on longevity, very high fat diets do not give the same protection as do high carbohydrate diets."

In other studies, restricting calories "typically and strongly lowers the incidence of most spontaneous and induced tumors, delays their onsets, and extends maximum life span in rodents." A recent article reviewing the research in this area stated, "Restriction of dietary energy maintains most physiologic systems in a youthful state and retards a broad spectrum of disease processes."

Some scientists believe that the benefits of this diet go beyond just preventing disease to actually slowing the process of aging. One researcher wrote, "In experimental animals, dietary restriction reduces the body weight increase due to aging, increases longevity and delays the onset of age-related physiological deterioration. A diet low in calories and high in fiber . . . [may] reduce age-related deterioration of brain functions." Eating fewer calories helps protect your cell membranes from aging as quickly. According to one group of researchers:

> Restricting the food intake of rodents extends the median length of life and the maximum life-span. It also retards most age-associated physiologic change and age-associated diseases. Our research indicates that the ability to retard disease processes is not the major reason for the extension of life-span or for the retardation of age change in most physiologic systems. Rather, it appears that most of the actions of food restriction are due to its ability to slow the primary aging processes.

## A RADICAL DIET?

A diet lower in calories and fat also reduces your body's production of what are called "free radicals." Your body creates free radicals as a by-product of normal metabolism and also in response to your diet, sunlight, X-rays, and air pollution such as cigarette smoke, car exhaust fumes, and ozone.

Free radicals are molecules that can damage your cells. They hasten aging and contribute to causing heart disease, cancer, lung disease, cataracts, and a variety of other illnesses. They impair the function of your immune system. When you reduce free radical formation, you may age more slowly and decrease your chances of many illnesses.

The diet I recommend is:

- low in oxidants that cause your body to produce free radicals
- high in antioxidants that help your body to remove free radicals

Dietary fat and iron are some of the major oxidants. These substances are found in the highest concentrations in animal products, especially in red meat. Since the diet I recommend is so low in animal products, it's also low in these oxidants.

For example, a recent series of studies found that iron is a potent risk factor for heart disease, because it oxidizes cholesterol. When cholesterol is oxidized, your body absorbs cholesterol into your arteries more easily. So when you eat a lot of meat, you eat the cholesterol that can cause heart disease, and you also consume the fat and iron that oxidize the cholesterol into a more harmful form.

Even when your body produces free radicals, the diet can help to remove them. This diet is rich in naturally occurring vitamins. Some vitamins act as antioxidants or scavengers of free radicals, thereby helping to prevent, forestall, or even reverse many diseases. For example, vitamins A (beta carotene), C, and E act as scavengers of free radical molecules that can harm DNA, your genetic blueprint, helping to prevent cancer. Also, they help prevent cholesterol from being changed into a form that is more likely to deposit in your arteries. Other vitamins, such as folic acid, help to stabilize chromosomes and may help to prevent cervical cancer and tumor formation.

The problems of a meat-centered diet—and the benefits of the diet I recommend—are especially easy to see in relation to preventing heart disease. Meat gives you a quadruple whammy:

- Meat is high in cholesterol, which clogs up your heart's arteries.
- Meat is high in saturated fat, which raises your blood cholesterol level.
- Meat is high in oxidants, like iron, which oxidize cholesterol to a form that is more easily deposited in your arteries.
- Meat is low in antioxidants.

In contrast, the diet I recommend gives you a quadruple benefit:

- It contains virtually no cholesterol.
- It is very low in saturated fat.
- It is very low in oxidants (even the iron in spinach is in a form that does not act as an oxidant).
- It is high in naturally occurring antioxidants.

In summary, then, this diet can help you to lose weight and keep it off—without hunger, without deprivation. You feel better. You have more energy. And eating this type of diet will also encourage a return to a style of eating—grazing—more in concert with your body's evolutionary history and predisposition.

# 4

# *Girth Control*

I would never be able to stay on a diet that required me to count calories and figure out what percentage of my calories came from fat, and I don't expect you to do so either. It takes too much time and effort, and it's not necessary. The diet I recommend consists of approximately 10 percent of calories as fat, but you don't have to carry around a calculator to keep track of complicated formulas, and you don't have to count calories as long as you eat only the foods that are part of this program. Your body needs only about 4 to 6 percent of calories as fat to provide the essential fatty acids, so this diet provides you with *enough* fat without providing you with *too much* fat.

As I mentioned in chapter 3, the *type* of calories you eat is more important than the *amount* of calories. On average, we consume fewer calories now than our ancestors did one hundred years ago. Yet even though we eat less than our ancestors did, we weigh more than ever.

What's different today is where the calories come from. In 1910, Americans got almost 60 percent of their calories from carbohydrates and about 20 percent from fat. By 1980, Americans consumed only about 40 percent of their calories from carbohydrates and almost 40 percent as fat. In other words, in the United States we consume almost twice as much fat in our diet as our great-grandparents did and, as a consequence, we weigh more than they did. Simply put, eating fat makes you fat, even if you take in fewer calories.

A study at Stanford made this point even more strongly. Researchers found that overweight men and thin men ate about the same number of calories. However, the overweight men ate more fat, and the thin ones ate less fat and more complex carbohydrates.

Similarly, T. Colin Campbell of Cornell University and J. Chen of China directed a comprehensive study of more than 6,500 Chinese living in sixty-five counties in China. They found that as the intake of fat and animal products increased, so did weight (and heart disease, many types of cancer, and other illnesses). This is further borne out by the fact that the average person in China eats 30 percent more total calories than the average American yet weighs less. Why? Because people in China consume 60 percent fewer calories from fat than Americans do.

## THE DIET

Taking into account that all calories are not the same, the diet I recommend is simple: Eat foods that are very low in fat, high in complex carbohydrates, and high in fiber. Avoid foods from animals, which are very high in fat, very low in complex carbohydrates, and very low in fiber (not to mention that they are high in cholesterol, which is only found in animal products, and saturated fat, which raises your blood level of cholesterol).

Foods from plants, with only a few exceptions, are very low in fat, high in complex carbohydrates, and high in fiber. Because of this, this diet is a low-fat vegetarian way of eating. If you don't want to be a vegetarian and don't have heart disease, then add moderate amounts of fish to your diet.

Here's all you really need to know: You can eat the following foods whenever you feel hungry until you are full (but not until you are stuffed):

- **Beans and legumes** (lentils, kidney beans, peas, black beans, red Mexican beans, split peas, soybeans, black-eyed peas, garbanzos, navy beans, and so on)
- **Fruits** (apples, apricots, bananas, strawberries, cherries, blueberries, oranges, peaches, raspberries, cantaloupes, watermelons, pears, honeydew melons, pineapples, tomatoes, and so on)
- **Grains** (corns, rice, oats, wheat, millet, barley, buckwheat, and so on)
- **Vegetables** (potatoes, zucchini, broccoli, carrots, lettuce, mushrooms, eggplant, celery, asparagus, onions, sweet potatoes, spinach, and so on)

You can eat the following foods in moderation:

- **Nonfat dairy products**, including skim milk, nonfat yogurt, nonfat cheeses, nonfat sour cream, and egg whites
- **Nonfat or very low-fat commercially available products**, including Advantage\10 frozen dinners, whole-grain breakfast cereals, Health Valley chili (and many other Health Valley products), Kraft Free nonfat mayonnaise and salad dressings, Guiltless Gourmet tortilla chips, Quaker Oats oatmeal, Nabisco fat-free crackers, Fleischmann's Egg Beaters, Pritikin or McDougall soups, Light n' Lively Free nonfat sour cream, Häagen-Dazs frozen yogurt bars, Entenmann's fat-free desserts (watch out for the sugar, though), and many others. According to *New Product News,* more than 1,024 reduced-fat products were introduced in 1990 and 1,198 in 1991. In 1991, 408 fat-free products were introduced. Many more are on the way, so it gets easier all the time.

Read labels (see Appendix 1). Some of the nonfat or very low-fat commercially available products are high in sugar, so avoid these when possible. Ingredients are listed on food labels in order of the amount contained in that food. In other words, if the first ingredient is sugar, then there's more sugar than anything else in that food. Also, on most packages you'll find the number of grams of fat, the number of calories, and the amount of cholesterol. Some of the nonfat commercial foods are loaded with chemicals, which you may wish to avoid.

If you're trying to lose weight and don't have other significant health problems, such as heart disease, then you have a spectrum of choices. It's not all or nothing. To the degree you reduce your intake of the following foods, then you'll lose more weight and improve your health and well-being:

- Meats (all kinds, including chicken and fish)
- Oils (all kinds) and oil-containing products, including margarines and most salad dressings, other than 3 grams per day of fish oil (to preserve omega-3 fatty acids)
- Avocados
- Olives
- Nuts and seeds
- High-fat or "low-fat" dairy, including whole milk, yogurt, butter, cheese, egg yolks, cream, and so on
- Sugar and simple sugar derivatives (honey, molasses, corn syrup, high fructose syrup, and the like), including white flour and white rice
- Alcohol
- Any commercially available product with more than two grams of fat per serving

That's really all there is to it. The rest of this chapter just fills in the details. If you eat according to these guidelines, you won't have to bring a calculator to your meals to ensure that you eat only 10 percent of your calories as fat.

## "IF YOU CAN'T *BE* A VEGETARIAN, THEN *EAT* ONE!"

Remember, being overweight is primarily due to how much fat you eat. Most of the fat you eat comes from two sources: animal products and oils. Because of this, the optimal diet is a low-fat vegetarian diet. The only vegetarian products to avoid are oils, avocados, olives, nuts, and seeds, because these are high in fat.

Many others have recognized the value of a vegetarian diet, so you'll be in good company, ranging from Renaissance genius Leonardo da Vinci to Russian genius Leo Tolstoy, Beatles Paul McCartney and George Harrison to actors Dennis Weaver and Lindsay Wagner, Nobel Prize-winning novelist Isaac Bashevis Singer to pediatrician Dr. Benjamin Spock, and playwright George Bernard Shaw to professional wrester Walter "Killer" Kowalski. And about four billion others.

*Nonfat* dairy products are high in protein, so consume these in moderation because too much protein is not healthful. Whole milk is second only to beef as the largest source of saturated fat in the American diet. "Low-fat" products sound fine, but they aren't. "Low-fat" milk is sometimes called "2 percent fat" milk, which sounds pretty good—but it's 2 percent of the total weight, and most of the weight in milk is water. Whole milk is 50 percent of calories as fat, "low-fat" milk is 38 percent of calories as fat, but nonfat milk (also called "skim milk" or "1% milk") is less than 2.5 percent of calories as fat. Or put another way, one cup of whole milk has eight grams of fat, one cup of "low-fat" milk has five grams of fat, and one cup of nonfat milk has less than one-half gram of fat—big difference.

Fish and chicken are, in general, lower in fat than beef, pork, or veal, but they still contain significantly more fat (and cholesterol) than most plant-based foods. Also, fish and chicken are often cooked in oil, butter, or margarine, which are very high in fat.

If you really want to be able to eat as much as you want until you are full and still lose weight, then you need to reduce fat down to around 10 percent of calories. In practical terms, this means excluding all meats, including fish and chicken, and all oils. In addition, fish and chicken (and for that matter, beef, pork, veal, and eggs) contain essentially no fiber and no complex carbohydrates which, as we discussed in chapter 3, are important.

If you decide to eat fish or chicken, then consume small amounts of roasted or grilled skinless chicken breast or fish such as perch, sole, cod, or flounder that are lower in fat than the more fatty fish such as mackerel or salmon (see Appendix 2). There are two kinds of shellfish: those that move and those that do not. The ones that don't move, such as clams, mussels, scallops, and oysters, are the vegetarians of the sea, and they consume the phytoplankton, or sea vegetables. Since these shellfish eat a vegetarian diet, their bodies are relatively low in fat and cholesterol. So, as Dr. William Castelli of the Framingham Heart Study is fond of saying, "If you can't *be* a vegetarian, then *eat* a vegetarian."

This diet also excludes oils, because all oils are liquid fat, including olive oil, safflower oil, and canola oil—100 percent fat. No matter what you may have heard, olive oil is not good for you. The more oil of any type that you consume, the more weight you will gain. You would likely lose weight if you were to do nothing more than eliminate oils and oil-containing products from your diet. Remember, frying food is going to load it with oils.

The table below makes it a little more clear that plant-based foods are very low in fat, high in complex carbohydrates, high in fiber, and have no cholesterol. In contrast, animal-based foods are high in fat and cholesterol, low in complex carbohydrates, and low in fiber. (On this diet, most people will consume approximately 20 to 25 grams of fat per day. Later in this chapter I'll show you how to calculate the right amount of fat for you.)

## Plant Products

| *Food* | *Amount* | *Fat* (*grams*) | *Carbo-hydrates* (*grams*) | *Fiber* (*grams*) | *Cholesterol* (*milligrams*) |
|---|---|---|---|---|---|
| apple | 1 whole | 0.5 | 21 | 2.8 | 0 |
| lettuce | 1 cup | 0.1 | 1.3 | 0.9 | 0 |
| carrots | 1 cup | 0.1 | 8.2 | 1.1 | 0 |
| baked potato | 1 whole | 0.2 | 33.6 | 2.7 | 0 |
| lentils | 1 cup | 0.8 | 39.8 | 5.4 | 0 |
| brown rice | ½ cup | 0.9 | 22.5 | 0.3 | 0 |
| oatmeal | 1 cup | 2.4 | 25.2 | 2.1 | 0 |

## Animal Products

| *Food* | *Amount* | *Fat* (*grams*) | *Carbo-hydrates* (*grams*) | *Fiber* (*grams*) | *Cholesterol* (*milligrams*) |
|---|---|---|---|---|---|
| scrambled egg | 1 | 7.1 | 1.4 | 0 | 282 |
| butter | 1 tsp | 3.8 | trace | 0 | 10 |
| cheeseburger | 4 oz | 15 | 28 | 0 | 50 |
| mackerel | 3.5 oz | 14 | 0 | 0 | 80 |
| goose, roasted | 1.3 lb | 75 | 0 | 0 | 569 |
| fried chicken | 10 oz | 52 | 26 | 0 | 247 |

More extensive listings of what is contained in foods can be found in several books, including *How Many Calories? How Much Fat?* by Rosemary Baskin and Consumer Reports (Yonkers, N.Y. Consumers Union, 1991), and *The Complete & Up-to-Date Fat Book,* by Karen Bellerson (Garden City Park, N.Y.: Avery Publishing Group, 1991).

Some people think that complex carbohydrates, such as bread and potatoes, are fattening, when it's really the company they keep that makes them high in fats. For example, as you can see above, a whole baked potato has almost no fat, no cholesterol, and is high in fiber. But if you load on the butter and sour cream, you're transforming an ideal food into one very high in fat and cholesterol. The recipes in this book will give you new ideas for flavoring and dressing up complex carbohydrates without adding fats. Also, you will find cooking techniques that will allow you to avoid fats without sacrificing taste or texture.

Different methods of preparing or dressing can transform ideal foods into ones that are very high in fat. For example:

| *Food* | *Amount* | *Fat* | *Calories* |
|---|---|---|---|
| baked potato | 3.5 oz | 0.1 grams | 92 calories |
| French fries | 3.5 oz | 17 grams | 322 calories |
| oil-free Italian dressing | 1 tbsp | 0 grams | 6 calories |
| regular Italian dressing | 1 tbsp | 8.6 grams | 67 calories |
| onions | 1 oz | 0.1 grams | 10 calories |
| onion rings | 1 oz | 7.5 grams | 115 calories |

## LIFE CHOICES

Of course, it's not all or nothing. You have a spectrum of choices in what you eat. The closer you move toward the low-fat vegetarian end of the spectrum, the greater will be the corresponding benefit. How much you want to do is completely up to you. It's your choice. As I will discuss more fully in chapter 6, by seeing this diet as a spectrum of choices, rather than as a set of rigid rules such as "Eat this!" and "Don't eat that!" you may find it easier to avoid giving yourself a hard time for not being perfect. The freer you feel, the easier it becomes to make changes and to maintain them.

## "*McCALL'S* TELLS ALL!"

Pick up just about any magazine in the supermarket check-out line, and you'll likely read something like this excerpt from the November 1992 issue of *McCall's*, one of my favorite medical journals:

How do actresses stay so enviably svelte? It's not just good genes and personal fitness gurus. Much of it has to do with a disciplined approach to eating healthfully, especially while working on movies. Take Madonna, for example. On the set of her upcoming movie *Body of Evidence,* the lithe megastar ate the same lunch every day: steamed asparagus, a plain baked potato, brown rice, and a salad.

More and more actresses are shunning traditional movie-set fare (such as rich beef stews and buttered mashed potatoes) for low-cal, nutritious cuisine, because they don't want to wrap a movie looking heavier than when they arrived. Michelle Pfeiffer, for instance, frequently dined on Caesar salad and pasta with pesto while working on the forthcoming movie, *Age of Innocence,* while Jennifer Jason Leigh acted her way through *Single White Female* bolstered by lots of vegetable lasagna.

**ACCORDING TO *MIRABELLA:***

"Madonna works out like a triathlete, splitting her three-hour workout between hardcore weights and a cardiovascular routine. Integral to Madonna's exercise program is her diet: 75 percent carbohydrates, 15 percent protein, and 10 percent fat."

Of course, I'm not suggesting that this program will make you look like a movie star, but you'll be in good company. Some people are so daunted by media images of perfectly shaped bodies that they give up trying to lose any weight. But my program is about *choices.* A movie star may choose to work with a personal trainer four hours a day to achieve and maintain his or her body. You may prefer to choose to spend that time with your friends and family, doing charitable work, advancing your career, or other activities. Either way, this program will allow you to reach—and maintain—a healthy weight that is appropriate for your frame.

## HOW SWEET IT *ISN'T*

*Complex carbohydrates* are starches in their natural, unrefined forms—potatoes, pasta, rice, beans, whole wheat bread, apples, and so on. As described in chapter 3, complex carbohydrates are low in calories, high in fiber, and they are bulky, so they fill you up before you eat too much. Besides filling you up, they biochemically signal your brain that you have had enough to eat. When you eat fat, on the other hand, it's very easy to consume too many calories before you feel full. In one study, for example, adding complex carbohydrates to food caused people to eat less (because the starches caused them to feel full), but adding fat to food did not cause them to eat less.

In contrast, *simple carbohydrates*—table sugar, alcohol, honey, molasses, corn syrup—do *not* fill you up. They have no fiber and are not at all bulky. When sugar is "refined," the fiber and warning signals that tell your brain you've had enough to eat are removed. Because of this, it becomes very easy to consume virtually unlimited amounts of it and thus a large number of calories without feeling full. Sugar is less important than fat, but you would be wise to limit how much of it you eat.

In the third year of the Lifestyle Heart Trial, for example, several of our study participants discovered and began devouring the then-new Entenmann's fat-free desserts. "They're fat-free, so they must be all right," they reasoned. But these desserts are very high in sugar, and many of the participants began regaining some of the weight they had lost. You can't eat more and weigh less if you consume a lot of sugar.

And Americans consume a *lot* of sugar. In 1985, an average of 127 pounds of sugar per person was consumed in the United States. That means the average American consumes more than a pound of sugar every three days! On average, that's about 620 calories per day as sugar. One twelve-ounce can of a soft drink, for example, has *ten teaspoons* of sugar!

The sugar in complex carbohydrates is absorbed slowly into your bloodstream, so your blood sugar level and your energy level remain more constant. This gives you sustained energy while giving your stomach the sensation of being full.

In contrast, simple sugars are absorbed quickly. (The same is true for alcohol, which your body quickly converts into sugar.) Your blood sugar rises fast. In response, your pancreas pumps out more insulin to lower your blood sugar, so it then quickly falls—often to a level below where you started. When this happens, you feel tired and intensely hungry. When your blood sugar gets too low, then your body says, "Hey, I need some more food so I can raise your blood sugar level back to normal!" Also, as we learned in chapter 3, when your body produces more insulin, you are more likely to convert dietary calories into body fat.

Here again, this is an adaptive mechanism—homeostasis—designed to protect you that becomes harmful in the context of a modern diet. Our bodies have not yet had time to evolve to eat large amounts of refined sugar. Until recently, large amounts of sugar were not readily available. You had to work hard to get it—raid a beehive, chop down some sugarcane and chew it, and so on. Only in modern times have vast amounts of sugar been so easily available and found in so many commercially prepared foods. And the warning signals that tell your brain, "OK, you've had enough to eat," have been refined away. For example, if you eat too much honey or sugarcane in its natural form, you begin to feel queasy after awhile. With refined sugar, that doesn't happen.

## WHY A BEER BELLY IS JUST THAT

*Alcohol suppresses your body's ability to burn fat.* When you drink alcohol, your body burns up fat much more slowly than usual. In one study, for example, researchers found that three ounces of alcohol reduced the body's ability to burn fat by about *one-third.* The unburned fat may go to your waist, creating a beer belly. So it is not just the calories and the fact that alcohol is converted into simple sugars that make it fattening, but also the way that alcohol throws off your body's normal disposal of fat in your diet.

## WHAT ABOUT SALT AND CAFFEINE?

When you eat a lot of salt, it may cause your body to retain fluid. Your body regulates the concentration of salt quite carefully. If you consume a lot of salt, then your body holds on to water to dilute the salt concentration to proper levels. Therefore, eating a lot of salt will make it more difficult for you to lose weight.

The effects of caffeine are unclear. Data from a study by Abdul Dulloo, a research nutritionist at the University of Geneva, Switzerland, suggest that caffeine may increase your metabolism. In some people, caffeine may also increase appetite, whereas in others, caffeine acts as an appetite suppressant. On the diet I recommend, though, you can increase your metabolism without the potential side effects of caffeine, which may include jumpiness, disturbed sleep, stomach distress, heart palpitations, and diarrhea. Also, a number of studies have connected caffeine to more serious health problems, including fibrocystic breast disease, high blood pressure, arrhythmias, and some forms of cancer. So if you drink coffee, try to limit the amount, and drink it without the cream or nondairy creamer (which is high in fat).

## PURE AND SIMPLE

In general, there is so little fat in naturally occurring fruits, vegetables, grains, and beans that if you eat a diet consisting primarily of these foods, and if you eat according to the above guidelines, then you don't have to count calories and deal with complex formulas. You don't even have to count grams of fat, unless you eat a lot of commercially prepared foods which may be higher in fat than you think—more on this later. If you want to be more precise about keeping track of how much fat to consume, here's how:

The Metropolitan Life Insurance Company issues tables that list the so-called ideal body weights. (Insurance companies are in the business of predicting who is going to die pre-

## Table 1
## 1983 Metropolitan Height and Weight Tables

### MEN

| Height *Feet* | *Inches* | Small Frame | Medium Frame | Large Frame |
|---|---|---|---|---|
| 5 | 2 | 128–134 | 131–141 | 138–150 |
| 5 | 3 | 130–136 | 133–143 | 140–153 |
| 5 | 4 | 132–138 | 135–145 | 142–156 |
| 5 | 5 | 134–140 | 137–148 | 144–160 |
| 5 | 6 | 136–142 | 139–151 | 146–164 |
| 5 | 7 | 138–145 | 142–154 | 149–168 |
| 5 | 8 | 140–148 | 145–157 | 152–172 |
| 5 | 9 | 142–151 | 148–160 | 155-176 |
| 5 | 10 | 144–154 | 151–163 | 158–180 |
| 5 | 11 | 146–157 | 154–166 | 161–184 |
| 6 | 0 | 149–160 | 157–170 | 164–188 |
| 6 | 1 | 152–164 | 160–174 | 168–192 |
| 6 | 2 | 155–168 | 164–178 | 172–197 |
| 6 | 3 | 158–172 | 167–182 | 176–202 |
| 6 | 4 | 162–176 | 171–187 | 181–207 |

Weights at ages 25–59 based on lowest mortality. Weight in pounds according to frame (in indoor clothing weighing 5 lbs., shoes with 1" heels).

Source of basic data: *1979 Build Study,* Society of Actuaries and Association of Life Insurance Medical Directors of America, 1980. Table courtesy of Metropolitan Life Insurance Company.

**Table 1**
**1983 Metropolitan Height and Weight Tables**

WOMEN

| **Height** *Feet* | *Inches* | Small Frame | Medium Frame | Large Frame |
|---|---|---|---|---|
| 4 | 10 | 102–111 | 109–121 | 118–131 |
| 4 | 11 | 103–113 | 111–123 | 120–134 |
| 5 | 0 | 104–115 | 113–126 | 122–137 |
| 5 | 1 | 106–118 | 115–129 | 125–140 |
| 5 | 2 | 108–121 | 118–132 | 128–143 |
| 5 | 3 | 111–124 | 121–135 | 131–147 |
| 5 | 4 | 114–127 | 124–138 | 134–151 |
| 5 | 5 | 117–130 | 127–141 | 137–155 |
| 5 | 6 | 120–133 | 130–144 | 140–159 |
| 5 | 7 | 123–136 | 133–147 | 143–163 |
| 5 | 8 | 126–139 | 136–150 | 146–167 |
| 5 | 9 | 129–142 | 139–153 | 149–170 |
| 5 | 10 | 132–145 | 142–156 | 152–173 |
| 5 | 11 | 135–148 | 145–159 | 155–176 |
| 6 | 0 | 138–151 | 148–162 | 158–179 |

Weights at ages 25–59 based on lowest mortality. Weight in pounds according to frame (in indoor clothing weighing 3 lbs., shoes with 1" heels).

maturely, and they use body weight as one of the forecasters of early mortality.) Keep in mind that these tables are not very precise. First, the tables are reissued every few years. The table issued in 1983 has heavier weights than the one issued in 1959, and that may not be to the advantage of your health. Second, there is a wide range of "ideal weight" based on frame size. Third, and most important, these charts do not take into account individual differences in physiology and metabolism.

Having said that, here's how to determine a little more precisely your daily quota of fat on a 10 percent fat diet:

First, find your "ideal" weight using Table 1, based on

**Table 2**
**Maximum Total Fat Intake: Men**

| *Ideal Body Weight* | *Inactive* | *Moderately Active* | *Very Active* |
|---|---|---|---|
| 90 | 14 | 15 | 16 |
| 100 | 16 | 17 | 18 |
| 110 | 17 | 18 | 20 |
| 120 | 19 | 20 | 21 |
| 130 | 20 | 22 | 23 |
| 140 | 22 | 23 | 25 |
| 150 | 23 | 25 | 27 |
| 160 | 25 | 27 | 28 |
| 170 | 26 | 28 | 30 |
| 180 | 28 | 30 | 32 |
| 190 | 30 | 32 | 34 |
| 200 | 31 | 33 | 36 |
| 210 | 33 | 35 | 37 |
| 220 | 34 | 37 | 39 |

Find the figure in the left-hand column that most closely corresponds to the desirable weight you identified in Step 1. Then move across the chart to the vertical column that corresponds to your physical activity level. At the point where your ideal weight and activity level intersect, you will find the maximum amount of total fat (in grams) that you should consume each day.

your height and frame size. A better alternative may be to decide how much *you* want to weigh—the weight at which you feel the most comfortable. I'm not talking about looking like a fashion model (more on this in chapters 6 and 7). At your ideal weight, you should feel energetic as well as happy with how you look in the mirror.

After finding your "ideal" weight in Table 1, then look at Table 2. Based on your desirable weight and activity level, Table 2 will indicate the recommended number of total grams of fat per day.

Finally, add up how many grams of fat you consume each day. There are a variety of pocket-sized fat gram counters

**Table 2**
**Maximum Total Fat Intake: Women**

| *Ideal Body Weight* | *Inactive* | *Moderately Active* | *Very Active* |
|---|---|---|---|
| 90 | 13 | 14 | 14 |
| 100 | 14 | 15 | 16 |
| 110 | 15 | 17 | 18 |
| 120 | 17 | 18 | 19 |
| 130 | 18 | 20 | 21 |
| 140 | 20 | 21 | 22 |
| 150 | 23 | 25 | 27 |
| 160 | 25 | 27 | 28 |
| 170 | 26 | 28 | 30 |
| 180 | 28 | 30 | 32 |
| 190 | 30 | 32 | 34 |
| 200 | 31 | 33 | 36 |
| 210 | 33 | 35 | 37 |
| 220 | 34 | 37 | 39 |

Find the figure in the left-hand column that most closely corresponds to the desirable weight you identified in Step 1. Then move across the chart to the vertical column that corresponds to your physical activity level. At the point where your ideal weight and activity level intersect, you will find the maximum amount of total fat (in grams) that you should consume each day.

now available. Just writing down everything you eat each day will increase your awareness of your diet.

Commercially available foods are required by law to list the number of grams of fat per serving. Be careful, though—sometimes, the manufacturer will make the serving size ridiculously small just to make the number of grams of fat seem small. Also, the law currently states that if a food contains less than one-half gram of fat per serving, the manufacturer can state that the food is "fat-free." (Similarly, if the food contains less than 2.5 milligrams of cholesterol per serving, the manufacturer can state that the food is "cholesterol-free.") So if food manufacturers make the serving size very small, they may claim that the foods are fat-free when they really aren't.

## GOOD TASTE

Four tastes are inherent to our tongue: sweet, sour, salty, and bitter. Even so, these tastes can be modified. For example, you may have had the experience of reducing your salt consumption. When you first reduce the salt in your diet, the food may taste too bland, but after about two weeks, your palate has readjusted. At that point, if you go out to a familiar restaurant, the food may taste too salty even though it seemed just fine only a few weeks earlier. A little salt brings out the taste in foods, but a lot of salt tends to mask the subtle flavors. And you don't even know what you're missing until you reduce your salt consumption.

The taste for fat is an acquired one, so it's even easier to modify than one of the inherent tastes like salt. You may have switched from drinking whole milk to low-fat or skim milk. At first, the milk may taste too watery. Again, after about two weeks, the milk will taste just fine and whole milk will taste too rich, almost like cream. The same readjustment occurs when you reduce fat consumption in the rest of your diet. Like salt, a lot of fat tends to mask the subtle flavors. Once you reduce your fat consumption, you'll discover how wonderful the natural flavors in food can taste.

Surprisingly, our research has demonstrated that it's often easier to become a complete vegetarian than to just cut back on the amount of fish, chicken, and beef you consume. Your palate never gets a chance to readjust if you keep eating meat, even in smaller quantities, because eating a little meat only makes you want more. And not only more meat, but also other high-fat foods—ice cream, butter, cakes, pies, and so on.

The same is true for the new artificial fats like Olestra and Simplesse and artificial sugars like Nutra-Sweet. They reinforce your taste for fat, sweet, and greasy foods. Also, as I will discuss more fully in chapter 6, when you make comprehensive changes in your diet and lifestyle, you feel so much better, so quickly, that the choices become much clearer and easier.

So give yourself at least two weeks on this program. First, your palate and food preferences will begin to change in that amount of time. Also, you may begin to feel so much better that the benefits will become much clearer and more personally meaningful.

This book contains more than two hundred and fifty recipes by some of the country's leading chefs, but you don't have to throw out your old recipe books and embrace something totally new. Instead, modify the foods you're used to eating, or find recipes in this book that are familiar to you. After all, most people recycle the same dozen or so recipes. For example, if you're used to having spaghetti and meatballs with lots of oil and butter, try having the same spaghetti but with your favorite vegetables on top instead of the meatballs, cooked without the oil and butter. Or try the pasta recipes on pages 303–314 and 325–327 for some new ideas on how to prepare the foods you enjoy.

## A FEW HELPFUL IDEAS

- Eat like a gourmet, with mindfulness, slowly savoring each bite. Pay attention to the variety of flavors and textures. More on this in chapter 7.

- Pay attention to how the food is affecting you, and why and when you are eating. Notice when you're no longer hungry—or even when you're full—but you're still eating. At those moments, put the food away, at least for a while, and pay attention to what emotional feelings you're having, without judging them or trying to push them down. Try to "feed" your emotional need in a more constructive way. Write out your feelings in a journal. Call a friend with whom you feel comfortable talking. Take a walk. Meditate.
- You may find it helpful to eat food in only one or two rooms in your home—for example, your kitchen and your dining room. When you limit where you eat food, then you make the act of eating more special, even sacred.
- Avoid keeping high-fat foods around the house.
- Create a support group. In chapter 6, I'll describe in more detail the healing power of social support.
- The community and connection of eating with friends feels healing, so it is very tempting to order the same food as everyone else. Drawing attention to the fact that you may be eating differently from your friends and colleagues may make you feel different and more isolated from them. But it's not necessary. If you don't make a big deal over what you're eating, chances are no one else will either. As Bob Finnell, one of the participants in the Lifestyle Heart Trial, noted:

  > I found many problems were nonproblems. Rather than announcing in a restaurant that nothing fit my choices or making an issue of a banquet plate with a piece of meat, I learned to order what I needed or only eat what I wanted from the plate. I found that not a single person noticed that I didn't eat the meat and, more so recently, that no waiter batted an eye about ordering a vegetarian dish.

- Similarly, when you go to someone's home for dinner or a party, offer to bring something that you can eat. You don't have to announce that you are on a special diet.

Chances are your host will not even notice that the dish you bring is low in fat. If the dinner is buffet, then focus on the side dishes.

- Eat only when you're *really* hungry—"gut hungry," in the words of Dr. John Foreyt—not just because it's time for a meal.
- Divide your food into smaller portions. Instead of wolfing down an apple, for example, cut it into small pieces and enjoy each one more leisurely.
- Eat breakfast. In one study, moderately overweight women who regularly skipped breakfast were randomly divided into two groups. One group was asked to start eating a low-fat breakfast every morning, and one group was asked to keep skipping breakfast. After twelve weeks, the women who were eating breakfast lost significantly more weight than the women who continued to skip breakfast. Why? A good breakfast gives you energy and reduces your hunger during the morning, so you'll feel less need to grab a donut during a coffee break. Also, breakfast is the easiest, simplest, and most familiar meal to make. I usually have a bowl of whole-grain cereal or oatmeal with cinnamon with skim milk or nonfat yogurt on top (with a dash of vanilla extract), some whole wheat toast with a little jam, apple butter, or fruit preserves (or just plain), some water or juice. You might include some decaffeinated coffee or herbal tea.

In the next chapter, I'll talk about exercise—what I say may pleasantly surprise you. The last two chapters will focus on new ways of nourishing the deeper hunger that we are often trying to feed.

# 5

# *No Pain, No Pain*

## WHY DO SOME PEOPLE CONSUME MORE ENERGY THAN THEY USE?

On many diets, people eat too high a percentage of calories as fat and then feel overwhelmed when they are told how much exercise is necessary to counterbalance that much fat intake. When they hear "no pain, no gain," they worry that they may have to exercise until they drop. It seems like too much effort, so they may just roll over in bed and hide under the covers. Partly because of this syndrome, less than 20 percent of adult Americans engage in regular, vigorous exercise. Over one-half of U.S. adults are self-described couch potatoes.

Exercise is helpful, but it takes much more effort to try to "burn off" fat calories by intensive exercise than it does to consume fewer fat calories in the first place. For example, a typical fast-food dinner consisting of a quarter-pound cheeseburger, milkshake, and a small order of French fries has about 1,100 calories. You'd have to run for eleven miles to burn off 1,100 calories!

## USE IT *AND* LOSE IT

Since you consume so much less fat on this program than on most other diets, you don't need to exercise excessively. Moderate exercise is an important part of the program. Just walking twenty to sixty minutes a day, and not even very fast, is often enough. Moderate exercise gives you most of the physiological and psychological health benefits of more intensive forms of exercise while minimizing the risks of injury, both to your musculoskeletal system and to your heart.

In fact, moderate exercise may be even *better* than intensive exercise for losing weight. For example, Dr. John Duncan divided 102 sedentary women into three groups. Each group was asked to walk three miles, five days per week. One group walked three miles in thirty-six minutes, one group walked that distance in forty-six minutes, and one group strolled the same three miles in one hour. To the surprise of many, he found that the strollers lost more weight than the women in the other two groups. In other words, those who walked slower lost more body fat than those who walked the same distance but faster.

Why? The *number* of calories they burned was the same, but the *type* of calories varied. For short, intense exercise, your body tends to burn carbohydrates, because it takes less time to convert carbohydrates into glucose, your body's fuel. Longer, slower exercise gives your body a chance to use body fat as fuel.

In other studies, researchers have found that regular, moderate exercise tends to decrease appetite, food intake, and body weight, whereas vigorous exercise tends to increase appetite and food intake. And if you exercise instead of snacking at the times when you're most tempted to overeat—for example, when you're stressed, lonely, or unhappy—then you'll get a double benefit.

Moderate exercise can improve your resting metabolism—that is, how fast your body burns energy (calories). Your metabolism is the greatest source of your energy expenditure, so anything that affects your metabolism has a profound effect on your weight. As we discussed in chapter 3, restricting calories may lower your metabolism (since your body thinks you're starving and tries to conserve energy), whereas the diet I recommend can maintain or even increase your metabolism (since you don't restrict the amount of food you consume). The benefits of moderate exercise go beyond the calories burned while you exercise; even more important may be the effects of moderate exercise on increasing your metabolism.

However, intense exercise may actually *decrease* your metabolism. Here again, this is an adaptive response: When you exercise intensely, you start to burn up calories so quickly that your body tries to conserve energy by slowing down your metabolism.

Moderate exercise may also improve your immune system's function, while excessive exercise may depress your immune system. A study of 2,300 marathon runners found that runners who ran the marathon had *six times* the incidence of colds and influenza when compared to those who decided at the last minute not to run.

Also, low to moderate levels of physical activity produce the greatest psychological benefits. Low to moderate levels of exercise can improve your mood, self-confidence, self-esteem, and sense of well-being while helping to decrease stress, anxiety, and depression. In contrast, high-intensity exercise may increase negative emotions, such as anxiety, tension, and fatigue, in some people. As Dr. Judith Rodin wrote in her excellent book, *Body Traps,* "For some exercise-dependent people, workouts cease to be a means of improving life. They become an escape from it."

Just as yo-yo dieting leads to the problems described in chapter 3, so does yo-yo exercising. In a moment of inspiration—New Year's Day, realizing your clothes no longer fit, or after a medical scare—you may resolve to run five miles a day. After a while, though, you may find it hard to stick with an intensive exercise program and find yourself doing it less and less, until one day you're not exercising at all. This may have a worse effect on your body than never having started an exercise program.

In one study, sedentary animals were divided into two groups. One group remained sedentary, while the other group was put on an exercise regimen. When the exercised animals were taken off their program, they overate and regained weight. Worse, they had a higher percentage of body fat, higher blood pressure, and slower metabolisms than the rats that had remained sedentary. Even athletes who start and stop exercise training develop more abdominal fat. Repeated weight loss and gain also causes animals to prefer eating more fat—but moderate exercise prevents this increased preference for dietary fat.

If you start an intensive exercise program, you may not stick with it. However, if you only need to walk thirty to sixty minutes a day, it's something you can maintain indefinitely without much difficulty. This is especially true if you are overweight, because it's hard to exercise vigorously when you weigh too much. In this sense, being sedentary is both a cause and a consequence of being overweight.

Lean body tissue (muscle) has a faster metabolism than fat tissue. When you exercise moderately, you lose fat tissue more than lean body tissue, so your metabolism increases. This is part of the reason why moderate exercise helps to increase your metabolism. And as your metabolism increases, you burn off calories faster, even when you're not exercising.

Combining moderate exercise, such as walking, with moderate resistance training (such as light weight lifting, low-impact aerobics, push-ups, rowing, or stair climbing) can be especially helpful in building and preserving muscle and lean body tissue. When you lose fat tissue and gain muscle tissue, you can begin to raise your metabolism permanently, thereby allowing you to eat more and weigh less (assuming, of course, that you're eating in a way consistent with the guidelines in the last chapter). You'll feel better and you'll look better.

Finally, some evidence indicates that moderate exercise may slow the aging process. According to Dr. William Evans, chief of the Human Physiology Laboratory at the Human Nutrition Research Center on Aging at Tufts University:

> Most of the decline in physical functioning is caused not by aging but by lack of exercise . . . We think we shouldn't exercise because we're getting older. So what we have here is a self-fulfilling prophecy: we do get weak and frail and we assume it's because we're getting old. And this just isn't true. . . . Aerobic capacity and percentage of body fat is related to time spent exercising, not to age.

Similarly, in the Lifestyle Heart Trial, we found that the best predictor of improvement was neither age nor disease severity but the degree that people adhered to the program. The more people changed, the better they got. So it's never too late to begin changing—and never too early.

In recognition of the value of low to moderate exercise (for example, strolling three miles in one hour), a recent paper by three leading researchers from Yale University concluded:

> The findings that moderate levels of exercise are sufficient for improved health and weight control suggest a re-orientation of exercise prescription for overweight persons. Specifically, we propose that the typical [vigorous] exercise prescription . . . be avoided with overweight persons . . . The best exercise prescription is one that the person can and will follow.

## SLOW BUT STEADY WINS THE RACE

If you haven't been exercising in a long time, then remember the concept of homeostasis. The magnitude and speed of change determines the amount of resistance to change due to homeostasis. If you decide to run five miles on the first day after years of being a couch potato, your mind may be willing, but your body will not be pleased. If you start a program too quickly or vigorously, then you might become injured, overly tired, and uncomfortable, all of which may discourage and dishearten you.

Start *slowly.* Build up your level of exercise *gradually.*

Decide what is gradual for you, and go half as much as that when you begin. Remember the tortoise and the hare: "Slow but steady wins the race."

If you have been overweight for a while, chances are you've had some unhappy experiences around exercise. You likely have gone on and off at least one exercise program. You may have had some negative experiences associated with exercise when you were growing up—gym class from hell, for example. These negative associations may make it harder to get started.

When I was a child, exercise was often the preferred form of punishment: "Ornish! Take a lap!" Having gone to public schools in Texas, where corporal punishment was not only allowed but encouraged, I was often given the choice between getting paddled or doing fifty push-ups. So, it took me a while to learn how much fun exercise can be.

Because exercise is important, both in losing weight and in gaining health, here are some ideas to help you design a program that's right for you. You may wish to choose to exercise in ways that are:

- *Fun.* If you like it, you're more likely to do it. Make it playful, not work, drudgery, or medicine. Do what you enjoy, not what you think you "should" be doing. If you like to walk, then walk. Walk somewhere you want to go. If you prefer another form of exercise, do that instead. Some studies show that even gardening gives you most of the benefits of more vigorous exercise.
- *Fast.* Incorporate exercise into your daily life. Find ways to make exercise part of your normal activities. Take the stairs instead of the elevator. Park a little further from the store. Take heart: If you did nothing more than walking up and down two flights of stairs a day, you would lose at least six pounds of weight per year.
- *Flexible.* If you miss a day of exercise—or even a week—don't use that as an excuse to flog yourself. Just tell yourself, "Oh, well, nobody's perfect," and start again.
- *Gradual.* Start slowly, exercise moderately, then cool down slowly. If you can't talk comfortably while exer-

cising, then you're working too hard. Slow down until you can.

- *Easy.* As we've been discussing, moderate exercise is better for you than being sedentary or exercising excessively. And if it's not too strenuous, you're more likely to keep it up.
- *Varied.* Cross-training—doing different types of exercise—has a double benefit. First, you can work on different groups of muscles. Second, it may prove to be more interesting—"variety is the spice of life." Even if you just walk, you may want to vary when and where you choose to walk—and with whom. Resistance training gives you added benefits by both building up your muscle tone (which further increases your metabolism) and firming up your body.
- *Low-impact.* Avoid exercises that require you to jump up and down, like jogging or running, at least in the initial stages of starting to exercise. Repetitive, high-impact exercises may increase the risk of joint injury, especially if you are overweight. Walking, swimming, and rowing are only a few examples of low-impact exercises.
- *Social.* You may find it easier to exercise with a friend or at a local club with other people. As described in chapters 6 and 7, social support is a powerful determinant of health and well-being.
- *Comfortable.* Wear loose-fitting, warm clothing, comfortable shoes, and drink lots of water before, during, and after exercise. If you hurt, then stop.
- *Meditative.* Exercise with awareness. Pay attention to how the exercise is making you feel, and you will both increase your enjoyment and decrease the likelihood of injury. Many meditative traditions recommend "walking meditations," especially when you are feeling too agitated to meditate while sitting still. For example, you can count your steps, focus on your breathing, or repeat a meditative sound while walking. Some people like to exercise while watching television or listening to a

Walkman, but they miss the opportunity to exercise with awareness.

- *Simple.* The bottom line is this: Doing something is a lot better than doing nothing. You don't have to keep track of complex formulas, maximal oxygen uptakes, and pulse rates (unless you have heart disease), and you don't have to exercise until you drop. Just do it!
- *Convenient.* Joining a health club may be a great step, but not if it's far away. Home exercise equipment is convenient. If you are uncomfortable with your appearance, you may be more comfortable exercising at home. On the other hand, some people find it easier to motivate themselves when other people are around.
- *Regular.* Walking five or six times a week will help keep your metabolism higher than if you walk less frequently. Also, the more regularly you walk, the more likely it will become a habit.
- *Pleasant.* If it's cold and raining outside or if it's too hot, then head for the nearest shopping mall. (Stroll past the fast-food places inside.) Or pull out your treadmill or stationary bicycle.
- *Yours.* You choose if you want to exercise, *how much* you want to exercise, and *in what way* you want to exercise. You are in control.

Now that we've talked about behaviors like diet and exercise, let's turn to the deeper issues that really motivate our actions. Getting health information is important, but it's not usually sufficient to motivate us to make *lasting* changes in our lives. In the next two chapters, I'll describe what does.

# 6

# *What's Eating You?*

## "DO YOU BRAINWASH YOUR PATIENTS?"

Recently, I presented our latest research findings at a major international scientific meeting held in Osaka, Japan. Afterward, an elderly, distinguished Japanese physician asked me, in all seriousness, "Dr. Ornish, do you brainwash your patients in order to get them to change their diets and lifestyles?"

And I thought to myself, "What an amazing question! I mean, here I am in Japan, a country that has been eating a very low-fat diet for thousands of years, a land with a long and rich tradition of meditation—and in only one generation, the idea of eating a low-fat diet and meditating is now considered so radical that this doctor thinks we must need to brainwash people for them to do that. Amazing!"

Ironically, a scientist who spoke just before me presented data showing that animal fat consumption in Japan has increased *800 percent* during the past twenty-five years. Not surprisingly, obesity is becoming quite common in Japan, whereas it used to be very unusual to see an overweight Japanese. Cholesterol levels in Japanese boys used to be among the lowest in the world and stayed low throughout life. Now, Japanese boys ages ten to twelve have cholesterol levels 75 percent higher than American boys the same age. The time bomb is ticking.

In Singapore, it's already exploding. In 1990, while lecturing at a symposium sponsored by the International Society and Federation of Cardiology, Singapore, I learned that heart disease is now the leading cause of death there. Thirty years ago, it was among the countries with the lowest incidence of heart disease. Soon, the same will happen in Japan and in much of the developing world.

It's not hard to understand why. All you have to do is walk down the street in Tokyo or Osaka or Singapore, or just about any place in Europe or Asia, and you are greeted by Colonel Sanders, Wendy's, Burger King, and McDonald's. Someone once said that McDonald's is America's revenge for Pearl Harbor.

We seem to have come to a point at which it is considered "normal" to eat a high-fat diet, to smoke, to feel stressed, to be sedentary, and to take powerful, expensive drugs for the rest of one's life (with known and unknown side effects), yet we think a person would have to be brainwashed to eat a low-fat diet, meditate, exercise, and stop smoking. It is the Japanese who are being "brainwashed" by Western advertising and fast food. The rest of the world is copying our mistakes rather than learning from them. There is a better way.

## WHY IS IT SO HARD TO CHANGE OUR BEHAVIORS? AND WHAT REALLY MOTIVATES US TO MAKE AND MAINTAIN *LASTING* CHANGES?

When my colleagues and I first began applying for grants to conduct research to see if heart disease could be reversed by making comprehensive changes in diet and lifestyle, we were initially unable to obtain funding from the major foundations and government agencies. As I mentioned in chapter 1, few people at that time believed that heart disease could be reversed.

More than that, though, a bigger obstacle was that, as I

was told by these institutions, "No one has ever demonstrated that people in the real world can change their diet and lifestyle for very long. Since they won't stay on your diet, then you can't test your theory."

In the Lifestyle Heart Trial, we were able to demonstrate that heart disease often can be reversed simply by making comprehensive changes in diet and lifestyle alone. Perhaps equally important, we showed that our study participants were able to make these changes in diet and lifestyle in a real-world environment. To the best of my knowledge, our study is the only one to demonstrate that it really is possible for many people to maintain comprehensive changes in diet and lifestyle for several years.

The study was originally designed as a one-year intervention in the lives of patients who had severe coronary heart disease. Based on our results after one year, we received foundation and government support to continue studying the same group of people for five years. As I described in chapter 1, almost all of the participants remained on the program very successfully during the first year. On average, they showed even more reversal after five years than after one year. In contrast, participants in the comparison group who followed the conventional diet and lifestyle recommendations, including a 30 percent fat diet and exercise, became even worse after five years than after one year.

We did not select these participants because they were the most motivated to change their lifestyles. Rather, they just happened to be in the hospital receiving a cardiology test called an angiogram on the days that we were looking for volunteers. We approached them and asked if they wanted to be in the study. About one-half agreed, even though it required them to have another angiogram after only one year, a painful and somewhat risky test. We accepted anyone who volunteered. Only one person dropped out during the first year. Because of this, I think that more people may be willing to make and maintain comprehensive changes in diet and lifestyle than many doctors believe possible. Also, as I mentioned in chapter 1, I have received thousands of letters from people who have been able to follow this program successfully simply from reading my previous books.

Why were we successful? In the course of conducting our research, we have been learning what really motivates people to change their diet and lifestyle and to be able to stay with it for long periods of time.

Before joining our study, many of the research participants had been on and off diets for many years without much success. I asked them why they were able to follow our program so successfully, and for so long. Here's what I learned from them:

- Most diets are too complex to follow for very long, the food doesn't taste good, and you feel hungry and deprived.
- Comprehensive changes are easier to make than moderate ones, because you feel healthier and so much more energetic, so quickly—instant gratification.
- Joy is a more powerful motivator than fear—change to feel better, not just to live longer.

Let's examine these in more depth.

## A SIMPLE DIET IS EASIER TO FOLLOW THAN A COMPLEX DIET

Most diets don't work for very long because they are too complex and rigid. Too many rules, too much effort, too time-consuming. If I needed to lose weight, I don't think I could ever stay on a diet that required me to count calories. Not for long, anyway.

In contrast, the diet I recommend is very simple. No calories to count, no food to weigh, no behavioral modification tricks to learn, no portion sizes to measure. In fact, this is not a "diet" in the usual sense of the word, but rather a new way of eating.

In this spirit, I have written this book to be short, simple, and practical, telling you what you need to know without a lot of extraneous information. Simply put, the food is delicious, the ingredients are easy to obtain and prepare, and you can eat whenever you're hungry.

## COMPREHENSIVE CHANGES ARE EASIER THAN MODERATE ONES

In our research, we learned that it is often easier for people to make comprehensive changes in diet and lifestyle than to make only moderate ones. At first, this may seem like a paradox, but it makes sense when you understand why.

If you make only *moderate* changes in lifestyle—for example, reducing fat intake from the typical American diet of about 40 percent of calories as fat to the conventional dietary guidelines of 30 percent fat—then you have the worst of both worlds. You feel deprived and hungry because you are not eating everything you want and are used to, but you're not making changes big enough to feel that much better or to significantly affect your weight or how you feel (or, for that matter, your cholesterol, blood pressure, or heart disease). In other words, you're clear about what you're giving up, but you aren't getting much positive reinforcement to make you feel like you're getting something back that's equal or better.

For example, patients in the comparison group of the Lifestyle Heart Trial made moderate changes in their diet (30 percent fat, 200 milligrams of cholesterol), yet they felt worse. The frequency of their chest pains increased by 165 percent. They did not lose weight. And their heart disease worsened.

In contrast, when you make *comprehensive* changes in diet and lifestyle—for instance, with the program—then you begin to feel so much better, so quickly, that the choices and benefits become much clearer. And you don't feel deprived or hungry.

*During the first week,* patients in the Lifestyle Heart Trial began to lose weight and reported more energy and a greater sense of well-being than they had experienced in years. They reported a 91 percent reduction in the average frequency of chest pains due to heart disease, and most of that improvement occurred during the first few days to few weeks after changing lifestyle.

These rapid improvements are a powerful motivator. When people who have had so much chest pain that they can't work, or make love, or even walk across the street without intense suffering find that they are able to do all of those things without pain in only a few weeks, then they often say, "Sure, I like eating meat and a rich diet, but not *that* much! These are choices worth making." These often dramatic improvements in people with heart disease help to illustrate the power of the program, but its benefits extend to those without heart disease.

"We're always making choices," said our research participants, "and we don't mind making choices when we understand the benefits." Like them, I don't believe in giving up something that I enjoy unless what I get back is better than what I'm giving up.

I grew up in Texas eating lots of cheeseburgers, chilis, and chalupas, and I still love the way meat tastes. (People say they lose their taste for meat, but it hasn't happened to me.) But I found that I feel much better when I don't eat meat, so for me it was a choice worth making even though I don't have any significant health problems. Since I began eating this way, I've never had to worry about my weight. I have more energy. I need less sleep. I think more clearly.

For people who want to lose weight or for those with health problems, the benefits should be even clearer. People who follow this program usually find that they not only *feel* better, they usually are better in ways that can be measured. Weight decreases, blood pressure falls, cholesterol levels decline (by an average of almost 40 percent in the Lifestyle Heart Trial—as much as if we had used cholesterol-lowering drugs), heart disease improves, and so on.

Another reason comprehensive changes are easier to make than minor changes is that big changes disrupt your old routines. What you eat is patterned by your habits, in the same way that it's familiar for some people to light a cigarette when they get on the telephone or to have a drink when they come home from work. You tend to eat the same foods because you're used to them. You may have fallen into a pattern, a rut, and that familiarity is comforting.

For this reason, it's easier to comprehensively change the type of foods that you eat rather than just reduce the amount of food you eat. For example, if you're in the habit of eating an eight-ounce steak, then it's hard to eat only four ounces. If you're used to eating eight ounces, then you're likely to feel deprived when you eat only half as much. When you eat some, you may want some more. In a real sense, it's easier not to eat any steak at all and to eat something totally different—because you're changing your patterns, your habits, not just eating less of the same foods. And it's simpler—you don't have to wonder, "Is it four ounces or five?" Most important, you don't feel hungry and deprived.

Fat is an *acquired* taste, not one of the four basic flavors (sweet, sour, salty, bitter). For example, if you change from whole milk to skim milk, the skim milk may taste too watery at first, but after a few weeks it tastes just fine. If you then drink whole milk, it may taste like cream, too rich, because your palate has adjusted to the skim milk. However, if you always drink some whole milk and some skim milk, then your palate never has a chance to make that shift, so the skim milk will always taste too watery. In a similar way, if you always eat some meat or chicken or fish, then your palate never has a chance to adjust, so you don't lose your taste for them.

Comprehensive changes can be stressful at first, exactly because they disrupt your old patterns and habits. In the long run, though, it's easier to maintain adherence to big changes precisely because they take you out of your old habits and help you form new ones.

## JOY IS A MORE POWERFUL MOTIVATOR THAN FEAR

If I tried to scare you into changing your behavior, it wouldn't work very well. At least not for long.

We all know that we will die someday. But it's such a terrifying thought that it's hard to think about for very long. So we don't. We block it out of our awareness. We deny the truth, even to ourselves. There is an old joke that "denial is not just a river in Egypt," and there is some wisdom to that. Most people do not really believe that they ever will die, even though they accept the concept intellectually. Therefore, efforts to motivate you to change based on fear of dying prematurely do not succeed for very long.

I first learned this from my father, who is a dentist. When I was in elementary school, he used to make a presentation at our school once a year. To encourage us not to smoke, he showed horrible slides of people with lip cancer, throat cancer, tongue cancer, and so on. The slides were so gross that all we could do was laugh nervously. Afterward, some of the students got so upset that they went directly to the bathroom to smoke!

During times of crisis—a heart attack, for example, or just standing on the scale in the morning—the denial may break down temporarily. For this reason, a crisis is often an opportunity for real transformation if we can see it in those terms. For a few weeks after a heart attack, most patients are scared enough to do just about anything that their doctors recommend. But if fear is the primary motivator, the denial soon returns and the patients tend to revert to their previous behaviors. Similarly, trying to lose weight because you're afraid of how you may look at a wedding, or a high school reunion, or in a swimsuit as summer approaches may make you motivated for a while. However, when the special event is over, or winter comes, then both denial and the lost weight tend to return.

Telling you that you may live to be eighty-six instead of eighty-five if you change your lifestyle is not very inspiring—unless you're eighty-five, and not always even then. Instead, I am more successful in motivating you when I emphasize the *short-term* gains that you may experience by making extensive changes in your diet and lifestyle. You can weigh less without feeling deprived and hungry. You feel better. You look better. You become better in measurable ways. Inspiring our research participants to change was more successful, I learned, when I appealed to their joy of living—their love and lust for life—rather than to their fear of dying.

## FEELING FREE IS OFTEN MORE IMPORTANT THAN FEELING HEALTHY

For many of us, feeling free is often more important than anything, even our health. Once you go on a diet that commands you, "Eat this!" and "Don't eat that!" and "Do this!" and "Don't do that!" then it's hard to feel free.

This goes back to Adam and Eve, when God said, "Don't eat the apple." We know how ineffective that was—and that was God talking! God didn't need to make apples if God really didn't want Adam and Eve to eat them, so there must be a lesson there.

You may find ways of undermining your diet to preserve what may be even more important to you than losing weight: your freedom. On the other hand, it's hard to feel very free when you have a difficult time staying on a diet, so you lose motivation either way. That doesn't feel very good, and it certainly doesn't help you lose weight.

Instead, my program is based on informed choice reinforced by results that you can experience and measure. The choices that help you lose excess weight will likely improve the *quality* of your life, and they may even prolong the length of it.

In this book, I don't tell you what *not* to do and what *not* to eat. My approach is to give you the facts and information that you can use to make informed and intelligent choices. I will support whatever you choose to do (or not do). *You* are the final authority on what is right for you.

These are *choices,* not *rules.* You don't have to break the rules to feel free, because there are no rules in this book, only options, selections, and preferences. You have a *spectrum* of choices at any moment, and what you choose is really up to you. You can be flexible and compassionate with yourself, because there are no rigid guidelines that may make you feel that you need to be perfect—and to feel guilt, fear, and shame when you are not. The more you change, the more you benefit. It's not all or nothing. I hope that the information in this book will enable you to choose wisely.

## JUST GETTING THROUGH THE DAY MAY BE MORE IMPORTANT THAN LIVING LONGER OR LOSING WEIGHT

Why do otherwise very smart people sometimes engage in behaviors that are self-destructive and self-defeating?

Providing people with health information, as important as it is, is not usually sufficient to motivate *lasting* changes in behavior. For example, everyone who smokes knows the health risks—they can just read the Surgeon General's warning. Yet one-third of Americans, and over one-half of Europeans, still smoke. (When I was a medical student, the chief of pulmonary medicine smoked and one of the head cancer specialists smoked! It wasn't because they didn't know any better.) Likewise, everyone who wants to lose weight or lower their cholesterol knows that a steady diet of cheeseburgers and hot fudge sundaes is not helpful in achieving that goal.

Many doctors think it's easy to get people to take a pill, but hard to motivate them to change their lifestyles, especially in comprehensive ways. "I can't even get my patients to eat less red meat—how do you expect them to eat a near-vegetarian diet, stop smoking, exercise, and manage stress, all at the same time? It's impossible!"

In fact, though, several studies have shown that only a small percentage of patients are taking their medications as prescribed after only one year. So it's not a choice between high adherence to small changes and low adherence to big ones. Comprehensive changes can be easier than moderate ones, but only if we address what really motivates us.

Most of my patients are intelligent, but they do not always make wise choices. My colleagues and I have been meeting with those in the Lifestyle Heart Trial twice weekly for several years. So we get to know each other very well, and we learn from each other.

In our research, we are learning that the experience of emotional pain and unhappiness—whether due to being overweight or due to an illness like heart disease—can be a powerful catalyst for transforming not only behaviors like diet and exercise but also for dealing with the deeper issues that really motivate us. We are most successful when we also address the emotional and spiritual dimensions that most influence what we choose to do or not do. This is just as true for losing weight as it is for reversing heart disease.

I asked the patients in my studies to help me understand their behaviors. "Why do you overeat? Why do you smoke? Why do you drink to excess?" They replied, "To you, as a doctor, these behaviors seem *maladaptive,* because they increase our risk of getting sick or dying early. But to us, these behaviors are very *adaptive,* at least temporarily, because they help us to make it through another day. They help us to cope with the emotional and spiritual pain of loneliness, isolation, and alienation."

For many people, just getting through the day is more important than losing weight or living longer. Telling people who feel emotionally isolated and spiritually alone that they may live longer if they just quit smoking, change their diet, and begin exercising is not always terribly motivating—for who wants to live longer when they feel chronically unhappy?

As we enter the twenty-first century, many people in our culture are experiencing a profound sense of isolation: isolation from their inner feelings, isolation from other people and a sense of community, isolation from the spiritual dimension of life. By "spiritual," I mean the experience of what it means to feel a part of something larger than ourselves, in whatever religious or secular context, rather than always feeling separate and apart from everyone and everything else.

Life in the 1990s can be very stressful, but not necessarily for the reasons you may think. I don't think that the pace of modern life is the major cause of stress. When you think about it, a hundred years ago life was pretty stressful, too.

For example, most Americans raised their own food. If it didn't rain, your harvest might fail and you wouldn't be able to feed yourself and your family. They might even starve. Worrying that your crops might not come in has to be at least as stressful as wondering if your latest fax or Federal Express delivery has come in.

What is different is that a hundred years ago more people in this country had a sense of community and connection. They were born, raised, lived, loved, worked, played, and died in the same place. They had the same neighbors and their children went to the same schools. They attended the same churches and synagogues. They often held the same job for many years, and people at work knew each other. They lived in communities in which people knew they needed each other.

These social networks help protect us from isolation, illness, and premature death. A sense of community and connection can directly address and help heal the emotional and physical pain of isolation. To me, this is one of the most interesting and exciting areas of research.

A number of studies, conducted by well-respected investigators in different parts of the world and published in the leading medical and scientific journals, are reporting the same important observation: *People who feel socially isolated have two to five times the incidence of disease and premature death due to all causes as those who feel a sense of community and connection.* These differences in rates of disease and early death are true for a large number of illnesses, ranging from heart disease to breast cancer to immune system abnormalities.

Social support is also a powerful factor in helping you to lose weight and to keep it off. Researchers writing in the *American Journal of Clinical Nutrition* studied three groups of women:

- formerly obese women who lost weight and kept it off
- those who had always remained at the same average, nonobese weight
- those who lost weight and regained it

Compared with the women who lost weight and regained it, the women in the first two groups who kept weight off were much more likely to use available social support. Also, women in the first two groups exercised regularly, were conscious of their behaviors, confronted problems directly, and used personally developed strategies to help themselves. Few women in the third group exercised, most ate unconsciously in response to emotions, few used available social support, and few confronted problems directly.

In one of the most recent and well-designed prospective studies, Dr. Lisa Berkman and her colleagues at the Yale School of Medicine studied men and women who had recently suffered a heart attack. She simply asked them, "Can you count on anyone to provide you with emotional support?"

The results were dramatic: People who answered "no" were almost three times as likely to die during the next six months after their heart attack as those who had at least one person from whom they had emotional support. Those who had more than one close relationship did even better. These differences were not related to their age, the severity of their heart attack, or any other identifiable factors.

In most studies, the protection provided by social support is independent of other risk factors, including diet, cholesterol, smoking, genetics, and so on. For example, much has been written lately about the so-called French paradox. In France, the rate of heart disease is 30 percent lower than in the United States, even though the traditional French diet is not very low in fat. (Heart disease is still the number-one cause of death in France, but it is lower than in the United States.) I would like to believe that there is something protective about eating pâté de foie gras, or olive oil, or red wine, but I believe that the French may live longer *despite* their diet, not because of it.

The major difference between France and the United States is cultural. Their social support helps protect them from their diet. They eat some fatty foods, but in small portions. They tend not to eat between meals. Fresh fruits, vegetables, grains, and beans play an important role in their diet. And, perhaps most significant, meals are important occasions for being with friends and having social support. When people eat together in an unhurried fashion, they receive nourishment and sustenance for their souls, not just food for their bodies. The isolation is bridged and healed, at least for a while.

In contrast, the majority of families in the United States do not eat even one meal together. Even within France, heart disease is much lower in the southwest region, where villagers have lived in stable communities for centuries, than in the northwestern Normandy region where the divorce rate is high and the communities are more disrupted and urbanized.

I'm not arguing for a return to a mythical, Norman Rockwell-idealized view of family and community. I know how dysfunctional many families can be. But a family is a place where you can bring down your walls, at least to some extent. They know you, they know some of your secrets, and they still care about you.

Why is social support so important? If you have no place that feels safe enough to let down your emotional walls and your defenses, then your barriers tend to remain up all the time. Unfortunately, the same walls that protect you can also isolate you if they are always up.

It's not that we shouldn't have defenses. The problem comes if you have no place that feels safe enough to let down the walls, no one with whom you feel close enough to risk opening up. For many people, the fear is, "If you *really* knew me, if you knew my secrets, my insecurities, my fears, my feelings of inadequacy, my shame, my guilt, my imperfections, then you'd reject me and I'd feel even more alone. So I'll only show you those parts of myself that I think are likable and lovable."

If you feel like this, then you may lose either way. For example, when I was an intern at the Massachusetts General Hospital in Boston, one of my patients (with heart disease *and* cancer) appeared very successful. He drove a very expensive car and wore two-thousand-dollar Italian suits. He confided to me that he'd declared bankruptcy, but he hadn't told anyone else except his attorney and accountant. Even his own wife didn't know! So he lost both ways. If he didn't get the love and respect he needed, then he felt isolated. But even when he got it, he couldn't really enjoy it—because, as he told me, "If they really knew I was bankrupt, then they'd be outta here."

In our research, our support groups began as a place for people to exchange recipes, shopping tips, and so on, but it evolved into something much more powerful: a community, a place that felt safe enough for people to talk about what was *really* going on in their lives, what they were truly feeling, without fear of being judged, rejected, or abandoned. In these groups, we learned to listen supportively, without offering advice or trying to fix the problem expressed. Giving advice, especially when it is not asked for, often tends to diminish the other person, who may think, "Gee, if it's *that* easy to fix, there must be something wrong with me," or, "They don't really understand how difficult my problem is or they wouldn't give such glib advice."

You may wish to find a group of friends and create a support group. Even if you have just one person with whom you can be yourself, share secrets, and openly discuss your feelings without fear of being criticized or rejected, then you can begin to experience how powerful and how healing real intimacy can be.

## HUNGRY FOR LOVE

In the 1990s, our social networks are breaking down. As recently as two generations ago, many people had extended families nearby to support them. Now, even the nuclear family is melting down, and the two-parent family is becoming uncommon. Single parents have extra burdens and stresses.

With the layoffs resulting from the recession and from corporate mergers and acquisitions, people often do not have a real community at work and they don't feel very safe there. They might lose their job if they're too open and honest. Or they might become close with another employee who may get fired, and that would be painful.

Increasing mobility and urban crime have turned many neighborhoods that were once real communities into places where people live who hardly know or care about one another. And many people don't find a feeling of community or meaning at church or synagogue, where the emphasis is often on the rituals rather than on the underlying spiritual meaning.

Along with this isolation comes chronic emotional pain. Many are on edge. Coping with the intensity of this pain is very difficult for many people—so they do what they can. Some eat too much. Some smoke. Some drink alcohol excessively. Some take drugs. Some work too hard. Some sit in front of cable television compulsively changing the channels, as attention spans shorten. After a while, these patterns can become addictive.

Here is what some of my patients have told me:

- "When something's eating me, I eat. When I'm lonely, which is much of the time, I eat. And then I eat some more. I keep trying to fill up the void with food, but the feelings of emptiness keep coming back. I use food to stuff my emotions, to keep the sadness from coming in. And to keep other people from coming in. I crave intimacy—you might say I'm *hungry* for love—but I'm also frightened of it. When I open myself up to someone else, they might hurt me. Food is my armor, and weighing too much is a barrier to intimacy. It helps me to keep people from getting too close. I've had some painful love affairs, but not now. Being fat makes me unattractive, so I don't have to deal with sex anymore. Food is my heroine—and my heroin. It numbs the pain. And now I weigh so much that I can't stand how I look. I don't even want to get out of bed, so I'm not exercising. I'm not as attractive to other people, which only makes me feel even more isolated and lonely. So I keep eating. And I don't care if I die sooner—in fact, it might be a relief!"
- "I smoke when I'm lonely. I've got twenty friends here in this pack of cigarettes, and they're always there for

me. Nobody else•is. They fill up the empty spaces. If you take away my twenty friends, what are you going to give me instead?"

- "I don't smoke, but I've got friends I see at the bar every day. Johnny Walker, Jim Beam. Old Grand Dad. They're always waiting for me. I drink to try to kill the pain. It works for a while, but it only makes things worse. My wife left me because she was tired of living with a drunk, and she took the kids with her. So now I'm all alone, which only makes me want to drink more. And I'm getting a beer belly, too."
- "I keep busy. I never have enough time in the day. I'm almost always working. It distracts me from how unhappy I am. I feel such a letdown when I finish a project because it never brings me what I most want. Vacations are even harder, because then I have the time to experience how lonely I feel."
- "I channel-surf in front of the cable TV, switching from one channel to another to distract myself from the loneliness and emotional pain."

My particular addiction is talking on the telephone. When I see telephone advertisements on television asking me to "reach out and touch someone," I know they're talking to me. My telephone bill each month is larger than the gross national product of some third world countries. I travel a lot, lecturing and attending scientific meetings in various places, and I have a small cellular telephone that I bring with me. In a hotel room in a strange city, my first inclination is to pick up the phone and call someone. Anyone. As a gentle reminder, a friend of mine once sent me a postcard with a drawing of a man who had a phone sutured to the side of his head "to leave his hands free." For me, long distance is not only the next best thing to being there—sometimes, it's even better. I can fill up the void and the loneliness without letting most people get *too* close.

Unfortunately, trying to heal our isolation by filling the void with food, or with the telephone, or with a cigarette, or whatever, provides only temporary relief. It may be fast, fast, fast relief, but it leaves us fast, too. Soon, we're left again not only with the feelings of loneliness and isolation but also with the consequences of our actions: weight gain, a big long-distance bill, even lung cancer or heart disease. We're looking in the wrong places.

To me, the real issue is to become more free of our compulsions and addictions. What makes the quick fix so seductive and addictive is that the relief seems so real. When we believe that relief in the short run comes from that which helps to destroy us in the long run, then we have a problem.

We become addicted to what makes us unconscious, so we don't feel the pain we create. The temporary pleasure is used to hide the chronic pain. Worse than that, when we blunt the capacity to feel pain, we also diminish the capacity to feel pleasure, joy, and love, both for ourselves and for others. When we can deal with the pain more directly, then we can increase our awareness and our joy rather than diminish it. The next chapter shows how.

So, when I'm alone in a hotel room in a strange city, I try to pay attention to my compulsion to call someone—and just observe it. I feel my loneliness and I begin to meditate until I remember what it feels like to be more peaceful. I remind myself that the meditation didn't bring me the peace, it only allowed me to stop disturbing it for a while. At that point, if I decide to call someone, then it's a choice, not a compulsion.

Perhaps one of the most painful aspects of being overweight is that it often creates more isolation, leading many people to overeat in a vicious cycle in a futile attempt to numb that pain or to fill the emptiness. The pain of that isolation is usually *very* intense. For example, in one study of forty-seven formerly overweight men and women, Dr. Colleen Rand and her colleagues at the University of Florida found that *every one of them* would rather have heart disease, diabetes, or be deaf than to be overweight again. About 90 percent would rather be legally blind or have a leg amputated! One patient reported, "When you're blind, people want to help you. No one wants to help you when you're fat." All patients said that they would rather be a normal weight than a very overweight millionaire.

## PHYSICAL, EMOTIONAL, AND SPIRITUAL HOMEOSTASIS

It is natural to resist change—for better and for worse. This resistance to change is called homeostasis, which we discussed on a physiological level in chapter 3.

On a physical level, for example, your body has billions of feedback loops that keep your physiological functions within a narrow, normal equilibrium. And it's a good thing, or you might die. For example, your body's thermostat keeps your temperature closely regulated. If your temperature goes up even a few degrees, then you feel feverish. When this happens, a number of intricate feedback mechanisms become activated that help cool you down.

The same is true on emotional and spiritual levels. We tend not to question our beliefs, our perceptions, and our patterns of behavior, even when they are causing problems for us. The same homeostasis that protects us from change also makes it more difficult for us to transform even when it's in our best interest to do so.

If you've been eating a high-fat diet for most of your life, then your mind will perceive this way of eating as normal and may interpret a change to a low-fat diet as threatening. As George Leonard wrote in his wonderful book, *Mastery,* "The problem is, homeostasis works to keep things as they are even if they aren't very good."

## FED UP WITH SUFFERING?

Part of the value of pain is to help motivate you to change. All change is stressful at first, because it disrupts the familiarity of the status quo. It perturbs homeostasis. When the status quo becomes painful enough, then changing begins to make more sense.

Getting in touch with the pain of isolation and loneliness can be a way of capturing your attention and motivating you to change old patterns. Even self-destructive habits—like overeating—can be hard to change, because change itself is stressful. When the pain of old patterns becomes intense enough, then change becomes easier.

## REAL HEALING

Anything that helps you transcend your isolation will help you lose excess weight and keep it off. More than that, though, transforming and transcending isolation is the essence of real healing. Even the word *heal* derives from the same Indo-European root as "to make whole" and "to become holy." Social support is only one of many approaches that can help you begin healing the pain of isolation. In the next chapter, I'll describe several other techniques, including meditation, that can help you to quiet down your mind and body enough to rediscover and reexperience what you may really be searching for when you overeat: an inner feeling of peace, joy, and well-being that transcends the pain of isolation. Even the word *yoga* comes from the Sanskrit root meaning "to yoke, to connect, to bring together," also translated as "union."

In the final analysis, this is a book as much about transformation as on weight loss. Being overweight is not just a physical problem, so it needs to be addressed in a broader context. If you are overweight, then you know what it means to be in emotional pain. When you're suffering, your distress can be a catalyst, a doorway to real healing.

In our research, we are finding that when people address their emotional and spiritual aspects, then they are more likely to make and to maintain lifestyle choices that are life-enhancing rather than ones that are self-destructive. Even on a physical level, they show greater improvements than if they only worked on changing their behaviors.

Their waistline improves. Their heart improves. But at that point, those improvements—as important as they are—

often mean less to them than their emotional and spiritual growth. Patients often say, "I may have started this program because I wanted to lose weight, or to unclog my arteries, but what's *kept* me in it is that my heart and soul are opening in ways that are more difficult to measure but ultimately are much more meaningful to me."

# 7

# *Who You Are Is Not What You Weigh*

## NOURISHING YOUR SOUL

Sometimes, you may find yourself eating when you are not really hungry. Or you may eat past the point when you feel full. When that happens, what are you really feeding, and what are you really feeling?

The social isolation that I described earlier is only part of something deeper: a spiritual isolation. When you eat, you are feeding more than just your body. You may also yearn for ways to nourish your soul. Food, which is such a basic source of nourishment, seems like it should be enough, but often it isn't.

When you were a baby, if you were lucky, you probably received nourishment both for your body and for your soul. While being fed, you were held, loved, and caressed. So, the association between food, intimacy, and love is powerful and often inextricable.

As a child, the experience of interacting with family may have revolved around the dining table. So the foods you are used to eating may be associated with these powerful memories of intimacy.

As you grew older, you may have begun to see yourself as separate and alone. No wonder that you may find yourself eating when what you really crave is deeper nourishment: the love and intimacy that once seemed so familiar and now may feel so distant.

Unless you address this deeper spiritual need, then all of the latest nutritional information in the world may be of only limited value to you. Because no matter how full your stomach feels, you may undermine your best efforts to alter your diet if your deeper hunger remains unsatisfied and unfulfilled.

The isolation from other people and a sense of community that I described in the last chapter may cause you to eat too much as a way of trying to fill up the emotional emptiness and the spiritual void. Along with this isolation from others comes something even more distressing: You may become isolated from *yourself,* from your inner feelings and your inner life.

This isolation from your inner self makes it hard to know when you've had enough to eat. Many of my overweight patients say that they are often unaware when they have eaten too much at a meal until it is too late and they notice how uncomfortably stuffed they feel. This lack of awareness often extends to other areas of their lives.

On the diet I recommend, you really can eat more and weigh less. You can eat until you're full and satisfied. But even on this diet, you can get too much of a good thing. You can't stuff yourself and lose weight.

So, before we talk about *what* to eat, let's first discuss *how* to eat.

## EATING WITH AWARENESS

This is more than just a diet, it's a new way of eating—a way of eating with awareness.

You probably lead a very busy life. You may have more

things you need to do than time in which to do them. A quiet, leisurely meal may seem like a luxury when you are only on page two of your twenty-page "to do" list. Gulping down breakfast while reading the newspaper, guzzling a luncheon sandwich in between phone calls, and gobbling a take-out dinner while watching television may be more familiar than having a relaxed, quiet meal with friends.

There is nothing wrong with eating this way, but you pay a real price for doing so. You ignore someone very important: you.

When you eat with awareness, you become reacquainted with yourself.

Here's what begins to happen:

- You enjoy food more fully
- You notice how food affects you and you are less likely to overeat
- You begin to become more aware of other aspects of your inner life, including your emotional and spiritual sides

## GOOD FOOD IS TO BE ENJOYED!

Have you ever eaten a meal while watching television? While talking on the phone? While driving? While reading? While engrossed in a dinner conversation? When this happens, you may look down at your plate at the end of a meal and find that your food is almost gone and you've hardly even tasted it.

Your mind can only focus on one activity at a time. It can shift back and forth quickly, but in any given moment your mind can only pay attention to one thing.

When you eat while doing something else, then you're distracted. You're not really focusing on what you're eating. So you lose twice: You don't enjoy your food as much and you are more likely to eat past the point when you are full. (And you're not enjoying the other activity as much either.) Feeling stuffed becomes a substitute for feeling satisfied, for having really enjoyed your meal.

When you really pay attention to what you are eating, then you can enjoy your food much more fully. Because of this, you don't need to consume the excessive amounts of food that cause you to gain weight. You can eat less and enjoy more.

Meditation is the art of paying attention. One way to develop your ability to give your undivided attention to what you are doing is to practice meditating. People often confuse meditation with withdrawing from the world, but it's actually a powerful technique for helping you to embrace the world more fully and to enjoy your life more completely. Even on a sensual level—*especially* on a sensual level—you can enjoy life so much more when you pay attention to what you are doing. Whether it's food, sex, music, massage, art, or anything involving your senses, you can enjoy what you are doing much more when you are fully present and not distracted.

For example, I would not be happy in a world without chocolate, so I have developed a Häagen-Dazs meditation. When I eat the teaspoon of ice cream, I close my eyes and meditate—on the rich flavor, the cold rush, the wonderful sensations as the ice cream melts on my tongue. I would prefer to have a small spoonful of Deep Chocolate Fudge Häagen-Dazs than a pint of a fake-fat frozen dessert. It's exquisitely satisfying. After all, the first bite is always the best and the last bite is the next best—so if you eat only a bite, then it can be heaven, but only if you really pay attention.

## PAYING ATTENTION TO HOW FOOD AFFECTS YOU

When you eat with awareness, you notice how food affects you. For example, soon after you eat a rich, fatty meal, you may notice how tired and sluggish you feel. Your mind is not quite as sharp. On the other hand, low-fat foods make you feel light, energetic, and clear thinking. When you begin to associate what you eat with how you feel, then it becomes easier to make more healthful choices. You begin acting out of your own experiences, not someone else's, and that is the best teacher and motivator.

The diet I recommend is rich in complex carbohydrates. In addition to other benefits, carbohydrates may increase the levels of serotonin, a neurotransmitter in your brain. Many antidepressants work by increasing brain levels of serotonin. Eating a diet rich in complex carbohydrates may help, too, but without the side-effects of these drugs.

When you eat while working or when you're under stress, you miss out in yet another way: You digest your food less effectively.

During times of stress, the fight-or-flight response described in chapter 3 affects not only your heart but also your digestive system. As part of the adaptive response designed to protect you from danger, your body shunts blood and energy away from your digestive system and to your arms and legs and other skeletal muscles—better enabling you to fight or to run.

Your body did not evolve to wolf down a sandwich while fighting tigers, but, metaphorically speaking, that's what you may be doing several times a day if you eat when you're working or feeling stressed. Here again, this is an example of an adaptive mechanism—the fight-or-flight response—that becomes maladaptive in modern times when it is chronically activated.

When blood is shunted away from your digestive tract, then you may be eating well but not digesting well. When this happens, even nutritional food loses much of its nutritional value.

The effects of emotional stress on digestion begins at the very first stage of eating. You may notice that your mouth feels dry when you feel stressed. Your saliva produces an enzyme, alpha-amylase, that starts the process of digestion. One group of researchers studied the effects of stress and of relaxation on digestion of complex carbohydrates. They found that emotional stress significantly decreased alpha-amylase activity, whereas relaxation techniques such as meditation significantly enhanced alpha-amylase activity.

So, if you're munching a sandwich while driving or while working, not only are you less likely to enjoy the food and more likely to overeat, but also your body is unlikely to extract the nutrients very efficiently.

## EATING AS MEDITATION

Virtually all religions and cultures have a tradition of meditating—for example, saying a prayer of thankfulness and gratitude for the meal—before eating. Among other benefits, this enables you to shift from fight-or-flight and eat-and-run to eating more peacefully, with joy and awareness. The ritual itself is comforting and provides both a sense of order and a sense of greater meaning. Some would say that meditation and prayer even affect the food at a more subtle level, even though most scientists would have a hard time believing this. But they clearly affect *us* at both physical and subtle levels.

Meditation is a powerful tool for increasing awareness. There is an old Zen saying, "How you do anything is how you do everything." When you rush through meals, you are likely to rush through life. When you feel nourished by food, you may allow yourself to feel nourished in other ways. When you choose to eat life-affirming foods, then you may choose to affirm your life in other areas. When you can practice eating with awareness, then you are more likely to begin living with greater awareness. In this context, meditation not only enhances the experience of eating; eating with awareness *becomes* a form of meditation.

## EXERCISING RESTRAINT

I once asked Dr. Jonas Salk, the renowned scientist, if he exercises. "I exercise restraint," he replied.

Besides mealtime prayers and meditations, dietary restrictions also exist in all cultures and in all religions—but not for the purpose of losing weight. They exist to bring us closer to our spiritual inner life.

Some religions forbid pork; others allow it. Some religions dictate fasting on certain days and feasting on others. Yet even though the specific dietary guidelines vary in each religion, all of them are designed to bring us closer to God. Does God care or are these dietary restrictions for us?

While there may be inherent benefit in each religion's recommendations, I believe that just the act of having voluntary restraints is beneficial to us. When we choose not to eat something when we might otherwise do so, the effect is to make the act of eating more special, more sacred, and thus more joyful. Also, voluntary restraint helps us to break free of our compulsions and our addictions.

Why not just do everything you want? Why impose limitations on your freedom? Because *self-imposed* limitations can help to free us.

For example, if a musician spends several hours a day practicing, it may seem as though she is limiting her freedom. She could be doing so many other things. But this self-discipline gives her the power and freedom to express herself through her music in ways that many others cannot. We all understand the value of self-discipline for an athlete who spends hours a day training intensely for the Olympics. Yet we may find it more difficult to understand the spiritual value of self-restraint.

When we understand the benefits of our choices, then they become easier to make. What appears like self-restraint can be self-empowerment. Ultimately, it's a choice between true freedom or being a slave to our compulsions. Meditation, which seems to some people like "doing nothing," is one of the most difficult—and one of the easiest—forms of self-discipline. When you meditate, you practice learning how to restrain and to control your own mind.

## WHY MEDITATE?

When you meditate, a number of desirable things begin to happen.

First, you increase your powers of concentration. When you can focus your attention on something, then you can accomplish it more effectively.

Second, meditation increases your awareness of what's going on around you.

Third, meditation increases your awareness of what's going on inside you. As described earlier, you can enjoy food much more fully when you pay attention to what you're eating. Also, you notice how food affects you and when you've had enough to eat, so you're less likely to eat too much.

Fourth, your mind becomes quieter when you meditate, allowing you to directly experience inner sources of peace, joy, and nourishment. The state of relaxation, both physical and mental, that meditation provides is deeper even than when you sleep.

Fifth, meditation can give you a clearer picture of yourself. When you don't pay attention, you may get a distorted view of yourself, your abilities, and your self-worth. For example, when I was a senior resident at the Massachusetts General Hospital and a clinical fellow in medicine at Harvard Medical School, I once picked up a Harvard catalog and saw a course entitled "Advanced Medicine and Clinical Problem Solving." I felt a little intimidated (could I keep up in such an advanced course?) and insecure (was I smart enough to do well in such a course?). After a while, I had to laugh at my lack of awareness—when I realized that these medical students would spend the entire course on the medical wards being taught by a senior medical resident. In other words, I was one of the people who would be *teaching* that course!

Sixth, meditation brings you into the present moment rather than dwelling on the past or worrying about the future. You begin to live life fully, as though each moment matters—which, of course, it does. The present moment frees us to change and to explore new patterns, pleasures, and possibilities.

Last, and perhaps most important, meditation can give you the direct experience of transcendence, perhaps the most powerful way to heal isolation. More on this later.

## HOW TO MEDITATE

There are as many ways to meditate as there are meditators. There is no one best way for everyone. What different forms of meditation have in common is this: Meditation is the art of paying attention.

If you choose to meditate, do it in a way that is comfortable for you, one that is compatible with your cultural, religious, or secular beliefs and traditions. One of the simplest forms of meditation (simple to learn, but difficult to master) is repeating a word, sound, prayer, or phrase over and over again.

If you are Christian, you might want to use the word *amen.* If you are Jewish, you might choose the word *shalom.* If you are Arabic, you might find *salaam* comforting. A traditional Buddhist or Hindu might meditate by repeating the word *om.* An agnostic or atheist might be more comfortable by repeating the word *one* or *peace.* Or you may want to choose a different word, sound, prayer, or phrase that *you* find more comforting.

Your mind is always thinking different thoughts, even when you are sleeping. And if you're like most people, those thoughts are not very organized and coherent. One moment you may be thinking about what you had for lunch; the next, what you did last night; then, what movie you're going to see later. My foot hurts. Sue says I look good, but I don't believe her. Where's my jacket? That guy looks like Fred. Sexy. Ah, my last vacation, when I ate the most *wonderful* . . . And so on.

Instead, when you repeat a sound over and over, your mind eventually begins to quiet down. When this happens, you may begin to experience an inner sense of peace and well-being. Those feelings didn't *come* from somewhere outside you. Meditation didn't *bring* it to you. That peace and well-being is always there if you simply quiet down your mind and body enough to experience it.

To meditate, find a comfortable place to sit, with your back reasonably straight. Closing your eyes will help to reduce distractions. Wear loose, comfortable clothing, if possible.

First, bring your awareness to your body. Begin with your feet: How do they feel? Do they feel comfortable? Tense? Allow your feet to relax, and imagine they are becoming healthier and feeling better. Then move to your ankles and repeat the same process. Then your legs. Then your knees. Then your thighs. Then your pelvis and buttocks. Then your abdomen. Check in with your stomach: Are you full? Stuffed? Hungry? Did you eat enough? Too much?

Now, pay attention to your breathing. Are you breathing fast and shallow, or slowly and deeply? Your breath both reflects your mental state and can help to change it. Place your left hand on your abdomen and your right hand on your chest. Inhale slowly and deeply through your nose. As you inhale, first allow the abdomen to expand and feel your left hand begin to rise. Then allow your chest to expand, and feel your right hand begin to rise. Take in as much air as you feel comfortable inhaling, and exhale slowly, first from your chest, then from your abdomen. Repeat this process of breathing a few times.

Then move your awareness to your back. Remember to pay attention to how you feel each time; allow that part to relax and imagine it's becoming healthier and feeling better. Then your shoulders. Then your neck. Then your face. Then your scalp.

Now, bring your awareness to your breathing. Without trying to change it, just notice yourself inhaling and exhaling. Whenever your mind wanders, bring it back to observing your breathing. Do this for about one minute.

At this time, keeping your eyes closed, begin repeating the sound, phrase, or prayer that you have chosen. When your mind wanders, gently but firmly bring your attention back, over and over and over again. At first, you may find it difficult to stay focused for more than a few seconds. Over time, with practice, this process will become easier and more pleasurable.

How long you meditate is up to you. Traditionally, many people recommend meditating for at least twenty or thirty minutes once or twice a day. More important than how *long* you meditate is how *regularly*. It's better to meditate for a few minutes every day than for an hour once or twice a week.

Sometimes, when I'm very busy, I'll tell myself that I only have time to meditate for three minutes. No matter how busy I am, three minutes sounds manageable. Once I start, though, I usually find the experience to be so pleasurable and peaceful that I allow myself to continue. Getting started is always the hardest.

After you have been meditating for a while, you are more open to receiving information from your body and from your mind. If you noticed a part of your body that felt uncomfortable or unhealthy when you began, return to that area and ask that part, "What do you need in order to heal?" If you listen carefully, you may "hear" that part of your body "talking" to you, as strange as it may sound. Or you may have an image of what you need to do. Or you may find nothing at all.

Sometimes, you may begin to hear your inner voice. Many religious and cultural traditions talk about "the still small voice within" that speaks softly but clearly and wisely. Usually, this inner wisdom is drowned out by the din and distractions of modern life. When you meditate, your mind may become quiet enough to begin hearing it. Listen carefully, for the information can be quite powerful and transformative. You may think of this inner voice as your own higher self, your inner teacher or guide, the God within, your intuition, or whatever seems right to you. If for whatever reason this process makes you uncomfortable, then skip it. (More information on this process can be found in Dr. Martin Rossman's book *Healing Yourself*.)

You may find that you can engage your inner wisdom in a

dialogue. If you ask specific questions and listen carefully, you may hear a wise reply, and that may lead to more questions and answers. For example, you might ask yourself, "When I overeat, what emptiness am I trying to fill? When I eat without being hungry, what empty place is the food filling? And how can I nourish myself and feel whole in other ways?"

Whenever I meditate, before stopping I ask myself, "What am I not paying attention to in my life that deserves attention?" At that point, I often will learn something very useful. I may not always put it into practice right away, but at least I have a better idea about what I need to be doing.

Ultimately, meditation is not just something you do for twenty minutes twice a day. It's an approach to living—living with awareness by paying attention to what you are experiencing.

More information on meditation is available from instructors certified by the Integral Yoga Institute (804-969-3121).

## SOUL FOOD

Meditation has become more popular as a way to cope with stress, to manage stress, to deal with stress. While it can be used in this way, and it is very useful, the ancient swamis, monks, nuns, rabbis, priests, and spiritual masters did not develop it for this purpose.

Meditation—in whatever form appeals to you—can give you the direct experience of transcendence. In this context, *meditation is food for your soul.* It satiates the hunger that is not satisfied by food alone. And when your soul is fed, you have less need to overeat. When you directly experience the fullness of life, then you have less need to attempt to fill the void with food.

Other ways of feeding your soul—that is, healing your isolation—include: altruism, compassion, massage, psychotherapy, and yoga. Learning communication skills and setting up support groups or developing friendships that feel safe enough to talk about what's really going on in your life also can help to heal loneliness and isolation.

Many people find that eating a low-fat vegetarian diet makes them feel more open, aware, and connected. I recently met with a well-known writer who had been eating this way for only two weeks. Here's what she told me:

> I feel so much better! And not just in my body. When I eat this way, I just notice that I'm much more open.
>
> I really think that, for me, eating high-fat food is what drinking would be for an alcoholic. It's really like a mind-altering drug. And drinking, by the way, can function in the same way for me. You know, a couple of glasses of wine is just as good as a hot fudge sundae. But what both do, it's almost like they coat the ends of the neurons and so I'm just not as receptive.
>
> Overeating high-fat foods, drinking, and (when I was young) drugs—all of them leave me feeling singular, alone. Numb, bloated, and lethargic. And I don't like feeling that way. It's no longer pleasurable, it's painful. I've found that when I numb the pain, I also numb the pleasure. I think numbing has its place in life, but I don't like it now in *my* life. For me, it feels like it's a set-up to live half a life. You know, just get lost for a while. Without numbing myself, I'm capable of connecting in profound ways with other people. And inwardly, too, with parts of myself that I'd covered over. It's such a *joy* to have that clarity and the feelings of interconnectedness.
>
> I have intimacy issues with so many people. I've always been well-defended. From the time that I learned how to become popular in junior high school, I was protected by an image. During high school, I was protected by the image of being an artist, and then during college I was known as a writer.
>
> And all along, the same person that wasn't taken care of, wasn't nurtured, wasn't recognized when I was growing up, is still walking around, going through the same thing. Earlier in life, eating a lot of fat probably saved my life; it may well have kept me from being a teenage suicide. Because eating that way helped to numb the pain.

When I was in high school and junior high school, around puberty, I started being obsessed about my body. I really loved ice cream, you know, high fat, high sugar. A hot fudge sundae was sort of like a cure-all. I think it lulled me. Last night, I took someone out to dinner at a seafood restaurant. We ate dessert, and I noticed afterwards that I felt a floaty sense of well-being and lethargy—very much like a drug, very much like an opiate.

And so you get to escape from having control of your own fate, whereas the thing that's really making you mad is that you clearly aren't in control. That's a pretty limited way of living life.

But I think that it's only through really stripping it all away that you begin to see it. And it's like lights going on—for example, in the middle of eating a handful of potato chips. "Wow. When I feel too much pain, I start reaching for fatty foods." Before, I might not have had the insight, or even if I had it I'd just put it aside and discard it.

There's a certain fearlessness to it. It's as if the excuses for not paying attention are laughable and I push them aside. Now, it's the dismissal that I dismiss, and the other stuff can stay there. And it seems like what I'm trying to do is figure out where the love is in each one of those incidents.

The moment of insight is a crossroads, and the indulging or rebelling against the insight is the familiar thing to do. And I think as people we choose the familiar whenever we have a chance. The other crossroad is to not indulge, and that's scary, because we don't have habits of nonindulgence.

I feel so much more open and clear. I feel like I'm waking up after being asleep for a long, long time.

## WHO YOU ARE IS NOT WHAT YOU WEIGH

Why do you want to lose weight? Do you think it will make you more lovable? Then you're setting yourself up to be unhappy.

In 1988, Patricia Farrell authored an extraordinary series

of articles for *The Washington Post* chronicling her struggle to lose weight. She wrote:

> All of my life I thought, "If only I could lose . . ." You know—you have said it a million times yourself. X number of pounds disappear and the whole world—work, relationships (romantic or otherwise), all will change for the better. Life will be grand! And what you feel about yourself will magically transform you into a butterfly. You will look good, you will like yourself and be likable.
>
> Well, I have run into a wall of my own construction. I know really, for the first time, that losing weight and keeping it off is a physical, health issue. Yes, I will indeed "look" better. And there will be an emotional payoff. But it will not change who I am or, more precisely, who I believe I am.

In the final analysis, even the inner peace of meditation and the love and social support from friends and family can only take us so far. What really frees us from our addictions, our habits, and our compulsions is the direct, transcendent experience that we are not isolated and we are not alone.

On one level, of course, we *are* separate from each other. You're you and I'm me. You have a body that needs to be fed and you have a mind that needs to think. But on another level, we are spiritual creatures. Our souls also need nourishment.

We *have* a body and a mind, but we are not *only* a body and a mind. We *are* separate from each other, but we are not *only* separate. This understanding is part of the perennial wisdom of virtually all religions, all faiths, and all cultures, once you move beyond the different rituals, doctrines, and forms. When we forget this truth, then we begin looking in the wrong places to try to fill the emptiness and to kill the pain: food, alcohol, cigarettes, telephones, overwork, and so on.

Our belief that we are separate and only separate is at the root of our suffering, our unworthiness, our shame, and our addictions. We use food not only to try to feed the emptiness but also to add to our pain by punishing ourselves when we seem unable to follow a diet. We attribute moral qualities to foods—"good foods" or "bad foods"—and thus to ourselves or others who eat those foods. These rigid judgments only serve to further isolate us from others and from ourselves. For once we think of foods as bad or forbidden, then we fear or desire them even more. Remember Adam and Eve? Making something forbidden only makes it more appealing and gives it power over us.

We give food the power to make us happy or sad, and in some cases, even to control our lives. The addiction comes from believing that it is the food (or the cigarette, or the phone, or whatever) that fills the void rather than realizing that we create the void by believing we're isolated and only isolated. And we create the disturbance by running after what we think will bring us peace, in the process disturbing what we already could have if we just stopped and looked inward.

At an extreme, when we can't measure up to our standards, we develop patterns of binging and bulimia, denial and depression. When you label foods as "bad," then it's only a small step to label yourself as bad for eating it, and then guilt and shame are close behind. Or you may find yourself eating the foods in secret, which only reinforces the power of the food. And when you eat food in secret, then you further isolate yourself from your inner voice and your intimate feelings.

But food has no power other than what we give to it. Food is just food, nothing more or less. Foods are neither good nor bad, and we are not good or bad when we eat them. Some foods are more healthful than others, but that is not a moral issue. (Some animal rights and ecology groups believe that food selections do present moral choices, but this is a different issue than whether or not certain foods are "good" or "bad" for your health.) We empower food when we believe it can bring us the peace and wholeness we have forgotten. We are afraid of food when we think it's bad. But we are looking in the wrong place. We don't need more willpower; we need more understanding.

You can experience the essence of this understanding, but

it is difficult to define it. Each spiritual and cultural tradition filters this knowledge through its own models, beliefs, and rituals. Some call it God, others Self, Allah, Jehovah, Christ, Buddha, Tao, and countless other names. One of the clearest and most beautiful descriptions can be found in the Mundaka Upanishads, written more than 2,500 years ago:

> Self is everywhere, shining forth from all beings,
> vaster than the vast, subtler than the most subtle,
> unreachable, yet nearer than breath, than heartbeat.
> Eye cannot see it, ear cannot hear it nor tongue
> utter it; only in deep absorption can the mind,
> grown pure and silent, merge with the formless truth.
> He who finds it is free; he has found himself;
> he has solved the great riddle; his heart is forever at peace.
> Whole, he enters the Whole. His personal self
> returns to its radiant, intimate, deathless source.
> As rivers lose name and form when they disappear
> into the sea, the sage leaves behind all traces
> when he disappears into the light. Perceiving the truth,
> he becomes the truth; he passes beyond all suffering,
> beyond death; all the knots of his heart are loosed.

# PART TWO

# *Introduction to the Recipes: Cooking the Nonfat Way*

I first met Dr. Dean Ornish and Dr. Shirley Brown when they came to see me about catering a luncheon at my restaurant, Square One. I had heard about their remarkable work with heart patients and was somewhat acquainted with their dietary program through some of my customers. In any case, I liked Dean and Shirley immediately. We met again to plan what I thought might be a simple but interesting menu. However, this luncheon was going to be unusual because three separate menus were needed. One was for guests who were on a nonrestricted diet and could have chicken, one was a vegetarian menu, and the third was a nonfat vegetarian menu.

I wanted a culinary theme that would carry over from one menu to another so that the differences, when food was served to the guests, would not be conspicuous. We started with vegetable pizzas and a few other finger foods. Then, at the tables, we served a garden tomato soup that everyone could eat. Onions were steamed in vegetable broth and the rest of the soup base came from the tomatoes. This was followed with a Moroccan-inspired roast chicken accompanied by couscous and a vegetable stew called a tagine. For the vegetarians, we served the couscous and a few different tagines, and for those on the fat-free diet, we prepared couscous and Moroccan vegetables without any fat at all. For dessert, we offered a choice of devil's food cake for those on an unrestricted diet and Angel Food Cake (page 381) for those who were restricting fat in their diet. The luncheon was a great success, we all had a good time, and Dean, Shirley, and I became friends.

Months later Dean called to ask if I would teach a cooking class to a group of his patients, people who had had major heart attacks, painful angina, bypass surgery and who had high cholesterol levels that required supervised diets. As a person whose life revolves around food, I enjoy a challenge and a learning experience. For more than thirty years, in one way or another, I've been in the food profession: teaching, writing, and running restaurants. As a restaurateur, I want to understand and second-guess what the public really wants to eat. I've had to keep up with all the latest dietary information so that my menus will reflect the requirements of vegetarian, vegan, and low-fat diets. So for me this was yet another culinary adventure.

Having lived with someone who was born with very high cholesterol levels, I'd had many years of experience in cooking low-fat foods. I had learned how to make do with as little oil as possible and how to cut back on fish and poultry portions until they were but the garnish in meals based on grains, pastas, and vegetables. The model for this is the versatile Mediterranean/Asian diet. But now I was faced with creating recipes that not only had no meat, fish, or chicken, and were not just low fat, but had no added fat at all!

I started to think about what taste and texture elements were sacrificed when you give up fat. In cooking, the fat is often the vehicle that traps the flavors. It also provides "mouth feel," a certain smoothness and clinginess that coats the leaves of lettuce in a salad vinaigrette, that binds the ingredients in pasta or sauces. A vinaigrette without fat means the vinegar and herbs slip off the leaves and sink to the bottom of the salad bowl. A sauce with no fat becomes a juice that also sits on the plate, but not on the food—sort of disappointing and not much fun to eat. I realized that I had to find ways both to dramatically increase flavor via spices and herbs and to provide sensual mouth feel or my recipes would be medically correct but otherwise stoic and spartan. Most important, what would keep people on a diet if it was unsatisfying?

I began to think about what could put the sex appeal back after the fat was removed. I started to think about cooking methods and procedures in a new way. If stock was used to steam onions, for instance, instead of sautéing them in oil, then it would have to be a very flavorful and intense stock. We developed a strong and "meaty" vegetable stock by roasting the vegetables in the oven without tossing them in oil first. If you couldn't use oil in salads, what would hold the acids, vinegar, or lemon juice in suspension? The answer was nonfat yogurt. We experimented with an ancient technique of hanging yogurt in a cheesecloth-lined strainer in the refrigerator for days and days until it thickened into a rich "cream" (page 148).

I began to think about cooking techniques differently. I started mentally revising recipes from my regular repertoire and soon moved from this intellectual stage to the true test, cooking the food. And eating it. With the help of Gerald, my sous chef, I proceeded to test the sixty-odd recipes I'd created for Dean's new book. We'd cook the dish, taste it, discuss it, adjust the seasoning, and then leave the pan on the back kitchen table. The cooks on the line would come back and take a taste. Our "experiments" vanished quickly, and the cooks said, "That was really good. When are we putting it on the menu?" We didn't tell them until afterward that these were fat-free "diet" dishes.

For you, the nonprofessional chef, after years of cooking food in butter and oil, of frying and braising, of eating large portions of meat, poultry, fish, and shellfish, to adapt to a totally new diet may seem daunting. I'm sure there are days when you think it's impossible to eat just vegetables and grains. You may have a fear that you'll be hungry all the time and feel unsatisfied. When cooking is not your life, a major change in diet and culinary procedures seems like a lot of extra trouble, just for a meal. There's the feeling that you're not going to be able to eat well and that mealtime now will be a necessary evil rather than a respite and a joy. Must you throw away all your old recipe cards and cookbooks? Must you remodel the kitchen? Do you need all new cooking equipment? No, what you need is a new turn of mind.

Look at those old recipes with new eyes. Wherever it says melt butter or warm oil in the pan to start the cooking process, erase that phrase from your mind. Start instead with vegetable stock. Instead of sautéing onions in oil, cook them in stock. Instead of frying green beans with garlic, cook them in stock. When you need something creamy to hold a brothy sauce together, forget the cream and remember nonfat yogurt. Want a vinaigrette that clings to the salad? No, the answer is no longer olive oil, it's nonfat yogurt or tomato puree. Most of your favorite recipes can be adapted—you don't have to start over.

Your basic pantry will change somewhat. You'll no longer need oils, canned soups, prepared salad dressings, and bottled sauces. You will still keep canned tomatoes, vinegars, spices, and herbs, but new items will appear in the cupboard. Dried mushrooms that can be soaked in hot water and added to soups and sauces for richness of flavor; nonfat dry milk; an ample supply of dry pasta, rice, couscous, polenta, and cracked wheat will join dried beans. You will now keep batches of vegetable stock in the refrigerator (and freezer) along with nonfat yogurt, in various degrees of thickness, and tofu. Egg whites will be collected and the yolks discarded or given away. And believe it or not, you will not feel hungry because you can eat as much as you want of these grains, legumes, fresh vegetables, and fruits. And, if you take the time to cook well for yourself, you won't feel emotionally hungry either.

Will you need any new cooking equipment? Not much. If you don't have any nonstick sauté pans, get a few. If you don't have a steamer or steamer rack that fits comfortably in another pan, this is a wise investment. The best multileveled steamers are available in hardware stores with a large Asian, especially Japanese, clientele. Will you need new cookbooks? Well, along with this one, books on Indian, Chinese,

Japanese, and Mediterranean cooking will give you recipe ideas that you can play with. When you read, "Heat a wok with oil," think vegetable stock. You see ghee, think stock—or yogurt. We all need new inspiration after cooking the same dishes over and over. And cookbooks can provide the impetus to try something new and adapt many dishes to your new methods.

In other words, this is not the end of fine dining for you but the start of dining and thinking about food in a new way. This book provides a good beginning because fine cooks and professional chefs have taken up the nonfat challenge and contributed the recipes.

Joyce Goldstein
Chef/Owner, Square One Restaurant
San Francisco

# *The Low-Fat Pantry and Equipment*

## PANTRY

***Agar-agar:*** This dried seaweed gelatin is also called kanten. Use it to thicken sauces and as a substitute for gelatin in dishes such as aspics, desserts, or molded salads. Wash, then soak the bars, sheets, granules, or flakes for 1 hour in cold water. If using bars and sheets, squeeze out any excess liquid. Add boiling water, sauce, stock, or juice and stir until dissolved. Use 1 teaspoon of agar flakes or granules per cup of cooking liquid and 2 cups of cooking liquid per stick of kanten.

***Bananas:*** Besides their more common uses, think of bananas when you want to thicken and add creaminess and flavor to pureed dressings and dips. They will also contribute moisture and sweetness to baked goods.

***Citrus Zest and Juice:*** Use either a small gauge grater or a citrus "zester" to remove just the brightly colored outer peel from any citrus fruit. You do not want to go as far as the "white" layer, the pith, which can be quite bitter. The fruit flavor is in the oil of the freshly grated peel and is much more intense than the juice from the fruit. If you substitute dried, bottled, or bagged citrus peel, you will miss out on the opportunity to turn an ordinary dish into something quite lively.

Reserve the juice from the lemon or the lime to use as a flavor enhancer. It is an essential element in recognized dishes from some countries and can act as a salt substitute. Use it to bring out the flavors of your salsas, dressings, and some vegetable stir-fries. Like the zest, fresh juice is much better tasting than the bottled or mass-produced kind.

***Cooking Oil Sprays:*** A teaspoon of any oil that you pour into a pan will contain almost 5 grams of fat (45 calories!). Cooking oil sprays are aerosolized oils and are formulated to help you use less oil than you ordinarily would when trying to coat a cooking surface with oil. They can be found in cans with propellant added or in simple pump bottles. The pump bottlers do not contain the propellant and deliver more oil per serving, and with it more grams of fat and calories. When you use any of these products, the goal is to spray as little as possible.

Most of the available products contain corn, safflower, canola, or olive oil, may or may not be "flavored" with butter, and deliver 2 grams of fat or less per serving. When reading the labels, be careful to note how the manufacturers define a "serving size." For example, if there are 2 grams of fat per serving and the manufacturer's serving is for only one-third of a 10-inch pan, then to coat a full pan you must deliver 6 grams of fat. There are "lite" varieties that have some water added and may deliver less than 1 gram per serving and work very well.

The sprays are useful to have in your pantry, but it is still best to purchase a few nonstick pans and limit your use of spray products.

***Daikon Radish:*** This looks like a very large white carrot and is used quite frequently in Japanese cooking. Look for it with the other fresh vegetables in supermarkets or in Japanese food markets. Pickled daikon, which is used as a condiment, is also available.

***Ginger:*** This root can be found in many supermarkets. Choose roots that have a smooth, papery skin and are not shriveled, which is a sign of dryness. The more mature the root, the more fibrous the texture and pungent the flavor will be. Much of the flavor of ginger is just below the skin, so it is best to peel away the most superficial layer only. If the root has begun to sprout, then most of the flavor will have already been lost. Young, green, and immature ginger is sometimes available in the spring. It is less fibrous and has a more delicate flavor. To use fresh ginger, peel and remove the knobby stumps, then slice, grate, chop, or shred it.

***Japanese "Basil" or Shiso:*** These leaves look very much like basil, and their flavor is frequently described as similar to that of basil or mint. The leaves may be red or green; the recipes in this book call for the green variety.

***Japanese Eggplant:*** This is much smaller than the usual eggplant, and like the Japanese cucumber has fewer seeds than its American counterpart. If you do not plan to cook the eggplant in its skin, cover it immediately with water after slicing it and then let it soak in water for 15 minutes to remove any bitterness and prevent discoloration.

***Japanese Noodles:*** The recipes in the book call for two widely available kinds of noodles: *soba noodles,* which are wide and flat and made from buckwheat flour, and *somen noodles,* which are made from wheat and are similar in thickness to vermicelli pasta. *Udon noodles* also are made from wheat and are widely available on both coasts, though you may have to go to specialty stores to find them. Cook Japanese noodles according to the package directions and use them as you would any pasta: in soups, stews, and salads. While Japanese noodles usually are egg- and oil-free, some of the "instant" noodles soups available in packages have added oils.

***Kabocha Squash:*** The edible part of this Japanese pumpkin has a very meaty texture and fine flavor. When cooked, it makes a smooth and creamy puree. It looks like a flattened drum and has a dark green thick skin. It's best to buy kabocha squash when the skin is very hard to scratch with your fingernail. Acorn or butternut squash can be substituted for kabocha.

***Kombu:*** This seaweed is frequently used for making stocks ("dashi" kombu) as well as eating. There are those who maintain that kombu aids in the digestion of legumes, and it is also rich in iodine. Look for it in markets specializing in Japanese foods or in health food stores. Lightly wipe the surface with a rag to clean kombu (too much washing or rinsing will wash away the flavor). Kombu is very flavorful and contains a small amount of naturally occurring glutamates. If you have had unpleasant reactions to monosodium glutamate, you may not be able to tolerate kombu either.

***Lemongrass:*** Like its name, this vegetable does taste quite a bit like a lemon. Finely chop and use the lower end of the stalk. Substitute the finely grated zest of half a lemon for a stalk of lemongrass if you cannot find it in your supermarket or in Asian markets.

***Mirin:*** Made from rice, this is sweetened sake and is used primarily for cooking. If you cannot find it in your local areas, you can make a substitute by adding 4 tablespoons of sugar to ¾ cup of sake, dry vermouth, or sherry (or substitute 1 tablespoon of sake and 1 teaspoon of sugar for each tablespoon of mirin required).

***Miso:*** This paste is made from fermented soybeans, salt, and various grains and comes in several varieties, from sweet and white (shiro) to yellow and salty (inaka) to red and salty (ala) to brown (hatcho). All are used to flavor soups, sauces, dressings, and stews and are high in protein (especially the hatcho variety). The flavors may change with prolonged cooking, so it is best to add miso near the end of cooking a dish. Generally, miso is high in sodium and should not be used in combination with salt. One tablespoon of miso is equal to approximately ½ teaspoon of table salt.

***Mustards:*** Mustard comes in a variety of flavors and textures. Its white, brown, or black seeds can be used to make spreads that can be used instead of spreads that contain higher amounts of fat and perhaps cholesterol. Mustards can also be used in dressings and sauces for extra flavor, as a thickening agent, and as an emulsifier. You can find them seasoned with herbs and spices, aromatic vegetables such as onions or garlic, and with other agents like honey or various wines.

The bright yellow "American" mustard is the easiest to find, but it is well worth the effort to find some of the others. "Dijon" mustard is also readily available, and its mild flavor is less likely to overwhelm the flavor of your sauce than some of the other mustards. "Chinese" mustard, because of its fiery heat, can be a real shocker for the uninitiated. You can purchase the powder yourself, mix it with cold water, and then use it in your dipping sauces. Some will find the "Jamaican" and "Bahamian" mustard-based sauces only slightly less "hot." All of these ethnic varieties can be found in stores catering to these populations.

Keep in mind that mustards can be high in sodium and a few contain eggs, so read the labels carefully.

***Nonfat Dairy and Cheeses:*** If you are thinking about weight loss and preventing a myriad of health problems, substituting nonfat for regular cheese is the commonsense choice. These cheeses melt, and some are quite flavorful. There are several brand names available, as are the familiar varieties such as Monterey Jack, Cheddar, Swiss, and American. Generally, 1 ounce of nonfat cheese has approximately the same amount of fat, cholesterol, and protein as a cup of nonfat or skim milk. The nondairy soy cheeses have too much fat to be considered nonfat and have more calories than nonfat cheeses.

The cheese made from draining yogurt (see page 148) is thick, creamy, and can be whipped quickly into rich desserts as well as used as a substitute for high-fat, high-cholesterol cheese fillings in savory dishes. (Nonfat yogurts containing gelatin will give you a less creamy, unsatisfying result.)

Undrained regular nonfat yogurt can be substituted for oil when making salad dressings. Recent additions to the dairy shelves also include nonfat versions of cottage cheese, cream cheese, and sour cream.

***Nori Seaweed:*** This particular type of seaweed is frequently sold in sheets and is used to wrap balls of rice and sushi. When toasted nori is called for, preheat the oven to 300 degrees, place the sheets on a middle rack, and bake for about 3 minutes. Or hold the nori directly over a flame, fanning it all the while, until the color changes from dark brown or black to green. Crush the toasted sheets between a towel or cut them with kitchen shears. Like other seaweeds, nori has a fishy odor and flavor.

***Ponzu Sauce:*** This vinegar-based dressing can be purchased, but it is easy to make your own. The basic ingredients are usually dashi stock (see the one on page 146), soy sauce, and vinegar or citrus juice in equal amounts.

***Potsticker Skins (Rounds):*** These wrappers, made from flour and water, can be made from scratch or found in the refrigerated cases of Chinese or Japanese groceries. Used classically for making dumplings that are either fried or steamed, they are circles 3½ inches in diameter with a thickness of 1⁄16 inch. They can be frozen for up to 2 months or refrigerated for up to 1 week. When you are working with them, they should be supple enough to be shaped without cracking.

***Quinoa:*** Unlike the vast majority of the other grains, this one is a complete protein. Native to Central and South America it has only in recent years been available in this country in many of the large supermarket chains as well as in health food stores. Besides being high in protein, it is also rich in many B vitamins, fiber, and iron, but compared with other grains it is moderately high in fat. Rinse quinoa well before cooking because its natural coating has a bitter taste. It can be used as you would use any other grain.

***Sake:*** A Japanese beverage made from fermented rice, sake is sometimes used in cooking to add flavor and remove odors. If you can't find it in your local liquor store, try an Asian or health food store, or substitute dry vermouth or sherry.

***Shiitake Mushrooms:*** These mushrooms come fresh or dried. The dried mushrooms have a very distinct flavor and can be stored for many months if kept in a tightly lidded jar. Soak them for 15 to 30 minutes in warm water. Longer soaking will remove much of their flavor. The soaking water should be reserved for use in stocks and sauces, or as braising liquid.

***Sun-dried Tomatoes:*** These come hard, dried, and leathery or dried and packed in oil with a slightly softer texture. Both are intensely flavored and will add considerable depth and richness to any dish. Loosely packed dried tomatoes have the lower fat content and calorie count, are also usually lower in price, and are widely available in the larger food chains and specialty shops. To prepare sun-dried tomatoes, remove any stems; then, using kitchen shears, cut them into chips or strips. If you are not planning to cook them in a sauce, stew, or soup, you should soak the pieces in boiling water for 10 minutes. You can then add them to various dishes and puree them for use in spreads and dips.

***Texturized Vegetable Protein:*** The protein extracted from soybeans is widely used commercially and is now available in the bulk food sections of many health food markets. Because it is derived from soybeans, it, like all other legumes, is an incomplete protein. Use it to add a meaty texture and boost the protein of your soups and stews. Be sure to read the label before you buy it to check if oils and salt have been added.

***Tofu:*** This soybean-based product is available widely throughout the United States. It spoils easily and therefore needs to be kept refrigerated and covered with water. After you open the package, change the water daily, then drain the tofu well before using it in your recipes. Wrap it in a clean dish towel and let it sit for 30 minutes before using. Silken tofu is firmer than "soft" tofu and does not need refrigeration. It is sold in paper boxes and lasts for up to six months in the unopened package.

***Vegetable Stocks:*** These are essential for adding flavor in the absence of cooking oils and meat or poultry bases. Use them instead of water as the main ingredient in soups, stews, sauces, and even dressings. They are particularly useful for braising vegetables, in that the richly concentrated flavors of the stock will act as a cooking medium and contribute to the flavor of the vegetables. Make a large quantity at once and freeze it in ice cube trays or small containers. You can then remove only the amount that you need to prepare the day's meals.

***Vinegars:*** The spectrum of available vinegars has grown much wider than the highly acidic and bitter white vinegar made from distilled alcohol that we depended on in the past. There are many now to choose from. Balsamic vinegar (made from grapes, then aged for several years) and the wine vinegars (red or white, sherry and champagne) are, like all of the vinegars, flavor enhancers, and each has its own distinctive flavor. Tarragon, sage, mint, thyme, or any of a variety of herbal vinegars are generally infusions of that herb into a vinegar base and will impart the flavor of that herb whenever used. Generally, all of these vinegars are mildly acidic and have a much more delicate flavor than standard white vinegar. Once you learn how to use them, you will be surprised at how excellent they are for adding a robust flavor to any meal when oils are not being used.

Use them sparingly, however, because too much can quickly overtake other flavors and ruin whatever you are preparing. Experiment with them by stirring a small amount into homemade dressings, chutneys, and relishes. Also, add a very little to soups or stews at the end of cooking to really enrich their flavor. Raspberry vinegar is particularly wonderful as a dressing in combination with mustard and honey, apple or even orange juice concentrate. Many of these vinegars can be found in your local markets. Two that are used frequently in the recipes in this book are worth saying a little more about:

*Rice vinegar* is a Japanese product found in specialty stores or in special sections of the larger supermarket chains as well as in many health food stores. It is made from fermented rice and has a very mild flavor. Use white wine vinegar or cider vinegar if you can't find it, although the flavor will not be as mild or sweet.

*Seasoned vinegar* can be used for the rice for any sushi, salads, and pickling vegetables. It can be purchased in the store on those shelves stocking international foods, or you can make your own by adding varying amounts of sugar and salt to a mild vinegar and heating it just enough to dissolve the sugar and salt. For a mildly seasoned vinegar, try ⅓ cup vinegar, 2 teaspoons of salt, and 2 teaspoons of sugar.

***Wasabi:*** Commonly called Japanese horseradish, this root vegetable is in fact a radish. Finely grated or paste-form wasabi is usually served with sushi or sashimi (raw fish). The fresh root is almost impossible to find in this country, but the powdered form is readily available. Mix the green powder with an equal amount of cold water. This pungent spice has a wonderful flavor but should be used sparingly until you decide how much of its "heat" you can tolerate.

***Water Chestnuts:*** This root vegetable is made predominantly of water and a fibrous starchy material. Since it is very low in calories and has a mild flavor, it makes a nice crunchy addition to just about any dish. Water chestnuts are most frequently used in Chinese cooking and can be found fresh or in cans in Chinese markets. If you are using fresh water chestnuts, remove the outer husks.

## EQUIPMENT

The low-fat kitchen does not require any fancy equipment to be successful, but a few simple items are very useful in keeping this menu plan simple and streamlined and eliminate a lot of work. A simple *blender* is invaluable for blending sauces and dressings and pureeing soups. A *food processor*—one of the inexpensive mini versions is fine for chopping fresh herbs, garlic, onions, and shallots easily; larger, good-quality models will handle all blending and pureeing chores if you do not have a blender. Small and large *nonstick sauté pans* make sautéing vegetables and preparing pasta sauces simple and fat-free. For the busy cook a *pressure cooker* can reduce the cooking time for legumes by 50 percent. Alternatively, and paradoxically, a *slow cooker,* one that you can turn on before you go to bed, run errands, or leave for work will also get dinner on the table a lot sooner. A simple cotton *cheesecloth* and a large *strainer* will help to keep your refrigerator stocked with yogurt cheese and clear vegetable stocks. A *microwave oven* is essential for reheating prepared entrées and steaming vegetables quickly. Place the raw vegetables in a microwave-safe container, sprinkle with a few teaspoons of water, and cover with suitable plastic wrap. The cooking time will vary with the vegetables. For even cooking, make sure that all vegetables cooked together are cut uniformly. And finally, small *covered containers* allow you to prepare condiments ahead of time and keep them handy in the refrigerator.

### *SNACKS*

Keep these healthful snacks handy to prevent you from straying to high-fat foods:

Air-popped popcorn
Bagels with sugar-free jam
Fat-free tortilla chips and homemade tomato salsa
Rice cakes with sugar-free jelly or jam
Steamed vegetables with fat-free dressings
Fresh fruit and vegetables
Salt-free pretzels
Nonfat frozen yogurt

# *The Low-Fat Staples: Legumes and Grains*

If you are on a vegetarian diet you must make sure that you meet all of your dietary protein requirements. To achieve this, combine dried beans and legumes with various grains, such as corn, rice, and wheat. Combining the legumes and grains or adding a small amount of a dairy product (such as nonfat milk) to either food group will not only provide complete proteins but will also add variety, texture, and satisfying hearty flavors to a vegetarian diet.

## GENERAL INFORMATION AND COOKING INSTRUCTIONS FOR LEGUMES

Legumes are the edible seeds of several plants in the Leguminosae family, varieties of which can be found worldwide: soybeans and their products in Japan and China; borlotti beans in Italy; flageolets and lentils in France and North Africa; black beans, kidney beans, and pigeon peas in the Caribbean; pinto beans in Central America; and navy beans in North America. The peanut, while usually thought of as a nut, is actually a legume and is widely used in Africa; it was brought to the Americas in the sixteenth century. The peanut is very high in fat and is not recommended for those attempting to lose weight and/or lower their cholesterol.

Legumes have universal appeal, and their popularity is growing in the United States. They are an excellent source of protein and many other nutrients, are high in fiber, low in fat, and have recently been proven to aid in lowering cholesterol. An added benefit is that legumes are far less expensive than animal sources of protein. In order to make best use of the protein available in legumes, you should eat them with grains, in a ratio of approximately 1 part legume to 3 parts grains. This is necessary because while legumes are a superb source of protein, they are missing a few protein building blocks, which are easily provided by the grains.

Legumes and grains are both quite versatile, so this ratio can be satisfied in many ways. Serve any legume with the grain of your choice in the form of breads, pastas, muffins, sweet or savory pancakes, tortillas, and pilafs. Beans and peas can be served in delicious soups, stews, salads, dips, and as stuffings for pastas and sandwich spreads. Mashed beans with sweeteners added are even used as the basis for desserts in China and Japan and for a pie sold in New York and California.

The chart below provides some general information about cooking times and yields for various legumes. Most legumes will need to soaked and rinsed before cooking. Lentils, split peas, and black-eyed peas do not need to be soaked.

***Soaking:*** Soaking the dried beans before cooking will reduce the cooking time by about half. Draining and further rinsing will also help to break down and remove some of the sugars that are responsible for the flatulence legumes cause in some people. Before soaking and cooking, rinse the beans to remove any sand and pick out any pebbles, twigs, and shriveled old beans that you can find. For soaking you can either:

| *Dried Bean (1 Cup)* | *Water or Stock* | *Cooking Duration* | *Yield* |
|---|---|---|---|
| Aduki beans | 3 cups | 2 hours | 2 cups |
| Anasazi beans | 4 cups | 1½ hours | 2 cups |
| Baby lima beans | 2 cups | 1½ hours | 1¾ cups |
| Black beans | 4 cups | 2 hours | 2 cups |
| Black-eyed peas | 3 cups | 1 hour | 2 cups |
| Chick-peas | 4 cups | 3 hours | 2½ cups |
| Cranberry beans | 3 cups | 1½ hours | 2½ cups |
| Fava beans | 3 cups | 3 hours | 2 cups |
| Great northern beans | 3½ cups | 2 hours | 2 cups |
| Kidney beans | 3 cups | 1½ hours | 2 cups |
| Lentils | 3 cups | 45 minutes | 2¼ cups |
| Mung beans | 2½ cups | 1½ hours | 2 cups |
| Navy beans | 3 cups | 2½ hours | 2 cups |
| Pigeon peas | 3 cups | 30 minutes | 2¼ cups |
| Pink beans | 4 cups | 1½ hours | 2 cups |
| Pinto beans | 3 cups | 2½ hours | 2 cups |
| Red beans | 3 cups | 3 hours | 2 cups |
| Soybeans | 4 cups | 2½ hours | 3 cups |
| Split peas | 3 cups | 45 minutes | 2¼ cups |

1. Soak the beans overnight in four times as much water, or
2. Quick-soak the beans by adding them to four times as much water in a large pot, bring to a boil, and boil for 2 minutes. Remove the pot from the heat, cover, and let stand for 1 hour.

Either way, drain off the soaking water, rinse, and continue with the recipe.

***Using Canned Beans:*** Substitute canned beans for dried ones if you do not want to start from scratch. The yield column on the cooking chart will tell you the approximate volume of canned beans you will need according to the amount of dried beans called for. Drain the beans and reserve the liquid if you want a thick bean sauce.

For salads simply rinse the beans with cool water, drain,

and add the remaining salad ingredients. For soups or stews, you can lightly braise the herbs, spices, and aromatic vegetables in vegetable broth and then add the canned beans along with any other vegetables. In any recipe in which you are cooking the beans along with a number of other vegetables, add the drained liquid from the can and enough additional liquid to provide one-third of the amount of cooking liquid required in the recipe.

## GENERAL INFORMATION AND COOKING INSTRUCTIONS FOR GRAINS

To get a balance of proteins the body needs, you must recognize which foods are legumes and which are grains. The charts for grains and legumes will help you identify the most common ones that are commercially available.

There is a large variety of grains with differing flavors and textures to choose from. These seeds of grasses or similar plants have fed the earth's population for thousands of years, for they are rich in calories and several essential nutrients. Refined grains tend to be lower in these nutrients unless the vitamins and minerals have been replenished after the grain has been ground into flour. The refining process also removes a large portion of the protein, vitamin E, and fiber. Low blood levels of vitamin E are being investigated for their role in cancer and heart disease. Low dietary fiber is thought to be related to rectal and other gastrointestinal cancers, hemorrhoids, constipation, and diverticulosis.

There are a few differences among various grains. Some listed below are not grains by the truest definition—amaranth, buckwheat, quinoa, and wild rice—but all can be prepared and enjoyed similarly. If you are looking for grains that are gluten-free, look to rice, corn, buckwheat, and millet. Avoid whole grain products that are not refrigerated in the grocery store, since the oil tends to become rancid more quickly. Whole grains can be kept for five to six months in a refrigerator or freezer. They can be kept in an airtight container in a cool spot in your home for up to one month.

Don't forget that grain products come in many forms. Pastas, breads including the whole wheat, white, and sprouted varieties, muffins, rice cakes, corn and wheat flour tortillas, breakfast cereals, oat and wheat bran are all there to add interest and variety to your meals as well as nutrition.

| *Grain (1 Cup)* | *Water or Stock* | *Cooking Duration* | *Yield* |
|---|---|---|---|
| Amaranth | 1½ cups | 20 minutes | 2 cups |
| Arborio rice | 2 cups | 25 minutes | 2½ cups |
| Barley | 3 cups | 45 minutes | 3½ cups |
| Basmati rice | 2½ cups | 20 minutes | 3 cups |
| Brown rice | 2 cups | 45 minutes | 3 cups |
| Bulgur | 2 cups | 15–20 minutes | 2½ cups |
| Hominy grits, quick-cooking | 3½ cups | 5 minutes | 3¼ cups |
| Kasha (buckwheat groats) | 2 cups | 15 minutes | 2½ cups |
| Millet | 2¾ cups | 40 minutes | 3½ cups |
| Oats, whole grain | 2 cups | 1 hour | 2½ cups |
| Quinoa | 2 cups | 15 minutes | 2½ cups |
| Rye berries | 2¾ cups | 1 hour | 2 cups |
| Wheat berries | 2¾ cups | 2 hours | 2¾ cups |
| White rice | 2 cups | 20 minutes | 3 cups |
| Wild rice | 2 cups | 50 minutes | 2⅔ cups |

# *Low-Fat Cooking Methods and Techniques*

***Al Dente:*** In Italian, *al dente* means "to the tooth"; in cooking it has a similar meaning—"crisp to the teeth" or "resistant to the bite"; "cooked, but still firm." Properly cooked pasta is the perfect example of *al dente.* The technique is also critical to well-made Chinese and Japanese dishes.

In addition to those foods that are best enjoyed before that bit of firmness is lost, dishes that are to be reheated or finished with a second stage of cooking should be slightly underdone initially, since they will continue to cook.

Cooking times vary according to the size and thickness of an item—for example, angel hair pasta will cook faster than fettuccine, julienned vegetables will cook faster than those left in larger pieces. Ripeness and quality also affect cooking times. Vegetables that are to be cooked together should be cut in similar shapes and thicknesses. Those of varying sizes should be cooked separately, for they will cook at different rates. (See *Parboiling.*)

***Baking:*** This should always be done in a preheated oven because the heat will seal and prevent juices from escaping from foods and thus keep foods from drying out. For low-fat baking, a nonstick pan is best, but you can also use a pan lightly sprayed with vegetable oil. If your pan is sprayed too heavily, the extra fat should be wiped off. Waxed paper can be used to line molds or baking sheets that are nonstick; the paper should be peeled off right after baking.

***Braising:*** With this method you can cook vegetables to the desired tenderness in enough liquid to form a sauce or you can use just a slight amount of liquid so that the vegetables can be added without sauce to another recipe.

Vegetables used in braising can be raw, oven-roasted, or sautéed. Cut them into uniform pieces to ensure even cooking. Partially cover the vegetables with liquid. Cover the pot and place it over a low to medium heat to prevent burning.

Using vegetable stock or wine will contribute to the flavor of the vegetables. If you are braising a wide variety of vegetables (such as onions, carrots, celery, and leeks), you may not need to start with a stock because the vegetables will provide enough flavor on their own.

If you are cooking with water, add dried herbs at the same time you add the vegetables. Fresh herbs should be added toward the end of cooking; they have a tendency to lose flavor with prolonged cooking. Salt should also be added toward the end of cooking because saltiness becomes concentrated as the liquid evaporates during cooking.

If you plan to use the braising liquid as a sauce and you find it has a weak flavor, strain the liquid away from the vegetables once they have been cooked. Return it to a high heat and boil to reduce it and concentrate its flavor. Then add fresh herbs, salt, pepper, and any thickening agents.

***Chiffonading Leaves (Spinach, Basil, or Other Large Flat Leaves):*** Roll the leaf tightly; slice the roll thinly. Each piece will form a ribbon when unrolled that is very decorative.

***Grilling:*** This technique retains all the juices and flavor of food because it seals them in with dry heat. Use a nonstick grill and make sure it is clean and very hot before placing the vegetables on it. Temperature and time depend on the type of vegetable used, ripeness, quality, and size of cut. Different vegetables grilled together should be cut to the same thickness to ensure equal cooking time. Salt should be used at the end of cooking or else it will extract moisture.

***Parboiling, or Blanching:*** Parboiling or blanching is a way of partially cooking ingredients. Blanching is also done to extract bitterness or too strong flavors from vegetables such as daikon. Beans can be blanched as an alternative to soaking them overnight, and this method has the added advantage of extracting some of their elements that can cause flatulence. To blanch beans, a ratio of ten times the amount of water to the amount of beans is recommended. Rinse and pick over the beans and place the beans in cold water, bring to a boil, then boil for 6 minutes, rinse and refresh under cold water before continuing with the recipe.

Blanching should always be done in a large amount of lightly salted boiling water. The salt can be omitted, but it does help to retain the colors of vegetables; 1 tablespoon per quart of water is recommended.

Green vegetables in particular contain elements that when subjected to heat change color and texture. Therefore, when blanching green vegetables, the following steps are recommended:

1. Use a nonreactive pot—enameled or stainless steel. Bring the water to a rolling boil. Do not cover. Taste often to determine doneness.
2. Once cooked, the vegetables should be drained and submerged in a large amount of ice cold water to stop the cooking process.

Blanching times for some vegetables:

| *Vegetable* | *Duration* |
|---|---|
| Carrot, julienned | 2 minutes |
| Celery stalk, julienned | 2 minutes |
| Fennel bulb, julienned | 2 minutes |
| Green beans (2-inch lengths) | 1 minute |
| Green onions | 30 seconds |

| *Vegetable* | *Duration* |
|---|---|
| Green peas, fresh | 1 minute |
| Leek, julienned | 30 seconds |
| Mushrooms, julienned | 30 seconds |
| Snow peas | 1 minute |
| Spinach | 10 seconds |
| Summer squash | 1 minute |

***Roasting:*** This is another way of cooking with dry heat. You can roast in a preheated oven on the rack or in a roasting pan. It is best to roast vegetables such as onions, squashes, peppers, and garlic in their own skins so that the meaty part of the vegetable will taste sweeter. The skin can then be discarded.

***Roasting Chili Peppers:*** Fresh chilies can be roasted under the broiler. Turn them frequently, and broil until the entire skin is somewhat blackened. Transfer the chilies to a container that can be sealed tightly. Once the chilies have cooled, remove them from the container and slide off the blackened skins. They are then ready to be used.

Dried chilies can be roasted in a dry skillet. While heating the pan and the chilies, agitate the pan to prevent the chilies from burning and blackening.

You may find the juice in these peppers quite irritating to your skin, and if the juice gets into your eyes, transferred by your fingers, you might experience itchy, burning eyes. Wearing gloves while preparing chilies can prevent irritation.

***Roasting Eggplants:*** Preheat the oven to 350 degrees. Prick the skin of a 1-pound eggplant several times. Place on a nonstick cooking sheet and bake for 1 hour, turning once after 30 minutes. Slice in half lengthwise and scoop out the pulp. For a very soft pulp, bake for 50 minutes.

***Roasting Garlic:*** Place the unpeeled garlic cloves on a nonstick baking sheet in a 375-degree preheated oven and bake for 30 to 35 minutes, or until the garlic is very tender.

Longer baking will continue to soften and caramelize the garlic, and the soft garlic flesh can then be squeezed out of its skin. Or roast peeled cloves for a somewhat shorter baking time.

***Roasting Onions:*** Preheat the oven to 450 degrees. Put an unpeeled whole onion on a nonstick baking sheet and bake for 45 to 60 minutes until the onion is tender. Turn the onion once halfway through the baking. Peel and coarsely chop the onion after it is roasted.

***Roasting Shallots:*** Preheat the oven to 375 degrees. Roast the unpeeled shallots by putting them on a nonstick baking sheet in the middle of the oven; bake for 30 to 40 minutes until tender. Peel them after roasting.

***Roasting Spices:*** This intensifies flavor and can be done in a preheated oven set to grill position or at maximum heat or in a sauté pan, preferably one with a thick bottom and a flat surface. Add the spices to a preheated skillet without any oil or liquid. The pan must be absolutely dry or the spices will stick to the pan and be more likely to burn. The pan should be preheated first over high heat. Add the spices and lower the heat to medium. The spices will lose their moisture during the first minute and then they will start to roast or toast, smoke lightly, and change color. Their smell will intensify. To avoid burning, shake the pan or stir the spices. Remove the pan from the flame before any released oil from the spice starts to smoke and burn. Spices should be roasted only until they become light brown, not dark, or they will develop a burning, bitter flavor. Roasting times vary according to the types, amounts, and ages of the spices being roasted.

To make a mixture of different spices, roast each spice separately before combining them. If the spices are to be ground after roasting, they should be cooled or their flavors will be lost.

***Roasting Sweet Bell Peppers Over an Open Flame:*** This will give you a roasted pepper more quickly than doing it in the oven. Simply set the whole pepper directly on a burner with the flame at medium height. Rotate the pepper over the flame as the skin becomes charred. When the skin is charred on all sides, place it in a paper bag for about 20 minutes. Pierce the pepper to allow the steam to escape. Hold the blackened pepper under cold water and with your thumbs slide the charred skin off. Slice the pepper open, trim the stem end, and scrape away the seeds.

***Roasting Tomatoes:*** Roasting fresh tomatoes works best when they are in season. Slice the ripe tomatoes at least ½ inch thick, and arrange the slices in a single layer on a parchment-lined baking sheet. Place in a 300-degree oven for approximately 45 minutes, or until most of the liquid has evaporated. The tomatoes are ready when they darken in color and lose their glossy appearance. They do not need to be roasted until they are charred. If tomatoes are not in season, try substituting soaked sun-dried tomatoes that have not been packed in oil in recipes. They will give excellent results, and the sun-dried variety does not need to be roasted. If delicious fresh or sun-dried tomatoes are not available, you can use canned whole tomatoes, which need to be sliced and then roasted as fresh ones are.

***Steaming:*** Like blanching, steaming seals foods with moist heat and helps to retain their nutrients, flavor, and texture. The water should be at a full boil to produce a high heat and full steam, but kept below the steaming rack and not in contact with the food. Watch the level of water carefully and add more water as needed.

***Tofu Pressing:*** This decreases much of the water content and should be done if you are trying to prepare tofu "cutlets" or "steaks." Slice the tofu into slabs no more than 1 inch thick. Wrap the tofu in a clean towel and place a cutting board or baking sheet on top of it. Place up to 2 pounds of weight on top of the cutting board or sheet and let the tofu sit for an hour this way. It should then be firm enough to use.

# *Sample Week's Menus*

The following week of vegetarian menus consists of flavorful, colorful, and healthy dishes for breakfast, lunch, and dinner that are all fat-free. These very diverse menus are designed to help you create your own menus. Do not get bogged down by trying to duplicate them on a daily basis. While many of the recipes in the menus and in the book require minimal preparation, some are a bit more labor intensive. For those recipes demanding more time use the weekends to chop and put away vegetables, as well as to prepare one or two entrées and a soup. Once made, all of the dishes can frequently be incorporated into other meals. For example, in this menu the Vegetarian Red Beans and Seven-Grain Dirty Rice is prepared for an evening meal on Day 2. It is then folded into whole wheat or corn tortillas and spiked with a tomato salsa for lunch on Day 3. For another shortcut, the Grilled Asparagus with Lemon, Peppers, and Caper Vinaigrette served on one night could be chopped and folded into some cooked rice for a tangy rice salad. Serve this with lunch or dinner on another day of the week.

When you are eliminating fat from your diet, you must be sure not to eliminate flavor as well. Intensely flavored ingredients and condiments keep the palate satisfied. Make sure your pantry is stocked with some or all of the items listed on pages 114–123. Zesty condiments and fillers such as the chutneys, pickles, salsas, and yogurt cheese can be made ahead of time and stored in small covered containers in the refrigerator. It is also a good idea to make a pot of vegetable stock for soups, sauces, and quick sautés. All should add flavor and interest to different dishes throughout the week without compromising your active lifestyle.

## Day 1

### BREAKFAST

Cold Cereal
Nonfat Yogurt
Fresh Berries
Orange Juice
Warm Beverage

### LUNCH

Stuffed Baked Potato
Broccoli, Potato, and Chick-pea Salad with Lemon-Tarragon Dressing
Tossed Green Salad
Fresh Fruit

### DINNER

Bruschetta with Sun-dried Tomatoes and Capers
Pasta with Red Peppers, Greens, White Beans, Garlic, and Lemon Zest
Grilled Asparagus with Lemon, Peppers, and Caper Vinaigrette
Tossed Green Salad
Peaches Cooked in Red Wine

## Day 2

**BREAKFAST**

Persimmon Spice Muffins
Nonfat Cottage Cheese
Cantaloupe
Fruit Preserves
Warm Beverage

**LUNCH**

Lentil, Celery, and Ginger Salad with Cucumber Vinaigrette
Roasted Eggplant Dip with Pita Chips
Cool Gazpacho with Couscous
Tossed Green Salad

**DINNER**

Vegetarian Red Beans and Seven-Grain Dirty Rice
Braised Okra with Tomatoes
Smoked Tomato and Asparagus
Tossed Green Salad
Banana Heart

## Day 3

**BREAKFAST**

Oatmeal with Cinnamon and Raisins
Nonfat Yogurt
Whole Wheat Toast
Preserves
Orange Juice
Warm Beverage

**LUNCH**

Whole Wheat Burrito with Vegetarian Red Beans and Seven-Grain Dirty Rice
Tomato Salsa or Chutney
Chopped Fresh Cilantro
Tossed Green Salad

**DINNER**

Spinach Ravioli
Creamed Lentil Soup with Celery
Garlic Croutons
Tossed Green Salad
Vanilla Poached Fruits

## Day 4

**BREAKFAST**

Cold Cereal
Nonfat Yogurt
Fresh Fruit or Juice
Whole Wheat Toast
Preserves
Warm Beverage

**LUNCH**

White Beans, Greens, and Sun-dried Tomato Crostini
Red Potato Soup with Garlic and Wild Greens
Tossed Green Salad

**DINNER**

Roasted Quesadillas with Chiquita Bananas
Pico de Gallo Salsa
Vegetarian Chili
Spanish Rice
Tossed Green Salad
Broiled Pineapple with Cinnamon and Rum

## Day 5

**BREAKFAST**

Scrambled Mexican Tofu
Pico de Gallo Salsa
Whole Wheat Toast
Orange Juice
Warm Beverage

#### LUNCH

Black Pepper Polenta with Bell Pepper Sauce and Shiitake Mushrooms
Italian Bean Salad
Tossed Green Salad
Melon Sorbet

#### DINNER

Roasted Tomato Aram Sandwiches
Anasazi Bean Soup with Corn and Chili
Oven-Roasted Potatoes with Fresh Herbs
Tossed Green Salad
Fresh Fruit
Apples and Raspberries in Apple-Ginger Consommé

### Day 6

#### BREAKFAST

Apple Pancakes with Cinnamon
Fresh Berries
Nonfat Yogurt
Whole Wheat Toast
Preserves
Warm Beverage

#### LUNCH

Bruschetta with Sun-dried Tomatoes and Capers
Rice, Lentil, and Spinach Pilaf
Tossed Green Salad
Fresh Fruit

#### DINNER

Tofu Gumbo
Basmati Rice with Peas
Black-eyed Pea Salad
Grilled Asparagus with Lemon, Red Peppers, and Caper Vinaigrette
Green Salad
Figs and Blueberries in Citrus Broth

## Day 7

**BREAKFAST**

Cheese Blintzes with Fresh Fruit
Juice
Whole Wheat Toast
Warm Beverage

**LUNCH**

Couscous Salad
Eggplant Toasts
Fennel Salad with Cucumber and Chick-peas
Fresh Fruit

**DINNER**

Brown Rice-Filled Chilies with Black Bean Sauce
Tomato Salsa
Pumpkin Salad
Corn, Orange, and Tomato Relish
Tossed Greens
Fresh Fruits

# PART THREE

# Basics

## VEGETABLE STOCK

Bradley Ogden

MAKES 4 CUPS

- **1 medium red onion, peeled and quartered**
- **3 medium carrots, peeled and halved**
- **2 celery stalks, halved**
- **4 medium ripe tomatoes, halved**
- **1 fennel bulb, coarsely chopped**
- **4 ears sweet corn, cut into pieces**
- **1 cup washed, coarsely chopped leeks**
- **½ bay leaf**
- **2 sprigs of fresh thyme**
- **1 sprig of fresh marjoram**
- **8 parsley stems**
- **½ teaspoon red pepper flakes**

Combine all the ingredients with 2 quarts cold water in a large stainless-steel stockpot. Bring to a boil over high heat, lower heat, and simmer gently for 45 minutes. Strain the stock through a fine-meshed strainer and cool to room temperature. Refrigerate until needed. If you are not using all of the stock right away, transfer it to 1-cup containers and refrigerate for up to 4 days. It can be frozen for up to 1 week.

*Serving size = 1 cup*
*28 calories*
*0.4 gram fat*
*0 milligrams cholesterol*
*13.0 milligrams sodium*

## BROWN VEGETABLE STOCK

Joyce Goldstein

*A good basic vegetable stock with intense flavor.*

MAKES 4 CUPS

**2 yellow onions, cut in quarters**
**1 red onion, cut in quarters**
**5 carrots, cut in chunks**
**3 leeks, cut in chunks**
**3 stalks celery, cut in chunks**
**1 garlic clove, cut in half**
**1 bay leaf**

Preheat the oven to 450 degrees. Put the cut vegetables in a heavy baking pan. Roast in the oven, uncovered, stirring occasionally, for about 1 hour.

Transfer the vegetables to a stockpot. Cover with 2 quarts water. Bring to a boil and simmer, covered, for 1 hour. Strain. Cool to room temperature and refrigerate for up to 4 days or freeze for up to 1 week.

*Serving size = 1 cup*
*29 calories*
*0.1 gram fat*
*0 milligrams cholesterol*
*13.4 milligrams sodium*

## CHINA MOON VEGETABLE INFUSION

Barbara Tropp

*This is a light vegetable stock with great flavor and a lovely sweetness. Add cooked pasta and slivered vegetables for a terrific main-dish soup.*

MAKES 3 QUARTS

**4 large, rock-hard heads garlic**
**6 large Chinese dried black mushrooms**
**2 yellow onions, thinly sliced**
**4 carrots, thinly sliced**
**10 quarter-size rounds fresh gingerroot, smashed**
**6 fat scallions, cut into 1-inch chunks, smashed**
**2 small green serrano chilies, halved and smashed**
**¼ cup Chinese rice wine or dry sherry**
**1 tablespoon black peppercorns**
**1½ tablespoons Szechuan peppercorns**
**12 cups cold water**
**1 fat stalk lemongrass, cut into 2-inch pieces, smashed**

Preheat the oven to 350 degrees. Arrange a rack in the middle position.

Roast the garlic, root side down, on a baking sheet until very soft, about 30 minutes. (Don't worry if some brown ooze bubbles volcanolike from the top.) Let cool, then smash the heads lightly to expose the pulp.

While the garlic roasts, cover the mushrooms in a shallow bowl with 1 cup cold water. Weight the caps down with a saucer and let soak until soft, about 30 minutes. Cut the caps into thick slices. Strain and retain the soaking liquid.

Heat a heavy nonaluminum stockpot over low heat until a bead of wine evaporates on contact. Add the garlic, mushrooms, onions, carrots, ginger, scallions, chilies, and wine, and stir to combine. Cover the pot and let the vegetables sweat until soupy, about 20 minutes. Don't rush the process; the fuller the sauna, the better tasting the stock.

Add the peppercorns, water, and reserved mushroom-soaking liquid. Stir to blend, raise the heat, and bring the mixture to a near boil. Adjust the heat to maintain a weak simmer and cook, uncovered, for 45 minutes. Add the lemongrass and simmer gently 15 minutes more.

Strain the stock and discard the solids. For best flavor, use the stock within 2 days.

*Serving size = 1 cup*
*41 calories*
*0.2 gram fat*
*0 milligrams cholesterol*
*164 milligrams sodium*

## DASHI VEGETABLE STOCK

Jean-Marc Fullsack

*This stock has an exceptionally rich flavor due largely to the kombu seaweed, which is classically used in Asian cooking this way. Kombu is a natural source of small amounts of the flavor enhancer monosodium glutamate.*

*The stock can be made and refrigerated for up to 1 week. It can also be kept frozen for up to 6 months.*

MAKES 1 QUART

**2 14-inch pieces dried kombu seaweed**
**6⅔ cups cold water**
**2 cups carrots, coarsely chopped**
**4 cups onions, coarsely chopped**
**4 cups celery, coarsely chopped**

Slice each 14-inch piece of kombu into 3 pieces. Using a damp cloth, wipe the excess salt from both sides of the kombu sheet. Place the kombu and 5 cups water in a large covered pan and bring to a boil. Cover, leaving a small opening, reduce the heat, and simmer over medium heat until the liquid is reduced by one-quarter, or to about 3¾ cups.

Add 1⅔ cups cold water, the carrots, onions, and celery to the kombu and broth. Allow the water to return to a boil.

Reduce the heat and simmer, covered, over medium heat for at least 30 minutes. Strain and discard the kombu and vegetables.

*Serving size = 1 cup*
*24 calories*
*0.3 gram fat*
*0 milligrams cholesterol*
*45.7 milligrams sodium*

## VEGETABLE CONSOMMÉ

Hubert Keller

MAKES APPROXIMATELY 1½ QUARTS
SERVES 4 TO 5

**2 medium leeks, white part only, diced**
**½ small celery root (or 2 celery stalks), peeled and diced**
**4 shallots, coarsely chopped**
**1 large tomato, peeled, and seeded**
**3 medium carrots, diced**
**3 garlic cloves, coarsely chopped**
**3 sprigs of parsley**
**8 to 10 basil leaves**
**10 white mushrooms, diced**
**1 sprig of thyme**
**2 bay leaves**
**2 sprigs of cilantro**
**2 pinches of chervil**
**Freshly ground pepper**

Combine all the ingredients in a stockpot, cover with 2 quarts cold water, and bring to a boil, then turn the heat down to a light simmer. Simmer for about 20 minutes. Turn off the heat, keep covered, and set aside to infuse for 20 more minutes. Strain the broth carefully through a fine strainer.

*Serving size = 1 cup*
*19 calories*
*0.2 gram fat*
*0 milligrams cholesterol*
*10.6 milligrams sodium*

## NONFAT YOGURT CHEESE

Michael McDermott

*This alternative to cream cheese can be used in dips, for desserts, or wherever a recipe calls for cream cheese. The freshest yogurt makes the sweetest cheese. Find out what day your favorite brand of yogurt is delivered and always check the freshness dates. The cheese will keep for up to 4 days covered and refrigerated.*

MAKES 1 CUP

**2 cups gelatin-free nonfat yogurt**

Line a strainer with a cloth napkin or coffee filter and set it over a bowl. Place the yogurt into the strainer. Cover the yogurt with plastic wrap and set it in the refrigerator to drain. It is yogurt "cheese" when it is reduced to 1 cup, which may take from 4 hours to overnight.

*Serving size = ½ cup*
*126 calories*
*0.4 gram fat*
*4.1 milligrams cholesterol*
*173.5 milligrams sodium*

## A LITTLE ITALIAN

Michael McDermott

*Use this herb and spice mixture in pasta sauces or with braised or roasted vegetables.*

MAKES A SCANT CUP

**2 tablespoons dried basil**
**2 tablespoons dried marjoram**
**2 tablespoons dried oregano**
**2 tablespoons ground coriander**
**2 tablespoons dried thyme**
**2 tablespoons dried rosemary**
**2 tablespoons dried savory**
**1 teaspoon hot red pepper flakes**

In the bowl of a food processor, combine all the ingredients. Process for 30 seconds until finely ground. Transfer to a tightly sealed container, label, and date. Store in a cool dark place for up to 3 months.

*Serving size = 1 tablespoon*
*12 calories*
*0.4 gram fat*
*0 milligrams cholesterol*
*1.5 milligrams sodium*

## BERBERÉ

Michael McDermott

*Except for the absence of ginger this is very typical of a spice mixture that is called Berberé in Ethiopia. This combination of spices is used throughout northern and southern Africa in various vegetable and meat dishes. Added to red lentils with garlic, onions, and tomatoes, it makes a satisfying lentil stew. It can also be used to flavor sweetened spice cakes or rice puddings.*

MAKES A SCANT ⅔ CUP

**1 tablespoon ground cardamom**
**1 tablespoon ground coriander**
**1 tablespoon fenugreek**
**1 tablespoon ground nutmeg**

**1 tablespoon ground cloves**
**1 tablespoon ground cinnamon**
**1 tablespoon ground allspice**
**1 tablespoon paprika**
**1 tablespoon turmeric**
**1 teaspoon cayenne**
**1 tablespoon ground black pepper**
**1 tablespoon ground sea salt**

In a medium bowl, combine all the ingredients and mix well. Transfer to a tightly sealed container, label, and date. Store in a cool dark place for up to 3 months.

*Serving size = 1 tablespoon*
*21 calories*
*0.78 gram fat*
*0 milligrams cholesterol*
*663 milligrams sodium*

## CAJUN SPICE

Jean-Marc Fullsack

*This has a much more exuberant flavor than the premixed spices from the grocery. It is best when the ingredients are fresh.*

MAKES ¾ CUP

**4 tablespoons paprika**
**2 tablespoons onion powder or flakes**
**2 tablespoons garlic powder or flakes**
**1 tablespoon gumbo filé**
**1 tablespoon ground cumin (or whole seeds, toasted and ground)**
**1 tablespoon ground coriander (or whole seeds, toasted and ground)**
**½ tablespoon dried thyme**
**½ tablespoon ground fenugreek (or whole seeds, toasted and ground)**

**½ tablespoon ground fennel (or whole seeds, toasted and ground)**
**½ tablespoon salt**
**¾ teaspoon cayenne**
**¾ teaspoon black pepper**

In the large bowl of a food processor, combine all the ingredients and pulse for 30 seconds or until finely ground. Store in an airtight container in a cool place. Use within 3 months.

*Serving size = 1 tablespoon*
*21 calories*
*0.6 gram fat*
*0 milligrams cholesterol*
*296 milligrams sodium*

## CROSTINI

*Eating Well* magazine

MAKES APPROXIMATELY 4 DOZEN

Preheat the oven to 350 degrees. Cut a 16-inch-long loaf of French bread (baguette) into ⅓-inch-thick slices. Arrange the bread slices on a baking sheet. Set another baking sheet over top of the bread and bake for 15 minutes. Turn the bread over, re-cover with the baking sheet, and bake for about 15 minutes longer, or until golden. Let cool. The crostini can be stored in an airtight container for up to 1 week.

*Serving size = 1 piece*
*21 calories*
*0.2 gram fat*
*0 milligrams cholesterol*
*0.2 milligram sodium*

## SEITAN

Victor Karpenko

*Usually made from wheat gluten, seitan is very high in protein, with a texture similar to meat or fowl. In the stores it is sometimes simply called "gluten." It is very versatile; its flavor depends on good stock. Slice it thinly or in small chunks to absorb the most flavor. It makes a good basic food item to have in your refrigerator. Use it in sandwiches, soups, stews, pasta dishes, and stuffings. Reserve the vegetable stock from this recipe for sauces, soups, and stews.*

Makes 4 cups

**1½ cups gluten flour**
**¼ teaspoon finely chopped assorted fresh herbs (thyme, oregano, sage, and so on)**
**¼ teaspoon freshly ground black pepper**
**2 tablespoons soy sauce**
**1 cup chopped onion**
**1 cup chopped carrot**
**½ teaspoon whole black peppercorns**
**2 bay leaves**

In a large bowl, combine the gluten flour, herbs, and ground black pepper.

In a small bowl, stir together 1 cup water and the soy sauce. Add this slowly to the dry ingredients, mixing with a sturdy wooden spoon until the mixture forms a ball. Turn the dough out onto a clean dry surface dusted with additional gluten flour. Knead the dough for 3 to 5 minutes. Remove the dough from the kneading surface and hold it under cold running water. Stretch the dough, keeping the water running, and use your fingertips to work any starch and remaining bran free of the dough. The rinsing water will appear cloudy. Form into a 2-inch-diameter roll.

In a large kettle, add to 3 quarts of water the onion, carrot, peppercorns, and bay leaves. Bring to a boil. Gently lower the gluten slices one at a time into the boiling stock. Simmer for 20 minutes. The gluten slices will rise to the top. Drain, reserving the stock. Slice the gluten into ¼-inch strips. Cover the gluten strips in enough stock to prevent them from drying out. Store refrigerated and covered with liquid for up to 1 week.

*Serving size = ½ cup*
*104 calories*
*0.6 gram fat*
*0 milligrams cholesterol*
*221.8 milligrams sodium*

# *Hors d'Oeuvres and Appetizers*

## GRAPEFRUIT TERRINE

Jean-Marc Fullsack

*A beautiful presentation for this appetizer would be to chill portions in individual martini glasses or other crystal and serve garnished with fresh mint. Serve early in the meal as an appetizer or between courses as a palate cleanser.*

MAKES 2 CUPS
SERVES 4 TO 8

- **4 large pink grapefruits, skinned and cut into segments with all membranes removed, juice reserved (there should be 1 cup)**
- **1 tablespoon agar powder (page 114), or 1 tablespoon gelatin powder**
- **1 red jalapeño pepper, seeded and diced**
- **1 tablespoon chiffonaded fresh basil**
- **1 teaspoon chiffonaded fresh mint**
- **1 teaspoon minced fresh gingerroot**

In a small saucepan, combine 1 cup grapefruit juice with the agar powder. Stir continuously to dissolve the agar. Bring to a boil, reduce the heat, and simmer for 2 to 3 minutes. Set aside to cool to room temperature.

In a large bowl, combine the grapefruit segments, grapefruit-agar mixture, jalepeño, basil, mint, and ginger. Transfer the mixture to a 2½-cup terrine. Refrigerate overnight or for at least 4 hours before serving. This will gel with cooling and can be served in ½-inch-thick slices.

*Serving size = ¼ cup*
*38 calories*
*0.1 gram fat*
*0 milligrams cholesterol*
*0.8 milligram sodium*

## WHITE BEANS, GREENS, AND SUN-DRIED TOMATO CROSTINI

Joyce Goldstein

*In southern Italy people know how to make satisfying meals out of very little. This crostini is a variation on* capriata, *a slice of grilled bread spread with a rich and garlicky white bean puree and topped with tart wilted greens. To replace the olive oil, which keeps the bean puree moist, use stock and yogurt.*

SERVES 8

**1 cup dried white beans, soaked overnight in the refrigerator**
**1 large onion, chopped**
**8 to 12 whole garlic cloves**
**Salt and pepper**
**½ cup sun-dried tomatoes (not packed in oil)**
**½ cup nonfat plain yogurt**
**10 cups assorted greens (escarole, arugula, dandelion, or radicchio), well rinsed and coarsely chopped**
**3 tablespoons red wine vinegar**
**½ teaspoon hot red pepper flakes or more to taste**
**8 slices whole grain bread**

Drain the beans, rinse, and cover with 4 to 6 cups fresh water. Add the onion and all but 1 of the garlic cloves, and bring to a boil. Reduce heat and simmer for about 1 hour, until the beans are very soft.

Drain the beans, onions, and garlic, and reserve the remaining bean liquid. Place the bean mixture in the container of a food processor and puree, adding enough cooking liquid to make a soft puree. Season with salt and pepper. Set aside.

Chop the sun-dried tomatoes and soak them for 15 to 30 minutes in just enough bean cooking liquid to soften and release their flavor. Fold the tomatoes into the beans. Fold in the yogurt.

In a large sauté pan over high heat, wilt the greens in the vinegar. Drain well and season with salt, pepper, hot pepper flakes, and additional vinegar if desired.

To assemble the crostini, grill or toast the whole grain bread. While warm, rub it with the remaining garlic clove, cut in half. Spread the bread slices with white bean puree and top each with chopped greens.

*Serving size = 1 slice*
*152 calories*
*1.5 grams fat*
*1.1 milligrams cholesterol*
*247.4 milligrams sodium without added salt*

## DOLMAS (VEGETARIAN STUFFED GRAPE LEAVES)

Joyce Goldstein

*Stuffed grape leaves, also known as dolmas, can be a satisfying meal when served warm, topped with a little yogurt. They are also an ideal finger food for a predinner appetizer, served at room temperature with a lemon wedge or yogurt dip. Tightly wrapped, dolmas will keep under refrigeration for a few days.*

MAKES 3 DOZEN

**1 cup long-grain rice, Basmati preferred**
**1 cup Vegetable Stock (page 143)**
**2 medium onions, chopped**
**3 garlic cloves, minced**
**1 cup seeded and diced canned or fresh plum tomatoes**
**½ cup currants, plumped in hot water**
**3 tablespoons chopped fresh dill**
**3 tablespoons chopped fresh mint**
**2 teaspoons salt**
**1 teaspoon freshly ground black pepper**
**1 teaspoon allspice**
**36 to 40 grape leaves, rinsed, drained, and patted dry, stems removed**
**3 ripe tomatoes, sliced ¼ inch thick (optional)**
**1 cup nonfat plain yogurt**
**Lemon wedges**

Soak the rice in cold water for about 30 minutes. Drain. Bring the vegetable stock to a simmer in a large sauté pan and add the onions. Simmer, covered, until the onions are tender, about 20 minutes. Add the garlic and cook a few minutes longer. Add the onions and garlic to the rice along with the diced tomatoes, currants, dill, mint, salt, pepper, and allspice. Mix well.

Place the grape leaves, smooth side down, on a work surface.

Preheat the oven to 350 degrees.

Place a heaping teaspoon of filling near the stem end of each leaf. Fold the sides of the leaf over the filling and roll the leaf into a long cylinder. Do not roll too tightly, as the rice expands in cooking.

Arrange the dolmas, seam side down, close together in a large sauté pan or baking dish. Pour very hot water over the leaves and weight them down with a plate so they don't unroll while cooking. Cover the pan and bake the dolmas for approximately 40 minutes. Remove one dolma from the pan and test the rice for doneness. Uncover the pan to quickly cool the dolmas. As soon as they can be handled, remove the pan and arrange on a platter. Serve warm or at room temperature garnished with generous dollops of yogurt or a good squeeze of lemon juice.

NOTE: In the summer you may line the baking pan with slices of fresh ripe tomatoes and place the stuffed grape leaves on the tomato slices. Continue as above.

*Serving size = 1 dolma*
*25 calories*
*0.2 gram fat*
*0.1 milligram cholesterol*
*139.2 milligrams sodium*

## EGGPLANT CAPONATA

Joyce Goldstein

*This Sicilian eggplant dish is familiar to most of us because it is often served as part of a classic antipasto assortment. If the caponata becomes too thick, add a little vegetable stock. Serve at room temperature accompanied by bread sticks or good whole-grain bread.*

MAKES APPROXIMATELY 1 QUART

**2 medium eggplants**
**½ cup vegetable stock**
**2 onions, sliced**
**1 cup diced celery**
**¾ cup tomato puree**
**½ cup vinegar**
**2 tablespoons sugar**
**2 tablespoons capers**
**4 tablespoons currants or raisins, plumped in hot water**
**Salt**
**Pepper**

Preheat the oven to 400 degrees. Place the eggplants on a baking sheet and prick with a fork. Bake until tender but not mushy, about 35 to 45 minutes. When the eggplants are cool enough to handle, remove the peel and dice the flesh into 1-inch cubes. Place the cubes in a strainer or drainer.

In a large sauté pan over moderate heat, bring the stock to a boil. Add the onions and cook until tender, about 10 minutes. Add the celery and cook for 5 minutes. Add the tomato puree, vinegar, and sugar and simmer a few minutes. Stir in the reserved eggplant, capers, and raisins and warm through. Adjust the seasoning with salt and pepper. Serve at room temperature. This can be made a few days ahead of time. Bring to room temperature for serving, check seasoning, and add vinegar and salt if desired.

*Serving size = ½ cup*
*55 calories*
*0.2 gram fat*
*0 milligrams cholesterol*
*46.4 milligrams sodium without added salt*

## ARTICHOKE PASTE
Deborah Madison

*Artichokes make a subtle and delicate spread to serve with crackers. The time to make this is when the large spring artichokes from California are available and inexpensive. If it's available, garnish the spread with chopped chervil or tarragon.*

MAKES APPROXIMATELY ¾ CUP

**4 to 5 giant artichokes**
**Juice of 1 lemon**
**3 large pieces of lemon peel**
**2 tablespoons finely diced onion or shallots**
**2 garlic cloves, thinly sliced**
**1 bay leaf**
**3 sprigs of thyme or a couple of pinches dried**
**1 small branch of tarragon or ¼ teaspoon dried**
**4 sprigs of parsley**

**Salt**
**Freshly ground black pepper**
**Fresh lemon juice or tarragon vinegar to taste**
**Chopped chervil or tarragon, for garnish**

Trim the artichokes down to their hearts (they can be quartered) and set them in a bowl of water acidulated with the lemon juice as you work. Use a pan large enough to hold the artichokes in a single layer. Add water just to cover and add the lemon peel, onion, garlic, bay leaf, thyme, tarragon, and parsley. Bring to a boil, then lower the heat and simmer, adding small amounts of water as needed, until the artichokes are tender and just a few tablespoons of liquid remain.

Remove the bay leaf, lemon, parsley, and thyme branches. Transfer the artichokes to a food processor and puree, adding the remaining pan juices as needed to thin the mixture. If any fibers from the artichokes remain, pass the puree through a food mill. Season to taste with salt and pepper. Add a little lemon juice or vinegar to sharpen the flavors (again, do this to taste—the puree may already be fine as is). Heap into a bowl and garnish with the chopped chervil or tarragon.

*Serving size = ¼ cup*
*54 calories*
*0.3 gram fat*
*0 milligrams cholesterol*
*175 milligrams sodium without added salt*

## BEAN AND SALSA DIP

Lydia Karpenko

*This is a very easy, very colorful, and very popular party dish.*

MAKES APPROXIMATELY 5 CUPS
SERVES 5

**1 15-ounce can pinto beans**
**3 tablespoons Louisiana hot sauce**
**2 teaspoons fresh lime juice**
**3 tablespoons sweetened Chinese chili sauce**
**¼ cup thinly sliced green onions**
**16 ounces fat-free sour cream**
**1½ cups store-bought fresh and chunky hot salsa, drained**
**Fresh cilantro or parsley**
**Corn tortilla chips**

Drain the liquid from the can of beans and discard. Place the beans in a food processor and process until almost smooth. Add the hot sauce and lime juice. Mix well. Spread the bean mixture over the bottom of a large platter. Spoon and spread the sweetened chili sauce over the beans, then sprinkle the green onions evenly over the top.

Cover the bean mixture and scallions with the sour cream and top it with the salsa. Garnish this with sprigs of fresh cilantro and serve with tortilla chips.

NOTE: If you don't find the sweetened Chinese chili sauce, use plain chili pepper sauce and add 1 tablespoon rice wine vinegar and 1 tablespoon sugar. Also, if you can't find prepared uncooked salsa try the Pico de Gallo Salsa (page 238). Add more chopped chili peppers if you wish.

*Serving size = 1 cup*
*149 calories*
*0.7 gram fat*
*1.6 milligrams cholesterol*
*476.2 milligrams sodium*

## ROASTED TOMATO ARAM SANDWICHES

Tina Salter and Christine Swett

*The flavors of this great hors d'oeuvre or party sandwich are quite rich and intense. It can be prepared up to 8 hours ahead of time if kept tightly wrapped in plastic and refrigerated.*

SERVES 4

**1 large Armenian cracker bread disk ("lavosh")**
**½ cup Nonfat Yogurt Cheese (page 148)**
**3 plum tomatoes, oven roasted (page 134) and sliced ¼ inch wide**
**1 onion, oven roasted (page 133) and chopped (to yield 1 cup)**
**½ cup fresh herbs (e.g., basil, oregano, parsley, or a combination)**
**Freshly ground black pepper**
**Salt**

Sprinkle the cracker bread liberally with cold water and layer it between 2 damp towels. Allow the bread to rest for 1 hour or more, until soft enough to roll without breaking.

Spread the yogurt cheese evenly over the cracker bread. Layer with the roasted tomatoes and onions. Sprinkle the herbs evenly over the onions. Season to taste with pepper and salt.

Roll tightly in a jelly-roll fashion, and then slice into 1-inch-wide slices.

*Serving size = 2 slices*
*56 calories*
*0.4 gram fat*
*0.5 milligram cholesterol*
*101.0 milligrams sodium without added salt*

## CHINESE DIM SUM

Jean-Marc Fullsack

*Do not stack these dumplings while forming or steaming or they will stick together. Serve these dumplings with a small bowl of Manchurian Sauce (page 354), Chinese barbecue (hoisin) sauce, and/or mustard.*

MAKES 32 DUMPLINGS
SERVES 8

**¼ cup mung beans, peeled and soaked for 4 hours**
**¾ cup Vegetable Stock (page 143)**
**½ cup blanched frozen or fresh peas (page 131)**
**½ cup sliced and blanched napa cabbage leaves**
**½ cup chopped green onion**
**½ cup oven-roasted and chopped onion**
**¼ cup egg whites**
**1 tablespoon soy sauce**
**1 tablespoon minced lemongrass**
**Salt**
**32 potsticker skins (rounds)**

In a small saucepan, combine the mung beans and stock. Bring to a boil and simmer, tightly covered, for 30 minutes, or until the beans are soft. Transfer the beans to a food processor or blender and puree until smooth. Transfer the beans to a medium-size bowl and add the peas, cabbage, green onion, roasted onion, egg whites, soy sauce, and lemongrass. Stir to combine. Season to taste with salt.

To form the dumplings, moisten the edge of a potsticker skin with water. Place a scant tablespoon of filling slightly off center on a skin, fold the dough over to form a half moon, and pinch the edges to seal. Place in a bamboo steamer and steam for 10 minutes. Serve immediately.

The filling can be prepared and refrigerated up to 6 hours ahead of time.

*Serving size = 4 dumplings*
*139 calories*
*1.7 grams fat*
*0 milligrams cholesterol*
*555.4 milligrams sodium without added salt*

## VIETNAMESE VEGETABLE ROLLS

Jean-Marc Fullsack

*This makes a beautiful and exciting start to an Asian dinner. Try it as an addition to an hors d'oeuvres tray or as part of a light meal with the m Sum (page 162) and/or "Shao Mai" Dumplings (page*

*variation, brush some of the dipping sauce over the rice paper before arranging the vegetables over it. Then use a soy-based sauce such as the Manchurian Sauce (page 354) for a dipping sauce.*

MAKES 16 TO 18 ROLLS WITH 1 CUP SAUCE
SERVES 6 TO 9

| | |
|---|---|
| **½** | **cup egg whites (about 4 eggs)** |
| **½** | **teaspoon honey** |
| **⅛** | **teaspoon turmeric** |
| | **Salt** |
| **16 to 18** | **sheets rice paper** |
| **1** | **cup blanched mung bean sprouts** |
| **½** | **cup julienned and blanched carrots** |
| **½** | **cup julienned and blanched celery** |
| **½** | **cup julienned pickled daikon** |
| **2** | **ounces smoked tofu, julienned** |
| **16** | **mint leaves, chiffonaded** |
| | **Dipping Sauce (recipe follows)** |

Preheat the oven to 325 degrees.

In a medium-sized bowl, place the egg whites, honey, turmeric, and salt to taste. Mix well without creating bubbles. Pour the mixture gently through a sieve into a 6-inch nonstick sauté pan with ovenproof handles and bake for 25 minutes. Alternatively, pour the mixture into microwaveable ramekins and cook at Medium in a microwave oven for 1 to 2 minutes, or until just set. Set aside to cool. Cut into julienne slices.

To moisten the rice papers, lay them out between 2 wet towels for approximately 5 minutes until soft. Arrange the vegetables and julienned egg cake in a line in the center of each rice paper sheet. Roll the sheets, tucking in the ends of the seal completely. Refrigerate for 1 hour before serving.

### DIPPING SAUCE

**2 stalks lemongrass, minced**
**½ cup vegetable stock**
**¼ cup diced red bell pepper**
**¼ cup peeled and quartered pear**
**¼ cup peeled, seeded, and diced tomato**
**1 tablespoon fresh lime juice**
**1 teaspoon minced fresh gingerroot**

In a small saucepan, combine the lemongrass and stock. Bring it to a boil and continue boiling for 5 minutes. Remove from the heat and set aside for 30 minutes. In a blender, combine the boiled stock with the red pepper, pear, tomato, lime juice, and ginger. Puree until smooth.

*Serving size = 2 to 3 rolls*
*38 calories*
*0.3 gram fat*
*0 milligrams cholesterol*
*69.8 milligrams sodium without added salt*

## "SHAO MAI" DUMPLINGS

Jean-Marc Fullsack

*These are very easy to do. For a sweet, creamier filling omit the water chestnuts, tofu, and pepper.*

MAKES 15 BUNS (APPROXIMATELY ½ CUP EACH)

**DOUGH**

**¾ cup warm water**
**½ cup warm nonfat milk**
**1 tablespoon sugar**
**½ packet (1½ teaspoons) granulated yeast or 1 whole package fresh**
**3½ cups unbleached white flour**
**½ teaspoon baking powder**

FILLING

- **1 ounce dried shiitake mushrooms**
- **1 cup warm water**
- **1 cup sweet potatoes, cut into small dice**
- **¼ cup mirin**
- **¼ cup sake**
- **2 tablespoons soy sauce**
- **1 tablespoon sugar**
- **2 tablespoons diced water chestnuts**
- **4 ounces smoked tofu, broken up with a fork**
- **Black pepper**

Make the dough. In a large bowl, combine the water, milk, and sugar. Add the yeast and dissolve. Add the flour and beat until smooth.

Transfer to a large bowl, cover with a damp towel or plastic wrap, and let the dough rise 1 hour, or until doubled in volume. Transfer the dough to a lightly floured work surface. Sprinkle the baking powder onto the dough. Knead again for 5 minutes, or until the dough is smooth. Set aside, covered with a kitchen towel, and let the dough rise again until doubled.

Meanwhile, make the filling. In a large bowl, soak the mushrooms in the water for approximately 20 minutes. Transfer the mushrooms and soaking liquid to a large saucepan. Add the sweet potatoes, mirin, sake, soy sauce, and sugar. Combine well and bring to a boil. Reduce the heat and simmer for 45 minutes, or until any liquid has become syrupy. Cool to room temperature. Combine with the water chestnuts, tofu, and pepper before forming the dumplings.

When ready to form the buns, roll the dough approximately ⅓ inch thick and cut 3½-inch-diameter circles, using a biscuit or cookie cutter. Place 1 teaspoon of filling at the center of each circle and pinch the edges of the dough together to make a sealed little ball.

Place the bun on a small square of parchment paper and steam in a bamboo steamer for 10 minutes.

NOTE: The dough can be prepared and frozen for up to 2 months; allow it to return to room temperature before forming the buns. The finished shao mai can be made up to 3 weeks in advance. Let the entire bun return to room temperature before serving. The filling can be prepared and refrigerated for up to 3 days ahead or frozen for 2 months.

*Serving size = 2 dumplings*
*140 calories*
*1.7 grams fat*
*0.3 milligram cholesterol*
*325 milligrams sodium*

## ROASTED AUBERGINE HERO

Hank and Phyllis Ginsberg

*If you like, roast as many garlic cloves as you wish on the same baking sheet as the eggplant. Once the garlic has softened, squeeze it out of its skin, and spread it over the baguette before the dressing. These sandwiches are great for a picnic or at a tailgate party.*

SERVES 4

**½ cup nonfat plain yogurt**
**1½ teaspoons Dijon mustard**
**1 eggplant (approximately 1 pound), sliced into ½-inch rounds**
**2 green bell peppers, cored and cut into ½-inch slices**
**1 tomato, cut into ½-inch slices**
**½ onion, cut into ½-inch slices**
**½ pound domestic mushrooms, cut in ¼-inch slices**
**1 24-inch-long thin French baguette**
**Salt (optional)**

Preheat the oven to 350 degrees.

In a small bowl, whisk together the yogurt and mustard. Refrigerate until ready to use.

On a large parchment-lined nonstick baking sheet, place the eggplant, green pepper, tomato, onion, and mushroom slices in a single layer. (It may be necessary to use 2 sheets.)

Roast the vegetables for 30 minutes, or until tender but not dry.

Slice the baguette lengthwise and spread each side with the yogurt and mustard mixture. Layer the roasted vegetables over the spread on half of the baguette. Lightly salt to taste. Cover with the second half of the baguette and cut the loaf into 4 6-inch sandwiches.

*Serving size = 1 serving*
*283 calories*
*2.9 grams fat*
*0.5 milligram cholesterol*
*463.5 milligrams sodium without added salt*

## STUFFED ESCAROLE LEAVES WITH MARINATED CHICK-PEAS

Donna Nicoletti

MAKES 12 TO 15 STUFFED LEAVES
SERVES 6 (APPETIZER PORTIONS)

**3 cups chick-peas**
**2 tablespoons dried sage**
**5 bay leaves**
**Salt**
**Freshly ground black pepper**
**4 medium tomatoes**
**2 teaspoons chopped garlic**
**2 tablespoons chopped fresh Italian parsley or basil**
**2 tablespoons white wine vinegar**
**1 large head escarole**

Sort through the chick-peas and remove any stones. Soak the chick-peas in 9 cups of cold water and refrigerate overnight. Bring a large pot of water to a boil with the sage and bay leaves. Drain the soaked chick-peas and rinse well. Add the chick-peas to the water and cook for approximately

30 to 45 minutes, or until they are completely soft. Drain them, reserving 2 cups of the cooking liquid. Spread the chick-peas out on a baking sheet and toss them with the salt and pepper; mash the chick-peas lightly with a fork. Set aside to cool completely.

Core, seed, and dice the tomatoes completely. Toss with salt, pepper, garlic, and chopped parsley.

Mix the cooled chick-peas and tomato mixture together and toss with just enough of the reserved chick-pea cooking liquid to moisten. Add the vinegar to taste.

Bring a small pot of salted water to a boil. Fill a large bowl with ice water and set aside. Core the escarole and discard any bruised outer leaves. Wash the leaves well and place them in a strainer that will fit inside the pot of water. Submerge the strainer into the boiling water for about 2 minutes. The leaves should be completely soft; immediately plunge them into the ice water to cool completely, then drain and pat dry. Lay the leaves out flat and season with salt and pepper. Place about 3 or 4 tablespoons of the chick-pea mixture at the broad end of each leaf and roll up like a cigar, turning in the ends so the stuffing is completely covered.

Serve at room temperature as an appetizer.

*Serving size = 2 to 3 stuffed leaves*
*242 calories*
*3.7 grams fat*
*0 milligrams cholesterol*
*94.6 milligrams sodium without added salt*

## MOSAIC OF YOUNG VEGETABLES IN FRESH HERB GELÉE

Hubert Keller

*This may look daunting at first, but it requires only a bit of time and care—and can be ready hours before you serve it. It is a special dish worth the effort for entertaining. For an added touch, accompany this terrine with Cucumber Vinaigrette.*

MAKES 12 CUPS
SERVES 12

**2 red bell peppers**
**2 yellow bell peppers**
**Vegetable oil spray**
**24 baby carrots, peeled**
**6 ounces green beans, trimmed**
**8 large romaine lettuce leaves**
**1 English cucumber, peeled, halved, seeded, and diced**
**2 tablespoons fresh or frozen corn kernels**
**1 dozen medium shiitake mushrooms, stemmed and left whole**
**1½ sticks agar-agar (page 114)**
**2 cups clear Vegetable Consommé (page 147)**
**2 tablespoons finely chopped chervil**
**2 tablespoons finely chopped chives**
**1 tablespoon finely chopped parsley**
**8 basil leaves, chopped**
**½ teaspoon coarse black pepper**
**3 hard-boiled egg whites, chopped**
**4 tomatoes, peeled, seeded, and diced**
**Cucumber Vinaigrette (recipe follows)**

Preheat the broiler. Coat the bell peppers very lightly with the vegetable oil pan coating. Place under the broiler and roast, turning frequently, until the skin is blackened on all sides. When the peppers are completely charred, cool until slightly comfortable to handle, then peel off the blackened skin. Remove the stems, cores, and seeds. Boil separately the baby carrots (5 minutes), green beans (6 minutes), and romaine lettuce leaves, English cucumbers, and corn kernels (6 minutes). Drain each cooked vegetable, and plunge immediately into ice water; drain again. Lightly spray a nonstick frying pan with vegetable oil coating and place over medium heat; sauté the shiitake mushrooms in the pan. Set aside.

Wash and soak the sticks of agar-agar in water for 30 minutes. Transfer the softened sticks to a small saucepan and dissolve over low heat; continue to cook for 5 minutes, stirring from time to time. Add the vegetable consommé, bring to a boil, and simmer 5 minutes. Remove from the heat, cover, and set aside to cool.

In a small bowl, mix together all the herbs, black pepper, and the chopped egg whites.

Line an 8-inch-long rectangular terrine or pâté mold with plastic wrap. Place a layer of romaine leaves over the plastic wrap.

Pour ¼ cup of the vegetable consommé mixture into the mold. Spread a layer of the egg white mixture over the consommé. Refrigerate for 15 minutes.

Arrange the blanched vegetables lengthwise over the egg white mixture, alternating colors. Spread a second egg white layer over this and sprinkle with the diced tomatoes. Spread on a third layer of herb mixture. Use the remaining vegetables to make another layer like the first. Finish with the last of the herb mixture.

Pour the vegetable consommé over the top and cover with romaine lettuce leaves.

Place the terrine in the refrigerator for 6 to 8 hours before unmolding. Fifteen minutes before serving, place the dinner plates in the refrigerator to chill. Just before serving, dip the bottom of the terrine into warm water and invert it onto a cutting board to unmold. Using a long sharp knife, cut the "mosaic" into 12 slices. Place 1 slice on each plate and serve with Cucumber Vinaigrette if desired.

### CUCUMBER VINAIGRETTE

Place 1 peeled, seeded, and diced cucumber in a blender, add a few drops of sherry, a small sprig of dill, ¼ teaspoon Dijon mustard, and ground pepper. Blend until very smooth. Chill until serving.

*Serving size = 1 cup*
*70 calories*
*0.7 gram fat*
*0 milligrams cholesterol*
*41.6 milligrams sodium*

## GRILLED ASPARAGUS WITH LEMON, RED PEPPERS, AND CAPER VINAIGRETTE

Bradley Ogden

SERVES 4

**1 pound asparagus, cut into 5-inch pieces**
**Kosher salt**
**Freshly ground black pepper**
**¼ cup chopped red onion**
**½ cup diced roasted red bell pepper**
**1 tablespoon capers, rinsed in cold water and drained**
**1 tablespoon champagne or balsamic vinegar**
**3 tablespoons lemon juice**

Prepare a charcoal grill.

Bring a large pot of salted water to a boil. Drop in the asparagus and cook for approximately 60 seconds, or until barely tender. Remove and place immediately into ice water. When cool, drain well. Season the asparagus lightly with salt and pepper and set aside. In a large bowl, mix together the rest of the ingredients to make a vinaigrette.

Place the asparagus on the hot grill. Turn the spears once so they are warmed through. Remove the asparagus and place in the large bowl with the vinaigrette and toss lightly. Divide the asparagus among 4 plates. Serve immediately.

*Serving size = ¼ pound asparagus*
*62 calories*
*2.9 grams fat*
*0 milligrams cholesterol*
*427.6 milligrams sodium without added salt*

## ROASTED QUESADILLAS WITH CHIQUITA BANANAS

Tracy Pikhart Ritter

*A surprisingly tasty sweet and spicy combination. The creamy texture of the bananas enhances the creaminess of the melted cheese and sets off the spicy flavors of the cilantro and jalapeños. Cut the quesadillas into wedges and serve with hot sauce or Tomato Salsa (page 358)*

MAKES 6 WHOLE TORTILLAS OR 36 TRIANGLES
SERVES 6 TO 8

**12 fat-free corn or whole wheat flour tortillas**
**6 ounces grated nonfat Monterey Jack or cheddar cheese**
**2 tablespoons chopped fresh cilantro or parsley**
**2 jalapeño peppers, seeded and minced**
**1 cup alfalfa sprouts**
**2 medium bananas, sliced into thin circles**

Preheat the oven to 350 degrees.

Place 6 tortillas on a nonstick baking sheet. Sprinkle with cheese, cilantro, chiles, sprouts, and bananas. Cover with the remaining tortillas and press down firmly.

Bake for 10 to 15 minutes, until the cheese is soft and melted.

Cut each quesadilla into 6 wedges and serve with hot sauce or salsa.

*Serving size = 1 whole quesadilla or 6 triangles*
*121 calories*
*1.5 grams fat*
*0.5 milligram cholesterol*
*82.6 milligrams sodium*

## PITA CHIPS WITH ROASTED EGGPLANT DIP

Jill O'Conner and Tracy Pikhart Ritter

SERVES 8

**1 medium eggplant**
**1 jalapeño pepper, membrane and seeds removed, minced**
**1 teaspoon lemon juice**
**1 teaspoon lime juice**
**1 shallot, minced**
**1 heaping teaspoon ground cumin**
**Pinch of ground cinnamon**
**Pinch of salt**
**2 whole wheat pita bread pockets**
**2 egg whites, lightly beaten**
**Cilantro garnish**

Slice the eggplant horizontally; place the flesh side down on a baking sheet lightly sprayed with oil or lined with parchment paper. Bake at 350 degrees for 45 minutes or until very soft. Cool.

Meanwhile, combine the jalapeño pepper, lemon and lime juices, shallot, cumin, cinnamon, and salt in a small bowl. Set aside.

Separate the pita bread pockets. Lightly beat the egg whites, and brush onto the smooth outer side of the pita halves. Cut each pocket into 8 sections for a total of 32 triangles. Bake at 350 degrees for 10 minutes or until crispy. Check often.

Place cooled eggplant and jalapeño mixture in a food processor. Blend until smooth. Transfer the dip to a bowl and garnish with chopped fresh cilantro. Serve with pita chips.

*Serving size = ½ cup dip and 4 pita triangles*
*45 calories*
*0.3 gram fat*
*0 milligrams cholesterol*
*69.8 milligrams sodium without added salt*

## BRUSCHETTA WITH SUN-DRIED TOMATOES AND CAPERS

Tracy Pikhart Ritter

*The robust flavors in this intense, concentrated spread are redolent of the Mediterranean. Try it also on vegetable sandwiches or add it to pasta.*

MAKES 24 SLICES OR 1½ CUPS SPREAD

**4 sun-dried tomatoes (not packed in oil)**
**3 ripe tomatoes, peeled, seeded, and finely chopped**
**3 tablespoons minced red onion**
**3 teaspoons capers, rinsed**
**3 garlic cloves, minced**
**2 teaspoons balsamic vinegar**
**1 tablespoon chopped fresh basil**
**1 tablespoon chopped fresh oregano**
**1 teaspoon freshly ground black pepper**
**½ teaspoon sea salt to taste**
**1 12-inch loaf Italian bread, cut into 24 slices**
**Grated nonfat Parmesan or Romano cheese (optional)**

Preheat the oven to 350 degrees.

Reconstitute the sun-dried tomatoes by placing them in a small bowl and pouring about 1 cup of boiling water over them. Let the tomatoes rest in the hot water until it cools. Drain the tomatoes and chop them finely.

Combine all ingredients, except the bread slices and the cheese, in a bowl and set aside for 1 hour at room temperature.

Toast the bread slices in the oven until lightly brown; cool slightly. Top with the tomato mixture. Sprinkle with Romano or Parmesan cheese if desired. Serve warm or at room temperature.

*Serving size = 1 slice with 1 tablespoon spread*
*92 calories*
*0.3 gram fat*
*0 milligrams cholesterol*
*239.1 milligrams sodium without added salt*

## SMOKED TOMATO AND ASPARAGUS

Michael McDermott

*An excellent first course—the deep flavor of the smoked tomatoes is a perfect match for the intense asparagus flavor. The sauce would also work well with artichokes. The sauce can be prepared and refrigerated up to 2 days ahead of time or frozen for up to 2 months.*

SERVES 4

**2 large tomatoes**
**1 tablespoon fresh lime juice**
**1 teaspoon honey**
**1 teaspoon minced jalapeño pepper**
**¼ teaspoon thyme**
**¼ teaspoon ground coriander**
**¼ teaspoon oregano**
**¼ teaspoon cumin**
**1 garlic clove, minced**
**1 pound asparagus, cooked, at room temperature**

Roast the tomatoes directly over a high gas flame until the skin becomes charred in spots, blistered, and loose. When cool enough to handle, carefully peel off the skin. Core and roughly chop.

In a large bowl, combine the chopped tomatoes, lime juice, honey, jalapeño, thyme, coriander, oregano, cumin, and garlic. Mix well. Serve at room temperature with the asparagus spears.

*Serving size = ⅜ cup sauce and ¼ pound asparagus*
*50 calories*
*0.6 gram fat*
*0 milligrams cholesterol*
*21 milligrams sodium*

## BLACK BEAN PANCAKES

Lydia Karpenko

*These savory pancakes would make a pleasing lunch served with a soup and salad. They could also be made into 2-inch pancakes and used as an hors d'oeuvre. Serve them with a papaya relish or salsa and a dollop of yogurt.*

MAKES 12 4-INCH PANCAKES
SERVES 4 TO 6

**2 15-ounce cans cooked black beans**
**1 cup nonfat buttermilk**
**1 tablespoon honey**
**2 teaspoons minced jalapeño pepper**
**2 teaspoons chopped fresh cilantro**
**1 cup unbleached white flour**
**1½ teaspoons baking powder**
**¾ teaspoon baking soda**
**3 egg whites**
**Vegetable oil spray**

Drain and rinse 1 can of the beans well. Drain very well, then add with the buttermilk and honey to a blender or food processor. Puree until smooth, then transfer to a large bowl. Drain, rinse, and drain well again the second can of beans, and add them along with the jalapeño and cilantro to the pureed mixture to combine.

In a medium-size bowl, combine the flour, baking powder, and baking soda. Set aside.

In another large bowl, beat the egg whites until stiff but not dry. Stir one-third of the beaten egg whites into the bean mixture to lighten it. Gently fold in the remaining egg whites.

Add the flour mixture to the bean puree in 3 parts, mixing carefully but taking care not to deflate the egg whites.

Preheat a large, nonstick griddle or sauté pan over medium-high heat and spray the griddle lightly with the vegetable oil. For each pancake, ladle ¼ cup batter onto the griddle and gently spread to about 4 inches. Cook until browned. Flip and repeat.

*Serving size = 3 pancakes*
*363 calories*
*1.0 gram fat*
*1.1 milligrams cholesterol*
*300.5 milligrams sodium*

## HUMMUS

Jean-Marc Fullsack

*Keep this in your refrigerator for quick snacks, sandwiches, and dips. It is frequently served as a dip with pita bread that has been cut into triangles, and salads such as tabbouleh or Couscous (page 197) and others. For a shortcut, start with 2½ cups of canned beans that have been drained and rinsed. The lemon juice and stock adds flavor and lightens the texture.*

MAKES 2¼ CUPS
SERVES 4 TO 8

**1 cup dried garbanzo beans, soaked overnight and drained**
**1 bay leaf**
**5 cups vegetable stock**
**¼ cup fresh lemon juice**
**6 garlic cloves, oven roasted, and 1 clove, chopped**
**Zest of 1 lemon**
**½ teaspoon ground cumin**
**½ teaspoon ground coriander**
**⅛ teaspoon cayenne**
**½ teaspoon freshly ground black pepper**
**½ cup fresh parsley, minced**
**Salt to taste**

Add the beans, bay leaf, and vegetable stock to a 2- or 3-quart pot. Bring to a boil, lower the heat, and simmer, covered, for 2½ hours, or until tender. After cooking, drain the beans of any remaining liquid and reserve the stock.

Transfer the beans to a food processor and puree. Add the lemon juice and continue to puree. Gradually add some of the reserved bean stock if a creamier texture is desired. Add the remaining ingredients and mix well. Add salt to taste and serve at room temperature or chilled.

*Serving size = ⅓ cup*
*140 calories*
*2.2 grams fat*
*0 milligrams cholesterol*
*21 milligrams sodium without added salt*

## ROASTED EGGPLANT COMPOTE

Mary Sue Milliken and Susan Feniger

SERVES 4 TO 6

**1 large or 2 medium eggplants**
**3 sweet red bell peppers**
**1 bunch scallions**
**½ cup balsamic vinegar**
**⅔ teaspoon salt**
**½ teaspoon freshly ground pepper**

On a charcoal grill or under a hot broiler roast the eggplant 10 to 12 minutes per side until the flesh is soft and the skin is charred black. Cook completely. Remove the stem and skin and chop the meat roughly. Roast the peppers under the broiler or over an open flame until uniformly black on all sides. Place them in a plastic bag or closed container to steam and cool. When cooled, remove and discard stem, seeds, and skin. Dice into ½-inch squares. Clean the scallions and remove and discard ends and dark tops. Slice thinly at an angle. Toss all ingredients together. Serve at room temperature.

*Serving size = ½ cup*
*40 calories*
*0.2 gram fat*
*0 milligrams cholesterol*
*265.8 milligrams sodium*

# Salads

## BROCCOLI, POTATO, AND CHICK-PEA SALAD WITH LEMON-TARRAGON DRESSING

Martha Rose Shulman

*This has a wonderful texture and bright, alive flavors. You could serve it with crusty French bread as a main course luncheon. It can be prepared up to 24 hours in advance but will lose some of its color as it sits.*

MAKES 6 CUPS
SERVES 6 TO 8

**1 pound new or russet potatoes, cut into 1-inch cubes or quarters**
**2 tablespoons dry white wine**
**1 tablespoon chopped fresh tarragon**
**Freshly ground black pepper**
**Salt**
**6 cups broccoli florets (approximately 2 pounds)**
**1 cup cooked chick-peas**
**½ cup nonfat plain yogurt**
**3 tablespoons fresh lemon juice**
**1 tablespoon red wine vinegar**
**1 teaspoon Dijon mustard**
**½ teaspoon minced garlic**

In a large saucepan, steam the potatoes until just tender. Drain and toss with the white wine and tarragon. Season to taste with pepper and salt.

Steam the broccoli florets until just tender. Drain and refresh under cold running water. Drain again and toss with the chick-peas, yogurt, lemon juice, red wine vinegar, mustard, and garlic. Adjust the flavor with additional pepper and salt.

In a large serving bowl, combine the potatoes and broccoli mixture. Toss gently to mix thoroughly. Serve warm or at room temperature.

*Serving size = 1 cup*
*158 calories*
*1.4 grams fat*
*0.3 milligram cholesterol*
*671.6 milligrams sodium without added salt*

## ARTICHOKE, MUSHROOM, FENNEL, AND ENDIVE SALAD WITH LEMON MUSTARD CREAM

Joyce Goldstein

*A generous, satisfying salad—serve for lunch, light supper, as an elegant first course or a festive dinner. The artichoke hearts should be somewhat firm, not cooked until soft and tender.*

SERVES 4

**2 large globe artichokes**
**12 to 16 large white mushrooms**
**2 fennel bulbs**
**4 heads Belgian endive**
**2 tablespoons Dijon mustard**
**3 tablespoons lemon juice**
**1 cup nonfat plain yogurt**
**Salt**
**Black pepper**

Trim the stems and cut across the top of the artichokes. Remove most of the leaves—down to the white ones—and set the artichokes in a pan with 3 inches of boiling salted water. Reduce the heat, cover the pan, and simmer until firm-tender, about 20 minutes; do not overcook. Remove the artichokes from the pan with a slotted spoon. Remove the remaining leaves and scoop out the fuzzy chokes. Slice the artichoke hearts into ¼-inch slices.

Slice the mushrooms thin, about ⅛ inch. Cut the fennel bulbs into quarters and cut away and remove the tough center core. Slice the fennel thinly. Remove the ends from the endive and separate the leaves. Whisk together the mustard, lemon juice, and yogurt.

Toss the fennel, mushrooms, and artichoke slices with half the dressing. Arrange the endive on 4 salad plates and drizzle over most of the remaining dressing. Top with the mushrooms, fennel, and artichokes mixture. Drizzle the remaining dressing over all.

NOTE: To simplify the process of trimming the artichokes, partially cook them first in boiling water for about 15 minutes. Drain and refresh under cold water; then remove the leaves and scoop out the fuzzy choke. If fennel is not in season, substitute celery, about 4 large stalks, strings removed.

*Serving size = 2½ cups*
*131 calories*
*1.5 grams fat*
*1 milligram cholesterol*
*523.7 milligrams sodium*

## CELERY ROOT, ORANGE, GRAPEFRUIT, AND SPINACH SALAD

Joyce Goldstein

*A refreshing winter salad. The citrus plays nicely off the starchy celery root and earthy leaves.*

SERVES 4

**3 tablespoons lemon juice**
**1 celery root (about 1 pound)**
**1 large pink or red grapefruit**
**2 oranges**
**½ cup orange juice**
**2 tablespoons thick tomato puree**
**1 teaspoon sugar**
**4 handfuls small spinach leaves, rinsed**

Place about 1 tablespoon of the lemon juice in a bowl of cold water. Trim and peel the celery root. Cut it into strips about ¼ inch wide and 1½ inches long, dropping them into the bowl of water to keep them from turning brown. Cook in boiling salted water until barely tender, 5 to 7 minutes. Drain and refresh under cold water, and drain again.

Remove the peel and all of the white pith from the grapefruit and oranges. Over a bowl to trap the juices, cut carefully between the membranes to remove the grapefruit and orange segments. Set aside. Combine the fruit juices, including what is in the bowl, with the tomato puree and sugar. Place the celery root and spinach leaves in a salad bowl and toss with the dressing. Place on 4 salad plates and top with the orange and grapefruit segments.

NOTE: For a version of celery root remoulade, prepare the celery as above, then toss with ½ to ¾ cup Yogurt "Tartar" Sauce (page 357), and sprinkle with chopped parsley.

*Serving size = 2 cups*
*123 calories*
*0.7 gram fat*
*0 milligrams cholesterol*
*169 milligrams sodium*

## INDONESIAN FRUIT SALAD

Joyce Goldstein

*This recipe yields quite a lot of fruit compote, but it will keep in the refrigerator for 2 to 3 days. You can serve it as is or over watercress.*

MAKES 13 CUPS

**1 cup brown sugar**
**3 cups water**
**2 teaspoons dried hot red pepper flakes**
**3 tablespoons fresh lemon juice**
**Segments from 3 large oranges, pith and membranes removed**
**Segments from 2 large grapefruit, pith and membranes removed**
**2 mangos, peeled and cut in slices or chunks**
**2 sliced cucumbers, peeled and seeded (unpeeled if English or Japanese)**
**1 medium pineapple, peeled, cored, and cut into chunks**
**3 tablespoons chopped Thai basil or basil and mint combined (optional)**

In a small saucepan over moderate heat, boil sugar and water for 5 minutes. Add the pepper flakes and lemon juice. Cool the syrup to lukewarm. Assemble all of the fruits and cucumbers in a bowl. Pour the warm syrup over the mixture. Chill well. Toss with greens if desired.

*Serving size = ½ cup*
*57 calories*
*0.2 gram fat*
*0 milligrams cholesterol*
*2.6 milligrams sodium*

## RUSSIAN POTATO AND BEET SALAD

Joyce Goldstein

*Earthy and satisfying, this salad can make a filling lunch, accompanied by some good black bread and a soup.*

SERVES 4

**1 pound small beets, well scrubbed**
**1½ pounds little new potatoes (rosefir, ruby crescents, yellow Finnish, bintjis, creamers)**
**1 small cucumber, peeled and seeded**
**6 green onions, finely chopped**
**½ teaspoon dry mustard**
**1 teaspoon sugar**
**1 teaspoon salt**
**½ teaspoon black pepper**
**2 tablespoons red wine vinegar**
**1 cup nonfat plain yogurt**
**2 tablespoons chopped dill (optional)**

Trim the leaves from the beets but leave about 1 inch of stem. Place the beets in a medium-sized saucepan and cover with cold water, bring to a boil, reduce heat, and simmer, covered, until tender, about 40 minutes. Drain and cover with lukewarm water. When cool enough to handle, slip the peel off the beets. Set them aside.

Scrub the potatoes, place them in a medium-sized saucepan, and cover with cold salted water. Bring to a boil, reduce heat to a simmer, and cook, covered, until firm-tender, about 15 to 20 minutes depending upon the size of the potatoes. Test one by cutting all the way through. Drain and place in ice water to stop the cooking. Drain again when cold.

Cut the cucumber into small chunks. Cut the potatoes into small chunks. Cut the beets into small chunks. The vegetables should all be about the same size.

Combine the potatoes, beets, cucumber, and green onions in a bowl. In a small bowl, whisk mustard, sugar, salt, and

pepper with the vinegar. Stir in the yogurt. Pour the d
over the vegetables and toss. Sprinkle with chopped d
desired.

*Serving size = 1 cup*
*116 calories*
*0.3 gram fat*
*0.5 milligram cholesterol*
*348 milligrams sodium*

## ITALIAN BEAN SALAD

Martha Rose Shulman

*Serve this delicious salad warm in the winter or chilled in the summer. It makes a wonderful main dish.*

MAKES 6 CUPS
SERVES 6 TO 8

- **1 pound dry white beans or borlotti beans, washed, picked over, and soaked overnight or for at least 6 hours**
- **1 large white or yellow onion, chopped**
- **3 garlic cloves, roughly chopped**
- **6 cups water**
- **1 bay leaf**
- **Salt**
- **2 garlic cloves, minced**
- **¼ cup red wine vinegar**
- **1 medium or large red onion, thinly sliced**
- **2 tablespoons lemon juice**
- **1 tablespoon balsamic vinegar**
- **1 teaspoon Dijon mustard**
- **1 red bell pepper, cut in thin 1-inch-long slices**
- **¼ cup chopped fresh basil or parsley, or a combination**
- **1 teaspoon chopped fresh sage**
- **Freshly ground black pepper**

Drain the beans and combine with the white or yellow onion, the chopped garlic, the water, and the bay leaf in a large, heavy-bottomed soup pot. Bring to a boil, reduce the heat, cover, and simmer for 1 hour. Add salt to taste and half the minced garlic, cover, and cook 30 minutes to an hour, or until tender. Drain, reserving the cooking liquid.

Meanwhile, combine 1 tablespoon red wine vinegar and 1 cup water in a bowl; add the red onion. Add more water to cover if necessary and soak 30 minutes. Drain.

Mix together the lemon juice, vinegars, remaining garlic, mustard, and ¾ cup cooking liquid from the beans. Add salt and pepper to taste and adjust the seasonings. Toss with the beans in a salad bowl, along with the red onion, bell pepper, herbs, pepper, and more salt to taste. Serve warm or chilled.

*Serving size = 1 cup*
*100 calories*
*0.5 gram fat*
*0 milligrams cholesterol*
*189 milligrams sodium without added salt*

## GREEN BEANS WITH SCALLION DRESSING

Mary Sue Milliken and Susan Feniger

SERVES 4 TO 6

**1 pound fresh green beans, stem ends removed**
**1 bunch scallions**
**3 garlic cloves**
**Juice of 1 lemon**
**1 teaspoon salt**
**½ teaspoon freshly ground black pepper**
**¾ cup nonfat plain yogurt**

In plenty of rapidly boiling salted water, cook the beans until tender but just a little crunchy. Drain and plunge into ice water to chill. Drain well, wrap in a towel, and refrigerate. Clean scallions; remove and discard ends and dark tops.

Slice as thinly as possible and place in blender. Chop garlic roughly and add to scallions. Add lemon juice, salt, pepper, and yogurt and puree at high speed 4 to 6 minutes until very smooth. Chill thoroughly. Remove beans from refrigerator and slice at an angle. Place on lettuce-lined plates and top with a dollop of dressing on each. Serve immediately.

*Serving size = 1 cup*
*57 calories*
*0.3 gram fat*
*0.5 milligram cholesterol*
*436.9 milligrams sodium*

## FENNEL AND WHITE BEAN SALAD

Bradley Ogden

SERVES 4

**1 cup small white beans, soaked overnight in cold water**
**¼ yellow onion, peeled**
**1 medium carrot, peeled and cut into large chunks**
**4 sprigs of fresh thyme**
**¼ bay leaf**
**3½ cups Vegetable Stock (page 143)**
**8 garlic cloves**
**½ tablespoon kosher salt**
**½ tablespoon freshly cracked black pepper**
**1 fresh firm fennel bulb, quartered, cored, and sliced crosswise ⅛ inch thick**
**1 large ripe tomato, diced**
**2 tablespoons chopped basil**
**2 tablespoons balsamic vinegar**
**4 tablespoons sliced green onions**
**2 tablespoons coarsely chopped Italian parsley**
**1 tablespoon freshly squeezed lemon juice**
**½ tablespoon finely chopped thyme**
**1 tablespoon rinsed capers, chopped**

Drain the beans. In a medium-sized saucepan, cover with cold water and bring to a boil, drain, return to the pan, and add the onion, carrot, thyme, bay leaf, stock, and garlic; add a pinch of the kosher salt and ½ teaspoon cracked black pepper. Bring to a boil. Reduce heat, cover, and simmer gently until the beans are tender—about two hours. Drain, remove the vegetables and aromatics and cool.

Combine the remaining ingredients in a large bowl, mix with the beans, and serve.

*Serving size = 1 cup*
*208 calories*
*1.4 gram fat*
*0 milligrams cholesterol*
*962.8 milligrams sodium*

## LENTIL, CELERY, AND GINGER SALAD WITH CUCUMBER VINAIGRETTE

Hubert Keller

SERVES 4

**1 large carrot**
**3 large ripe tomatoes, cored, peeled, and seeded**
**1 cup green lentils (8 to 9 ounces)**
**1 small yellow onion**
**1 celery stalk, finely chopped**
**½ small red onion, finely chopped**
**¼ teaspoon peeled and finely chopped gingerroot**
**1½ tablespoons lemon juice**
**1½ tablespoons soy sauce**
**Freshly ground black pepper**
**Salt**
**1 English cucumber, peeled, seeded, and diced**
**1 teaspoon sherry vinegar**
**1 small branch of fresh dill**
**½ teaspoon Dijon mustard**
**1 ounce onion or bean sprouts, for garnish**

Bring a medium-sized pot of salted water to a boil. Peel the carrot and cut it lengthwise into 8 strips about ⅛ inch thick, ¾ inch wide, and 5 inches long. Blanch the strips in boiling water for 1 minute and plunge them into cold water. Drain and dry on a cloth or paper towels.

Chop the tomatoes very finely. Drain them in a fine sieve over a bowl. Wash the lentils and cook them gently for about 45 minutes in water with 1 small yellow onion. Drain the lentils and cool. Transfer the cooked lentils to a mixing bowl and add the finely chopped celery, red onion, ginger, lemon juice, soy sauce, pepper, and salt. Mix together and check the seasoning. Set aside.

Place the diced cucumber in a blender, add the sherry vinegar, dill, Dijon mustard, pepper, and salt. Process until very smooth.

The lentils can be mounded on the center of a plate, smoothed, topped with tomatoes, and surrounded by the vinaigrette. Garnish with the sprouts and blanched carrot.

*Serving size = 1 cup*
*65 calories*
*0.4 gram fat*
*0 milligrams cholesterol*
*239.6 milligrams sodium without added salt*

## SPICED LENTIL AND FAVA BEAN SALAD WITH FENNEL

Hubert Keller

SERVES 4

**1 cup green or "French" lentils**
**1 small yellow onion**
**Freshly ground black pepper**
**¾ cup shelled fava beans**
**1 fennel bulb, trimmed, cored, and thinly sliced**
**1 tomato, peeled, seeded, and diced**
**1 to 2 hot green chilies, cored and minced**

- **¼ teaspoon fresh gingerroot, peeled and minced**
- **2 tablespoons chopped fresh coriander**
- **2 tablespoons chopped parsley**
- **1½ tablespoons lemon juice**
- **1½ tablespoons soy sauce**
- **12 Bibb lettuce leaves, washed and dried**
- **12 endive leaves**

Wash the lentils under running water and boil them for 1 minute. Place the lentils in a saucepan, add 1½ quarts of water, and bring to a boil over high heat. Add the whole onion and season with freshly ground pepper. Reduce the heat to a simmer, cover, and cook gently for about 45 minutes, or until cooked through but not soft. Drain the lentils, rinse, and set aside to cool. Discard the onion. Transfer the cooked lentils into a mixing bowl.

Meanwhile, boil the fava beans for 3 minutes; drain and refresh them under cold water. Press the beans gently between your thumb and index finger to remove their tough skins. Add the fava beans to the lentils along with the fennel, tomato, chilies, ginger, coriander, parsley, lemon juice, soy sauce, and pepper. Toss together very gently. Chill until you are ready to serve.

Arrange the Bibb lettuce and endive leaves on each plate and scoop the chilled lentil salad in the center.

*Serving size = approximately 1 cup*
*150 calories*
*1.3 grams fat*
*0 milligrams cholesterol*
*407.3 milligrams sodium*

## SPICY MELON AND GRAPEFRUIT SALAD

Hubert Keller

*The combination of mint, grapefruit, and melon is bright and refreshing and looks particularly beautiful when served in black china bowls.*

SERVES 4 TO 8

**1 ripe cantaloupe**
**½ ripe honeydew melon**
**1 grapefruit**
**12 fresh mint leaves**
**Freshly ground black pepper**
**½ cup dessert wine, such as sauternes or California late harvested Sauvignon Blanc or Semillion**

Cut the cantaloupe in half. Seed both varieties of melons. Using a melon baller, scoop out the melon flesh and place into a mixing bowl.

Using a serrated knife, peel the grapefruit and remove the white membrane around each segment; remove the seeds. Add the grapefruit segments, 4 mint leaves, black pepper, and dessert wine to the melon balls. Gently combine all ingredients. Cover with plastic wrap and refrigerate for 1 hour.

Divide the salad among 4 bowls. Spoon the liquid over the fruit and garnish each serving with 2 mint leaves.

*Serving size = 1 cup*
*53 calories*
*0.2 gram fat*
*0 milligrams cholesterol*
*8.3 milligrams sodium*

## HERB SALAD (SABZEE)

Deborah Madison

*The usual nature of this salad is one of emphatic tastes. The word* sabzee *refers to greens in Afghani and seems always to include dill, parsley, and cilantro mixed with a heartier green like spinach. These proportions are approximate and are, to a degree, suggestions. If one or two ingredients are lacking, improvise with other things that you like. There are so many tastes here that the dressing need only be a squeeze of lemon juice. This is wonderful tucked into pita bread along with a spoonful of yogurt and some succulent roasted peppers.*

SERVES 2 TO 4

**4 cups arugula or spinach greens, or a mixture**
**Handful of radish or basil sprouts**
**¼ cup each Italian parsley, cilantro, and dill leaves**
**2 tablespoons chopped mint**
**2 scallions**
**Several celery or lovage leaves**
**Salt**
**Lemon juice to taste**

Wash and dry all the ingredients. Tear the arugula or spinach into bite-size pieces and roughly chop the herbs; trim and slice the scallions. Toss everything together with a few pinches of salt, then add lemon juice to taste.

*Serving size = approximately 1½ cups*
*39 calories*
*0.7 gram fat*
*0 milligrams cholesterol*
*368.2 milligrams sodium without salt*

## FENNEL SALAD WITH CUCUMBER AND CHICK-PEAS

Deborah Madison

*The broth from the chick-peas, reduced until thick, acts as a substitute for the usual olive oil. White beans would be good also.*

SERVES 4

**1 small fennel bulb, core removed, finely diced**
**1 cucumber, peeled, seeded, and diced**
**½ bunch scallions, the whites and some of the greens, trimmed and thinly sliced**

**1 cup cooked chick-peas or white beans (page 124)**
**3 tablespoons reduced bean broth (page 346)**
**¼ cup nonfat plain yogurt**
**1 teaspoon finely grated lemon zest**
**Juice of 1 lemon**
**¼ cup finely chopped Italian parsley**
**2 tablespoons finely chopped fennel greens**
**2 tablespoons finely chopped tarragon**
**Salt**
**Freshly ground black pepper**

Combine the fennel, cucumber, scallions, and chick-peas in a bowl and toss together. In a smaller bowl, whisk the bean broth with the yogurt, lemon zest, lemon juice, and fresh herbs. Season well with salt and pepper. Pour over the vegetables and toss together. Serve on a bed of lettuce.

NOTE: If the fennel isn't available, use 1 cup diced celery in its place; include some of the light-colored leaves as well, finely chopped.

*Serving size = 1 cup*
*116 calories*
*1.2 grams fat*
*0.3 milligram cholesterol*
*524.6 milligrams sodium without added salt*

## MANGO OR PAPAYA AND BEET SALAD

Jean-Marc Fullsack

*This visually stunning salad must be made just before serving or the beets will discolor the entire dish. Prepare the ingredients 1 hour or so before serving, but don't toss them together until just before the meal.*

MAKES 4 CUPS
SERVES 4 TO 8

**2 cups cubed and cooked beets (about 1 pound)**
**1 cup cubed mango or papaya**

**½ cup minced red onion**
**½ cup fresh lime juice**
**2 tablespoons pickled ginger**
**2 tablespoons ginger vinegar (from the pickled ginger)**

In a medium bowl, combine all the ingredients and toss very gently. Serve immediately on a bed of lettuce.

NOTE: The beets can be quickly cooked in a microwave oven. Place them in a microwaveable dish, add 1 inch of water, and cook on High for 10 to 15 minutes, or until tender.

*Serving size = ½ cup*
*56 calories*
*0.2 gram fat*
*0 milligrams cholesterol*
*24 milligrams sodium*

## MOROCCAN EGGPLANT SALAD

Catherine Pantsios

*This is a great hors d'oeuvre on toasted slices of bread, or as a salad or side dish.*

MAKES 1 QUART
SERVES 8 AS A SIDE DISH

**2 large firm eggplants, about 2 pounds total**
**2 large ripe red tomatoes, peeled, seeded, and chopped**
**2 teaspoons minced garlic**
**1 teaspoon paprika**
**½ teaspoon ground cumin**
**Pinch of cayenne**
**Juice of 1 lemon**
**Salt**

Roast the eggplants in the oven at 400 degrees or over a gas flame until the skin puffs up; let the eggplants cool until they can be handled, and then, using a small knife, peel away the skin. Cut the flesh into ½-inch dice.

Put all the ingredients except the lemon juice and salt into a large skillet and cook over medium heat, stirring often, until the eggplant is soft and cooked through and most of the liquid has evaporated. Cool to room temperature and season with salt and lemon juice.

*Serving size = 1½ cups*
*79 calories*
*0.9 gram fat*
*0 milligrams cholesterol*
*16.6 milligrams sodium without added salt*

## COUSCOUS SALAD

Jean-Marc Fullsack

*Prepare the couscous in vegetable stock instead of water for more flavor. This can be prepared and refrigerated for up to 8 hours ahead of time.*

MAKES 6 CUPS
SERVES 4 TO 8

**2½ cups cooked couscous**
**2 cups diced fresh tomato**
**¾ cup chopped fresh mint**
**½ cup minced onion**
**½ cup diced cucumber**
**½ cup chopped fresh parsley**
**4 tablespoons lemon juice**
**1 garlic clove, minced**
**½ teaspoon ground cumin**
**½ teaspoon ground coriander**
**Freshly ground black pepper**
**Salt**

Prepare the couscous according to package directions. In a large bowl, combine the couscous, tomato, mint, onion, cucumber, parsley, lemon juice, garlic, cumin, and coriander. Season to taste with pepper and salt.

*Serving size = 1 cup*
*113 calories*
*0.5 gram fat*
*0 milligrams cholesterol*
*61.9 milligrams sodium without added salt*

## BLACK-EYED PEA SALAD

Jean-Marc Fullsack

*This very colorful and extremely tasty salad would serve well as an entrée. Prepare and refrigerate it up to 24 hours ahead of time.*

MAKES 6 CUPS
SERVES 6 TO 8

**2½ cups frozen black-eyed peas**
**1 large ear of corn to yield 1 cup fresh corn kernels**
**1 cup finely diced carrots**
**1 cup finely diced celery**
**1 cup finely diced red bell pepper**
**1½ teaspoons minced red onion**
**¼ cup seasoned rice vinegar**
**½ cup whole cilantro leaves**
**Freshly ground black pepper**
**Salt**

Bring 6 cups of water to a boil. Add the black-eyed peas. Allow the water to return to a boil and cook for 20 minutes, or until just tender. Drain and refresh under cold running water. Drain well and set aside.

In another pot, bring 6 cups of water to a boil. Add the corn, carrots, and celery. Blanch for approximately 1 minute, or until just tender. Drain and refresh under cold water. Drain well.

In a large bowl, combine the peas, corn, carrots, celery, red bell pepper, and onion. Pour the vinegar over and toss well. Allow to stand for at least 30 minutes at room temperature.

Thirty minutes before serving, add the cilantro and toss well. Season to taste with pepper and salt. Serve.

*Serving size = 1 cup*
*145 calories*
*1 gram fat*
*0 milligrams cholesterol*
*342.1 milligrams sodium without added salt*

## POTATO SALAD

Don Vaupel

MAKES 4 CUPS
SERVES 4 TO 6

**3 medium red-skinned potatoes**
**2 hard-boiled egg whites, diced**
**¾ cup diced onions**
**1 cup diced celery**
**1 cup egg-free, oil-free mayonnaise**
**2 tablespoons mustard**
**2 tablespoons dill pickle relish**
**1 teaspoon garlic powder**
**Freshly ground black pepper**
**Salt**

Wash the potatoes, remove any blemishes, and place in a large saucepan. Cover with water and bring to a boil. Reduce the heat and simmer for 25 minutes, or until just tender. Drain and refresh under cold running water. Drain and cut into ½-inch cubes and set aside in a large bowl.

Add the egg whites to the potatoes, along with the onions, celery, mayonnaise, mustard, pickle relish, and garlic. Toss well.

Season to taste with pepper and salt. Refrigerate for at least 2 hours before serving.

Serving size = 1 cup
*152 calories*
*0.5 gram fat*
*0 milligrams cholesterol*
*1,010 milligrams sodium without added salt*

## PUMPKIN SALAD

Jean-Marc Fullsack

*The cilantro and lime juice hint of Mexico.*

SERVES 4

**1 cup pumpkin, peeled and cut in ½-inch dice**
**1 cup chayote squash, peeled and cut in ½-inch dice**
**1 cup fresh corn kernels (approximately 1 large ear)**
**2 tablespoons lime juice**
**1 tablespoon seasoned rice vinegar**
**2 fresh green chilies, roasted and chopped (approximately ¼ cup)**
**½ cup chopped green onions**
**1 tablespoon minced fresh cilantro**

In a large saucepan with a steamer insert, steam the pumpkin and chayote for 2 minutes. Add the corn and continue to steam for 2 to 3 minutes, or until all the vegetables are just tender.

In a medium bowl, combine the lime juice and vinegar. Add the pumpkin, chayote, corn, chilies, onions, and cilantro. Toss well and serve at room temperature or chilled.

NOTE: Canned, roasted chilies can be substituted for fresh. Any hard orange-yellow squash, such as acorn or butternut, can be substituted for the pumpkin.

*Serving size = ¾ cup*
*81 calories*
*0.6 gram fat*
*0 milligrams cholesterol*
*4.7 milligrams sodium*

## COLESLAW WITH GREEN APPLES

Tracy Pikhart Ritter

MAKES APPROXIMATELY 6 CUPS
SERVES 6

**4 cups shredded green and red cabbage**
**1 large carrot, shredded**
**2 green apples, shredded with their skin**
**3 tablespoons nonfat plain yogurt**
**1 tablespoon grainy-style or honey mustard**
**2 tablespoons apple cider vinegar**
**1 tablespoon apple juice concentrate**
**1 teaspoon honey**
**¼ teaspoon salt**
**¼ teaspoon freshly cracked black pepper**

Shred the cabbage, carrot, and apples in a food processor or with a hand grater over a large bowl.

Whisk together the remaining ingredients. When well blended, pour over the cabbage mixture. Allow to marinate for 30 to 40 minutes or longer. This can be made up to 1 day in advance.

*Serving size = 1 cup*
*60 calories*
*0.5 gram fat*
*0.1 milligram cholesterol*
*152 milligrams sodium*

## ENGLISH CUCUMBER SALAD

Jean-Marc Fullsack

*There are many variations for this refreshing salad. A few are listed below. For all variations, including your own, keep the basil, cucumber, tomato, and yogurt measurements and methods the same. Prepare and refrigerate the salad up to 3 hours ahead of time.*

MAKES 3 CUPS
SERVES 4 TO 6

**1 cup nonfat plain yogurt**
**1 garlic clove, finely minced**
**1 teaspoon fresh gingerroot, minced**
**½ teaspoon ground cumin**
**1 English cucumber, peeled, quartered, and sliced ¼ inch thick**
**1 cup tomato (1 to 2 large tomatoes), seeded and diced**
**1 jalapeño pepper, seeded and minced**
**1 tablespoon fresh mint, chopped**
**1 tablespoon fresh cilantro, chopped**
**1 teaspoon sugar**
**Freshly ground black pepper**
**Salt (optional)**

In a small bowl, whisk together the yogurt, garlic, ginger, and cumin.

In a large bowl, combine the cucumber, tomato, jalapeño pepper, mint, cilantro, and sugar. Pour the yogurt mixture over the vegetables and toss well. Season to taste with freshly ground black pepper and salt. Serve at room temperature.

*Variations:* 1. Omit the ginger. 2. Omit the jalapeño pepper, cumin, and mint. 3. Omit the jalapeño pepper, cilantro, and ginger and add 1 tablespoon dried tarragon. 4. Omit the jalapeño pepper, cumin, cilantro, and ginger and add ½ cup golden raisins. 5. Omit the jalapeño pepper, cumin, cilantro, mint, and ginger and add 1 tablespoon dried dill and ½ cup golden raisins.

*Serving size = ½ cup*
*39 calories*
*0.3 gram fat*
*0.7 milligram cholesterol*
*82.9 milligrams sodium*

## WILD RICE SALAD

Jean-Marc Fullsack

*This bright array of color is an easy-to-make, tasty, and very satisfying salad. You can prepare and refrigerate it for a few hours before serving. Try it as part of a salad plate with Pumpkin Salad (page 200) and the Roasted and Rustic Sweet Peppers (page 300). It could also be served as part of brunch with the Scrambled Mexican Tofu (page 232) and salsa.*

MAKES 4 CUPS
SERVES 4 TO 6

**2 cups wild rice, cooked**
**½ cup cooked corn kernels**
**½ cup diced red bell pepper**
**½ cup chopped tomato**
**¼ cup cooked green peas**
**¼ cup diced red onion**
**¼ cup green beans, cut into pieces and cooked**
**4 tablespoons frozen apple juice concentrate**
**2 tablespoons red wine vinegar**
**2 tablespoons chopped fresh basil**
**1 tablespoon chopped fresh parsley**
**1 tablespoon chopped fresh tarragon**
**1 tablespoon fresh lime juice**
**Freshly ground black pepper**
**Salt**

In a large bowl, combine all the ingredients. Toss well and season to taste with freshly ground black pepper and salt.

*Serving size = 1 cup*
*175 calories*
*0.8 gram fat*
*0 milligrams cholesterol*
*130.6 milligrams sodium without added salt*

# Soups

## TOMATO CONSOMMÉ

Jean-Marc Fullsack

*This might look intimidating at first glance, but it is actually quite easy and a lot of fun to make. Serve it over Pea and Corn Pancakes (page 250) along with its garnish for a delightful first course. For an interesting flavor, try 1 tablespoon pepper vodka stirred into each serving. This consommé can also be used as a soup stock or braising liquid. Prepare it and refrigerate for up to 1 week or freeze for up to 6 months.*

MAKES 4 CUPS
SERVES 3 TO 4

**1 pound tomatoes, peeled, seeded, and quartered**
**3 cups tomato juice or vegetable juice cocktail**
**¾ cup chopped celery**
**¾ cup chopped leeks**
**½ cup chopped fresh parsley**
**2 whole cloves**
**1 garlic clove**
**½ bay leaf**
**1½ tablespoons tomato paste**
**1 teaspoon dried thyme**
**1 teaspoon coriander seeds**
**2 cups vegetable stock**

**6 egg whites with their shells**
**Cayenne**
**Salt**
**1 small tomato, peeled, seeded, and cut in ¼-inch dice**
**1 tablespoon chiffonaded basil or chopped tarragon leaves**

In a food processor or blender, combine the tomatoes, tomato juice, celery, leeks, parsley, cloves, garlic, bay leaf, tomato paste, thyme, and coriander seeds. Puree thoroughly.

Pour the pureed mixture into a large nonreactive pot. Warm the vegetable stock and add it to the puree. Bring to a boil, then simmer, covered, on low heat for 12 to 15 minutes. Turn off the heat and allow the soup to cool for 30 minutes.

Add the eggshells and whites to a large stainless steel bowl. Crush the eggshells and beat the egg whites just enough to break them down. Slowly pour small amounts of the shells and whites into the warm soup, whisking continually to prevent the eggs from cooking.

Place the pot over medium-high heat and continue to whisk as it comes to a boil. When the soup reaches a boil, stop whisking and simmer, uncovered, for 5 to 10 minutes. Stir periodically so that the eggshells have contact with the soup.

As a white foam rises to the surface, ladle it into a cheesecloth-lined strainer or a large coffee filter. After all or most of the foam has been removed, strain the hot soup through the foam into a clean bowl. Season to taste with the cayenne and salt. Pour into individuals serving bowls and garnish with the chopped tomato and herbs. Serve hot.

*Serving size = 1 cup*
*66 calories*
*0.5 gram fat*
*0 milligrams cholesterol*
*557.8 milligrams sodium without added salt*

## RED POTATO SOUP WITH GARLIC AND WILD GREENS

Bradley Ogden

SERVES 6

**1 pound red potatoes, rinsed in cold water**
**1 leek, including just a little of the green, chopped and washed well**
**1 medium Spanish onion, peeled and diced**
**4 garlic cloves, peeled**
**2 jalapeño peppers, seeded and finely minced**
**3 cups coarsely chopped red Swiss chard, mustard greens, and turnip greens (stems removed)**
**4 medium vine-ripened tomatoes, coarsely chopped**
**2 cups chopped canned plum tomatoes**
**1 quart Vegetable Stock (page 143) and water**
**1 teaspoon kosher salt**
**1 teaspoon cracked black pepper**
**3 tablespoons balsamic vinegar**

Combine all the ingredients in a heavy stockpot and cover. Place over high heat and bring to a boil; reduce heat, cover, and simmer slowly for 35 minutes, or until the potatoes are soft. Cool slightly and puree in a blender or food processor. Adjust seasoning if necessary.

*Serving size = 1½ cups*
*144 calories*
*0.8 gram fat*
*0 milligrams cholesterol*
*589.6 milligrams sodium*

## COOL GAZPACHO WITH COUSCOUS

Michael Lomonaco

SERVES 4

**6 ounces quick-cooking or instant couscous**
**Black pepper**
**Cilantro (optional)**
**1 22-ounce can plum tomatoes**
**6 ounces salt-free tomato juice**
**1 cup peeled and seeded cucumber slices**
**1 red bell pepper, diced**
**1 green bell pepper, diced**
**1 small onion, chopped**
**1 tablespoon chopped garlic**
**2 tablespoons balsamic vinegar**
**1 tablespoon fresh seeded and diced jalapeño pepper**
**Chopped scallions (optional)**

Cook the couscous according to the package directions. Season with pepper and chopped fresh cilantro if desired and set aside.

Combine the soup ingredients in a blender or food processor and process just until coarse and chunky in texture. Refrigerate until cold. Serve in a bowl with 3 tablespoons prepared couscous, additional chopped cilantro, and scallions if desired.

*Serving size = 2 cups*
*103 calories*
*0.6 gram fat*
*0 milligrams cholesterol*
*308.4 milligrams sodium*

## CHILLED TOMATO AND RED BELL PEPPER SOUP

Hubert Keller

SERVES 4

**4 red bell peppers**
**Vegetable oil spray**
**1 medium onion, peeled and chopped**
**2 garlic cloves, peeled and chopped**
**4 large tomatoes, peeled, seeded, and chopped**
**Pinch of thyme**
**8 fresh basil leaves**
**1 teaspoon honey**
**Freshly ground pepper**
**Salt (optional)**
**6 cups Vegetable Consommé (page 147)**
**1 tablespoon sherry or champagne vinegar**
**¾ cup nonfat plain yogurt**
**20 watercress leaves, or 4 pinches of chervil**

Preheat the broiler.

Spray the bell peppers very lightly with the pan coating. Place under the broiler and let them roast, turning frequently, until the skin is blackened on all sides. When the peppers are charred, cool them slightly and peel off the blackened skin. Remove the stems; remove the core and seeds. Chop the peppers and set aside.

Spray the bottom of a stockpot lightly with the pan coating. Over medium heat, add the chopped onion and sauté, stirring until translucent, about 1½ minutes. Add the garlic, tomatoes, bell peppers, thyme, basil, honey, pepper, and optional salt. Cook slowly for 5 minutes. Add the vegetable consommé and bring to a boil. Reduce heat and simmer for 15 to 20 minutes. Transfer to a blender or food processor and puree until completely smooth, in batches if necessary. Cool to room temperature and refrigerate.

Just before serving, stir in the vinegar and yogurt and taste for seasoning. Thin if necessary with additional yogurt.

Ladle the soup into shallow-rimmed soup plates and sprinkle with the watercress leaves or chervil.

*Serving size = 2 cups*
*82 calories*
*0.6 gram fat*
*0.8 milligram cholesterol*
*44.1 milligrams sodium without added salt*

## CHILLED CUCUMBER AND DILL SOUP

Hubert Keller

*This is a simple soup with great taste and definitely an eye-catcher. When it comes to choosing what kind of cucumber to use. I prefer the long European variety, which has almost no bitterness in the skin. They must be young.*

SERVES 4

**3 medium cucumbers**
**1 teaspoon chopped fresh dill**
**1 teaspoon Dijon mustard**
**½ teaspoon sherry or champagne vinegar**
**2 tablespoons nonfat plain yogurt**
**Freshly ground black pepper**
**1 teaspoon black mustard seeds**
**10 red radishes, trimmed and chopped**
**Sprigs of dill**

Peel the cucumbers and cut them in half lengthwise. Scoop out the seeds with a teaspoon and dice the cucumbers. Transfer the cucumbers to a blender. Add the dill, mustard, vinegar, yogurt, and pepper. Puree until completely smooth. Transfer to a mixing bowl and refrigerate.

Heat a small Teflon sauté pan over medium heat. Add the mustard seeds and toast them until they turn gray; take care that they do not burn. Partially cover the sauté pan to keep the seeds from jumping out. Remove from the heat and cool.

Just before serving, stir half the chopped radishes into the soup. Ladle the cucumber soup into shallow-rimmed soup plates and sprinkle with the remaining chopped radishes. Garnish with the dill sprigs and the toasted mustard seeds.

*Serving size = 1 cup*
*25 calories*
*0.5 gram fat*
*0.1 milligram cholesterol*
*26.2 milligrams sodium without added salt*

## BLACK BEAN AND SPINACH SOUP

Hubert Keller

SERVES 4

**⅔ cup black beans**
**3 tablespoons chopped onion**
**2 tablespoons chopped celery**
**1 teaspoon finely chopped garlic**
**1 teaspoon peeled and finely shredded fresh gingerroot**
**1 tablespoon orange zest**
**Freshly grated black pepper**
**5 ounces spinach leaves (about one bunch), stemmed and rinsed**
**4 tablespoons nonfat plain yogurt**
**8 orange segments, all white membrane removed**
**1 tablespoon coarsely chopped cilantro**

Sort, wash, and drain the black beans. In a heavy sauce pot, combine the beans, onion, celery, garlic, ginger, orange zest, and pepper to taste. Add 6 cups of water and bring to a boil, stirring occasionally. Lower the heat, cover, and simmer for 1 hour, or until the beans are fully cooked (the cooking time varies with the type and the age of the beans).

Meanwhile, carefully wash the spinach leaves to remove all sand and grit. Place the washed leaves in a heated Teflon sauté pan. Stir until they are wilted but still bright green, 2 to 3 minutes. Add ground pepper and cool. Mince the cooked spinach and set it aside.

Spoon one-third of the black beans into a blender or food processor. Puree until completely smooth and transfer back to the soup. Stir the spinach into the soup, return to a simmer, and serve immediately.

Ladle the soup into shallow rimmed soup plates. Spoon nonfat yogurt into the center of each, garnish with 2 orange segments, and sprinkle with fresh cilantro.

*Serving size = 1½ cups*
*133 calories*
*0.4 gram fat*
*0.3 milligram cholesterol*
*41.0 milligrams sodium*

## CREAMED LENTIL SOUP WITH CELERY

Deborah Madison

*This is a robust cold-weather soup. The celery makes a fresh contrast to the rich lentils. Use plenty of the light green leaves for the garnish.*

SERVES 6

**1½ cups brown or green French lentils**
**1 onion, diced**
**1 large leek, white part only, cleaned well and chopped**
**1 cup chopped celery**
**2 garlic cloves, mashed**
**2 bay leaves**
**¼ cup chopped parsley**
**1½ teaspoons salt**
**7 cups water or vegetable stock**
**2 teaspoons Dijon mustard**
**1 tablespoon strong red wine vinegar**
**Additional vegetable stock or water, as needed**

**Freshly cracked pepper**
**Chopped celery leaves**
**½ cup toasted croutons (page 151)**

Sort through the lentils and rinse them well. Combine the lentils, onion, leek, celery, garlic, herbs, salt, and water or vegetable stock in a stockpot. Bring to a boil, lower the heat, and simmer, partially covered, until the lentils are completely tender, about 45 minutes. Stir the soup occasionally.

When done, cool the soup a bit, puree it in a blender (this will have to be done in batches), then pass the puree through a food mill to remove the lentil skins. Return to the heat and stir in the mustard and vinegar. Taste and adjust the seasonings. Stir in additional stock or water to thin the soup, if needed. Serve garnished with pepper, celery leaves, and croutons.

*Serving size = 1½ cups*
*115 calories*
*0.9 gram fat*
*0 milligrams cholesterol*
*675.5 milligrams sodium*

## CURRIED SPLIT PEA SOUP

Martha Rose Shulman

*Split peas take on a whole new dimension in this subtly spiced Indian soup. It can be prepared and refrigerated up to 2 days ahead of time or frozen for up to 2 months. Do not add the yogurt or lemon juice until reheating it.*

MAKES 9 CUPS
SERVES 6 TO 9

**8 cups vegetable stock**
**2 cups yellow split peas**
**1 cup minced onion (approximately ½ pound)**

2 garlic cloves, minced
1 teaspoon curry powder
½ teaspoon turmeric
1 tablespoon black peppercorns
12 whole cloves
1 bay leaf
1 teaspoon mustard seeds
½ cup nonfat plain yogurt
2 tablespoons lemon juice
Freshly ground black pepper
Salt
Nonfat plain yogurt, for garnish
Garlic Croutons (recipe follows)
Cilantro, for garnish

In a large saucepan, combine the vegetable stock, peas, onion, garlic, curry powder, and turmeric. In a piece of cheesecloth, tie together the peppercorns, cloves, bay leaf, and mustard seeds. Add the spice bag to the saucepan and bring to a boil. Reduce the heat and simmer, covered, 45 minutes to 1 hour, or until the peas are just tender. Squeeze the liquid from the spice bag and discard it.

Cool the soup a bit, then process in a blender or food processor; process to a coarse rather than smooth puree. Return the soup to the saucepan. Just before serving, heat through and stir in the yogurt and lemon juice. Season to taste with pepper and salt. Garnish each serving with a dollop of yogurt, a few toasted garlic croutons, and chopped cilantro.

## GARLIC CROUTONS

Rub toasted thin slices of country or sourdough bread with the cut side of a garlic clove. Cut each slice into small cubes. Small baguette slices are pretty when left whole. For a more intense garlic flavor, press the garlic through a garlic press and puree with a small amount of salt before rubbing into the toasts.

*Serving size = 1 cup soup without croutons or garnish*
*94 calories*
*0.7 gram fat*

*0.2 milligram cholesterol*
*54.5 milligrams sodium without added salt*

## "FOUR-ONION" SOUP WITH GARLIC CROUTONS

Catherine Pantsios

*Cooking the onions in the water until the water evaporates brings out their sweetness without sautéing in fat. Vegetable stock can be used instead of the water for a richer flavor.*

SERVES 6

**2 medium onions**
**1 bunch medium leeks (about 6)**
**12 shallots**
**7 cups water or vegetable stock**
**Salt**
**White pepper**
**1 garlic clove**
**6 slices whole wheat sourdough bread**
**1 bunch chives, snipped fine**

Peel the onions, cut them in half lengthwise, then into very thin lengthwise slices. Cut the leeks in half lengthwise and wash them well. Cut the leeks into ¼-inch crosswise slices (the green tops can be saved for stock).

Peel and slice the shallots into thin slices. Place the onions, shallots, and leeks in a heavy pot with 1 cup of water or vegetable stock. Over medium heat, cook the vegetables until the water has evaporated and the vegetables have begun to soften without coloring. At this point add 6 cups of water or vegetable stock and salt and white pepper to taste. Simmer for ½ hour.

Remove 2 cups of liquid and vegetables to a blender or food processor. Puree well and return the puree to the remaining soup. Cut the garlic clove in half and rub the bread slices with the cut side of the clove. Toast under a broiler.

Put 1 slice of bread into each of 6 bowls, pour the soup over, and garnish with the chives.

*Serving size = 1 cup with croutons*
*194 calories*
*1.1 grams fat*
*0.2 milligram cholesterol*
*94.4 milligrams sodium without added salt*

## JAPANESE NOODLE SOUP

Jean-Marc Fullsack

*This very simple soup can be made with soba or somen noodles, which can be found in the Asian food section of your supermarket. However, thin Italian pasta, such as linguine or vermicelli, can also be substituted.*

MAKES 4 CUPS
SERVES 4

**4 ounces somen or soba noodles**
**2 cups Dashi Vegetable Stock (page 146)**
**8 fresh shiitake mushrooms, sliced ⅛ inch thick**
**1 tablespoon soy sauce**
**2 teaspoons sake**
**1½ teaspoons red miso paste**
**½ cup fresh, carefully washed spinach leaves, loosely packed**
**Zest of ¼ lemon**
**1 green onion, thinly sliced on the diagonal**

Cook the noodles according to the package directions. Drain, turn into a bowl, and cover with cold water.

In a large saucepan, combine the dashi stock and mushrooms. Bring to a boil. Add the soy sauce and sake. Reduce the heat and simmer for 2 minutes. Add the miso paste and stir to dissolve completely.

Drain the cooked noodles and add to the soup. Add the

spinach leaves and serve immediately. Garnish with the lemon zest and green onion.

*Serving size = 1 cup*
*72 calories*
*0.4 gram fat*
*0 milligrams cholesterol*
*126.8 milligrams sodium*

## ANASAZI BEAN SOUP WITH CORN AND CHILI

Deborah Madison

*Anasazi beans, the pretty purple and white mottled ones, are similar in flavor to pintos, which could be used in their place. They tend to cook a little more quickly than other beans.*

SERVES 6

**2 cups anasazi beans, cleaned and soaked overnight**
**1 large onion, cut into small pieces**
**2 carrots, peeled and diced**
**1 large celery stalk, finely diced**
**1 teaspoon dried oregano**
**3 garlic cloves, minced**
**1 teaspoon salt**
**1 16-ounce can crushed tomatoes, or 1 pound fresh tomatoes, peeled, seeded, and chopped**
**2 cups fresh or frozen corn kernels**
**1 to 2 tablespoons soy sauce**
**3 large green chilies, Anaheims or poblanos, roasted (page 132), seeded, and diced, or 1 4-ounce can, drained and chopped**
**1 bunch chopped cilantro**
**2 cups finely shredded cabbage**

Drain the beans, cover with fresh water, and bring to a boil; boil for 5 minutes. Drain. Cover again with 10 cups of fresh water, add the onion, carrots, and celery, and bring to a boil. Lower the heat, partially cover, and simmer for 1 hour. Pound or mash the oregano with the garlic and salt and add to the beans along with the tomatoes. Simmer until the beans are tender, then add the corn and cook until the corn is tender. Stir in the soy sauce to taste, then add the chilies and cilantro. Serve the soup garnished with a small mound of shredded cabbage in each bowl.

*Serving size = 1¼ cups*
*228 calories*
*1.1 grams fat*
*0 milligrams cholesterol*
*535.4 milligrams sodium*

## GREEN LENTIL AND SORREL SOUP

Hubert Keller

*The acidic sorrel makes a delightful balance with the rich lentils.*

SERVES 6 TO 8

**⅔ cup green (or "French") lentils**
**5 cups water**
**Freshly ground pepper**
**1 bouquet garni of parsley stems, sprigs of thyme, bay leaf, and celery leaves, securely tied with a string**
**1 small onion, finely chopped**
**2 garlic cloves, finely chopped**
**1 small carrot, finely chopped**
**¼ pound sorrel**
**1 tablespoon honey**
**2 tablespoons finely chopped chives**

Wash the lentils under running water and blanch them for 1 minute. Place them in a saucepan, add 5 cups of water, and bring to a boil over high heat. Season with freshly ground pepper and add the bouquet garni. Reduce the heat to a simmer, cover, and cook for 15 to 20 minutes. Add the onion, garlic, and carrot and cook until the lentils are tender, 20 to 25 minutes more.

Meanwhile, carefully wash and chop the sorrel. Place the sorrel in a preheated nonstick sauté pan and stir until wilted, 2 to 3 minutes. Set aside.

When the lentils are tender, discard the bouquet garni and stir in the sorrel and honey. Add the chopped chives. If the soup is too thick, add more water. Adjust the seasoning to taste and serve immediately.

*Serving size = 1½ cups*
*123 calories*
*0.8 gram fat*
*0 milligrams cholesterol*
*65.5 milligrams sodium*

## MISO SOUP

Michael McDermott

*Like any soup, this one is versatile and lends itself to many variations. On its own, it is full of flavor. But it can also be poured over endless combinations of tofu, steamed rice, noodles, fresh cilantro, pickled ginger, steamed and chopped spinach, or daikon for a heartier dish. Stir in an additional ½ teaspoon rice wine vinegar per serving for an even brighter taste. It can be frozen for up to 2 months.*

SERVES 4

**1 tablespoon rice wine vinegar**
**2 teaspoons minced fresh gingerroot**
**1 teaspoon honey**
**¼ teaspoon minced jalapeño pepper**
**4 cups Dashi Vegetable Stock (page 146)**
**¾ cup green onions, thinly sliced (approximately 4 green onions)**
**1 teaspoon minced garlic**
**4 tablespoons red miso paste**

In a small bowl, combine the vinegar, ginger, honey, and jalapeño. Mix well and set aside at room temperature.

In a large stainless-steel saucepan, bring ¼ cup vegetable stock to a boil. Reduce the heat to a simmer. Add the green onions and garlic. Cover for 1 minute. Add half the remaining vegetable stock and whisk in the miso until dissolved. Add the rest of the vegetable stock and heat just until the stock begins to simmer. Do not allow the soup to boil. Continue to simmer for 10 to 15 minutes.

Serve hot, with 1½ teaspoons of the vinegar-ginger mixture stirred into each serving.

*Serving size = 1 cup*
*79 calories*
*1.5 grams fat*
*0 milligrams cholesterol*
*648.1 milligrams sodium*

## TOMATO BEAN CORN CHOWDER

Tracy Pikhart Ritter

MAKES 6 CUPS
SERVES 6

**1 teaspoon minced garlic**
**½ white onion, peeled and cut into ¼-inch dice**
**1 stalk celery, trimmed and cut into ¼-inch dice**
**3 tablespoons vegetable stock plus 4 cups**
**3 large ripe tomatoes, cut into ½-inch cubes**
**1 large potato, peeled and cut into ¼-inch dice**
**1 cup cooked white beans**
**1 cup Corn, Orange, and Tomato Relish (page 371)**
**3 dashes of Tabasco sauce**
**Pinch of black pepper**
**Salt (optional)**

Sauté the garlic, onion, and celery in 3 tablespoons vegetable stock for 3 minutes over medium heat. Add the tomatoes and 4 cups of vegetable stock. Continue to cook for 10 minutes.

Add the remaining ingredients and cook for 10 more minutes, until the potato is soft. Adjust seasoning and serve.

*Serving size = 1 cup*
*188 calories*
*1.6 grams fat*
*0 milligram cholesterol*
*104.4 milligrams sodium without added salt*

## COLD CELERY SOUP WITH PINK RADISHES

Daniel Boulud

*This healthful and low-calorie soup combines character with an attractive presentation. The refreshing flavor of celery and the peppery taste of radish are enhanced by the curry powder. The soup can be prepared 6 to 8 hours in advance, cooled, covered with a plastic wrap, and refrigerated until ready to serve.*

SERVES 4

**Vegetable oil spray**
**2 cups leeks (about 2 medium), white part only, washed and thinly sliced**
**2 teaspoons mild curry powder**
**4 cups celery ribs, green part only, cleaned and finely sliced; reserve 8 celery leaves, chopped for decoration**
**5 cups Vegetable Stock (page 143) or water**
**½ cup potato, peeled and roughly chopped**
**Salt**
**Pepper**
**1 bunch small round pink radishes (about 6 pieces), cleaned, greens discarded, finely sliced with a vegetable cutter or mandoline (reserve 12 slices for decoration)**
**10 sprigs of parsley, stems only, cleaned**
**3 drops Tabasco**

Spray the inside of a large soup or stock pot with vegetable oil spray and place over medium heat. Add the sliced leeks, curry powder, and sliced celery. Stir with a wooden spoon for 5 to 6 minutes. Add the vegetable stock and diced potatoes and salt and pepper to taste. Bring to a boil and simmer gently for 15 minutes. Add the sliced radishes and parsley stems to the soup. Boil for 3 to 4 minutes. Pour the soup into the container of a blender and blend until very smooth. Add the Tabasco and mix well. Put the soup into a bowl and chill it on ice water to cool rapidly. When cold, season to taste, and refrigerate until needed.

Chill a soup tureen or bowl. Transfer the cold soup to the chilled soup tureen and decorate with the reserved slices of pink radishes. Sprinkle with the chopped celery leaves.

*Serving size = 1 cup*
*65 calories*
*0.5 gram fat*
*0 milligrams cholesterol*
*221.4 milligrams salt*

# Main-Course Vegetable Dishes

## BAKED BEANS, BOSTON STYLE

Deborah Madison

*Molasses, mustard, and long, slow cooking give Boston baked beans their characteristic flavor. Salt pork is traditional, too, but here, Bakon yeast contributes the smoky flavor instead. These beans spend many hours in a slow oven. A Crockpot would work fine, too.*

MAKES 6 CUPS
SERVES 6

**2½ cups dried navy or kidney beans, soaked 5 hours**
**⅓ cup molasses**
**¼ cup brown sugar**
**1 tablespoon dry mustard**
**¼ teaspoon cayenne**
**1 teaspoon Bakon yeast (available at health food stores)**
**2 teaspoons tamari**
**2 medium onions, chopped in large pieces**
**2 bay leaves**
**3 garlic cloves, minced**
**1 teaspoon salt**
**Freshly cracked pepper**

Preheat the oven to 300 degrees.

Drain the beans, cover with fresh water, and bring to a boil for 5 minutes, then drain again. Whisk together the molasses, sugar, mustard, cayenne, Bakon yeast, and tamari in a bowl, then mix with the beans and add the onions, bay leaves, garlic, salt, and pepper.

Place in a bean pot or 2-quart baking dish and add water to cover the beans. Cover and bake until the beans are very soft, 7 to 8 hours. Check periodically and add more water, if needed, to keep the beans from drying out. Remove the cover during the last half hour of cooking so a crust can form. Serve with corn bread and a salad.

*Serving size = 1 cup*
*401 calories*
*1.7 gram fat*
*0 milligrams cholesterol*
*21.7 milligrams sodium*

## ARTICHOKE HEART "BARIGOULE" ON A BED OF VEGETABLES ACCENTED WITH A BASIL AND GARLIC BROTH

Hubert Keller

*I always serve the artichokes in a shallow soup plate and give the diners a spoon with which to enjoy the broth. This dish has a pretty contrast of colors and a delightful taste that comes from the richness of the artichokes blended with all the fresh herbs and vegetables.*

SERVES 4

**4 medium artichokes**
**Juice of 1 lemon**
**1 onion, peeled**
**1 carrot, peeled**
**4 garlic cloves**
**6 basil leaves**

**1 small leek**
**3 cups Vegetable Consommé (page 147)**
**1 cup dry white wine**
**2 bay leaves**
**1 sprig of thyme**
**Freshly ground pepper**
**12 snow peas, blanched (page 131)**
**12 asparagus tips, blanched (page 131)**
**1 tomato, peeled, seeded, and diced**
**1 teaspoon finely chopped parsley**
**1 teaspoon finely chopped chives**
**4 sprigs of chervil, chopped**

Cut the stems off the artichokes. Cut away all the leaves and remove the choke with a spoon. Trim the bottoms, but leave a bit of the stem end attached. As you work, dip the cut edges of the artichoke bottoms into a bowl of water mixed with the lemon juice to keep them from darkening. Leave the artichokes in this acidulated water until you are ready to cook them. Slice the onion and carrot into thin slices. Finely chop 2 garlic cloves with the basil leaves and set aside. Cut the leek into julienne and wash.

Heat the vegetable consommé and white wine in a stockpot. Add the carrot, onion, and leek. Bring to a boil and lower the heat to barely simmering. Add the artichoke hearts, bay leaves, thyme, 2 whole garlic cloves, and pepper. Cook for 20 to 25 minutes. While this is simmering, blanch the peas and asparagus tips. Also peel, seed, and dice the tomato. Carefully transfer the artichokes to a warm serving platter and cover with aluminum foil to keep them hot.

Add the chopped garlic and basil, parsley, chives, tomato, asparagus tips, and snow peas to the broth and vegetable mixture. Bring to a boil over high heat and stir slightly. Taste and add pepper if necessary. Gently spoon the broth and vegetable ragout over the artichoke hearts. Serve hot or warm. Sprinkle with chervil.

*Serving size = 1 artichoke + 1 cup of vegetable stew*
*129 calories*

*0.6 gram fat*
*0 milligrams cholesterol*
*77.5 milligrams sodium*

## PHYLLO WITH SPINACH, RAISINS, AND ROSEMARY

Donna Nicoletti

*This is a typical Mediterranean combination of ingredients. The phyllo, which bakes golden brown, crisp, and light without fat, can be served as an elegant main course.*

SERVES 4

**3 large bunches of spinach**
**½ cup white wine or vegetable stock**
**1 teaspoon chopped garlic**
**2 teaspoons chopped fresh rosemary**
**Salt**
**Freshly ground pepper**
**⅓ cup raisins**
**1 tablespoon chopped onion**
**¼ cup water**
**½ pound oil-free, fat-free phyllo dough**
**Fine bread crumbs**
**1 tablespoon chopped parsley**
**1 egg white, lightly beaten**

Cut off the stems of the spinach, and wash and dry well. In a large sauté pan, put the wine or stock and garlic, add the spinach, simmer, and braise in batches if necessary until wilted. Drain completely and squeeze out excess liquid. It is important to remove as much liquid as possible or the dish will become soggy. Toss the spinach with the rosemary and season with salt and pepper. In a blender, mix the raisins, onion, and water together and blend to a puree.

Preheat oven to 350 degrees.

While working with the phyllo dough, keep it covered with a clean, damp cloth, as it dries out very quickly. Lay out one sheet of phyllo and brush lightly with the raisin and onion mixture. Make sure you cover the entire piece of phyllo to the corners but that the mixture is not thick. Sprinkle about 2 teaspoons of the bread crumbs over the sheet, then sprinkle ¼ of the parsley. Lay out another sheet of phyllo over the first and repeat. Continue until 5 sheets have been laid down, but do not cover the fifth sheet with the raisin mixture.

On the fifth sheet, scatter the spinach over the sheet, leaving a 1-inch border all around. Roll the phyllo tightly lengthwise like a jelly roll and use a bit of the raisin mixture to seal the end seam. Twist the edges to prevent the filling from leaking out. Put the roll on a very lightly oiled cookie sheet and brush the top with egg white. Bake in the oven for approximately 30 minutes or until golden brown. Allow the roll to cool slightly for 15 minutes before cutting. Cut on a diagonal in ½-inch-wide slices. Serve immediately or at room temperature.

*Serving size = ¾ cup*
*167 calories*
*1.2 grams fat*
*0 milligram cholesterol*
*329.8 milligrams sodium without added salt*

## A SUCCULENT TRUFFLED POTATO STEW

Hubert Keller

*Always remember that truffles are not a vegetable but a miracle! Nevertheless, this is a wonderful potato stew even without them.*

SERVES 6 TO 8

**3 pounds young potatoes**
**2 garlic cloves, finely chopped**
**1 onion, diced**
**3 tablespoons coarsely chopped carrot**

**3 tablespoons coarsely chopped celery**
**1 small leek, white part only, finely julienned**
**1 cup dry white wine**
**2½ cups Vegetable Consommé (page 147)**
**1 sprig of thyme**
**Freshly ground pepper**
**16 blanched asparagus tips**
**1½ ounces fresh black or white truffles**
**2 tablespoons finely chopped chives**

Peel the potatoes and cut them into ½-inch dice. Transfer to a heavy pot and add the garlic, onion, carrot, celery, leek, wine, consommé, thyme, and pepper. If the potatoes are not covered completely, add water. Cover and cook until the potatoes are fork-tender and the liquid has nearly cooked off. If the stew becomes too dry before the potatoes are ready, add additional consommé or water. Turn the stew into a deep warm platter and garnish with the warmed asparagus tips. Shave the truffles over the potatoes and sprinkle with chives. Serve immediately.

NOTE: The season for fresh truffles is usually from mid-December to mid-March. Frozen truffles, which are much more aromatic and flavorful than canned, can be substituted for fresh.

*Serving size = 1½ cups*
*190 calories*
*0.3 gram fat*
*0 milligrams cholesterol*
*21.8 milligrams sodium*

## SPRING VEGETABLE RAGOUT ACCENTED WITH AN HERBAL CONSOMMÉ

Hubert Keller

SERVES 4

**CONSOMMÉ**

**1 medium leek, white part only, washed and dried**
**1 celery stalk, diced**
**3 medium carrots, diced**
**4 shallots, coarsely chopped**
**1 large tomato, peeled, seeded, and roughly chopped**
**3 garlic cloves, coarsely chopped**
**10 white mushrooms, diced**
**3 sprigs of parsley**
**1 small bunch of chervil**
**8 basil leaves**
**1 sprig of thyme**
**2 bay leaves**
**2 sprigs of cilantro**
**12 whole peppercorns**

**VEGETABLE RAGOUT**

**4 cauliflower florets**
**4 broccoli florets**
**8 baby turnips with tops, peeled**
**8 asparagus tips, cut 2 inches long**
**16 baby carrots with tops, peeled**
**8 small spring onions, peeled**
**4 tablespoons freshly shelled peas**
**1 tomato, peeled, seeded, and diced**
**Freshly ground pepper**
**Several sprigs of fresh chervil**

Prepare the herbal consommé.

Combine all the ingredients in a nonreactive pot. Cover with cold water. Bring to a boil, then turn the heat down to a light simmer. Cover tightly. Simmer very slowly for 35 minutes. Turn off the heat, keep the cover on, and cool completely. Strain the broth carefully through a fine strainer; do not press down on the vegetables. Set aside.

Next, make the ragout.

Cook each vegetable separately in small amounts of the consommé until tender. Cool. Arrange the vegetables decoratively in individual shallow soup plates. Spoon the heated herbal consommé over the vegetables, season with pepper, and sprinkle with chervil.

*Serving size = 1 cup*
*104 calories*
*0.8 gram fat*
*0 milligrams cholesterol*
*84 milligrams sodium*

## BAKED TOFU CUTLETS

Lydia Karpenko

*This cutlet is a wonderful meat substitute. It stands well on its own merit and works even better in a sandwich. Serve it on a piece of good country bread with nonfat mayonnaise, lettuce, tomatoes, and shredded green onions.*

SERVES 4

**16 ounces firm tofu**
**4 tablespoons fresh lime juice**
**4 tablespoons soy sauce**
**1 teaspoon honey**
**1 teaspoon minced fresh gingerroot**
**1 teaspoon minced garlic**
**1 teaspoon chili sauce**

Slice the tofu into 4 slices lengthwise. Set aside.

In a flat pan or nonstick baking dish just large enough to hold the slices in a single layer, combine the lime juice, soy sauce, honey, ginger, garlic, and chili sauce. Place the tofu in the marinade and refrigerate for at least 2 or up to 6 hours, turning occasionally.

Preheat the oven to 350 degrees.

Remove the dish from the refrigerator and bring to room temperature. Bake for 45 minutes.

*Serving size = 1 cutlet*
*108 calories*
*2 grams fat*
*0 milligrams cholesterol*
*1,054 milligrams sodium*

## STUFFED TOMATOES WITH FRENCH LENTILS

Jean-Marc Fullsack

*Serve with a salad and some crusty bread for a delicious lunch or light dinner.*

SERVES 6

**3 cups vegetable stock**
**1 cup dried lentils**
**1 cup chopped onions**
**¼ cup chopped celery**
**1 tablespoon minced garlic**
**6 tomatoes, peeled, seeded, and hollowed out**
**1 bunch spinach, blanched and refreshed**
**White Bean Sauce (page 352)**

Preheat the oven to 350 degrees.

In a large saucepan, combine the vegetable stock, lentils, onions, celery, and garlic. Bring to a boil. Reduce the heat and simmer for 35 minutes, or until the lentils are just tender but not mushy. Set aside for 15 minutes.

Fill each hollowed-out tomato with the lentil stuffing and top with blanched spinach.

Ladle the White Bean Sauce into a large nonstick baking dish and set the tomatoes on top. Bake, covered, at 350 degrees for 10 minutes, or until heated through.

*Serving size = 1 tomato and ½ cup White Bean Sauce*
*198 calories*
*1.4 grams fat*
*0 milligrams cholesterol*
*322 milligrams sodium*

## VEGETABLE BROCHETTES

Jean-Marc Fullsack

*Serve these over rice or Kashe (page 334). Orzo with Lemon and Herbs (page 314) would go particularly well.*

SERVES 4

**3 tablespoons soy sauce**
**2 tablespoons mirin**
**1 teaspoon minced garlic**
**⅛ teaspoon black pepper**
**½ pound firm tofu, cubed**
**½ pound kabocha squash, cut into 1-inch chunks and boiled 5 minutes (or substitute acorn or butternut squash)**
**1 red bell pepper, seeded and cut into 1-inch pieces**
**1 yellow bell pepper, seeded and cut into 1-inch pieces**
**1 zucchini, sliced 1 inch thick**
**1 yellow zucchini, sliced 1 inch thick**
**4 cherry tomatoes**
**Carrot and Ginger Sauce (page 352)**

In a medium-sized bowl, combine the soy sauce, mirin, garlic, and pepper; add the tofu. Marinate for 30 minutes.

In a large nonstick pan, sauté each vegetable (except the tomatoes) separately until brightly colored and partially cooked. Drain the tofu and sauté.

Thread the vegetables and tofu with the tomatoes onto bamboo skewers and grill until tender but not overcooked. Serve with the Carrot and Ginger Sauce.

NOTE: If you do not have access to a grill, the skewers can be placed under an oven broiler.

*Serving size = 1 cup*
*107 calories*
*1.5 grams fat*
*0 milligrams cholesterol*
*838.9 milligrams sodium*

## SCRAMBLED MEXICAN TOFU

Jean-Marc Fullsack

*Serve over a tortilla and with a side of chili and salsa for brunch for a wonderful version of* huevos rancheros. *Once you have had these, you'll find no reason ever to serve scrambled eggs again.*

MAKES 6 CUPS
SERVES 6

**3 cups egg whites, about 24 eggs' worth**
**½ pound soft tofu**
**3 tablespoons soy sauce**
**1 teaspoon turmeric**
**¼ teaspoon ground black pepper**
**1 fresh tomato, peeled, seeded, and diced**
**½ cup diced onions**
**2 garlic cloves, minced**
**2 tablespoons chopped roasted green chili**
**⅛ teaspoon ground cumin**
**6 tablespoons chopped fresh chives or cilantro**

In a small bowl, beat the egg whites until broken up and just beginning to foam. Crumble the tofu finely and add to the egg mixture. Add the soy sauce, turmeric, and pepper. Set aside.

In a large nonstick skillet, sweat the tomato, onions, garlic, chili, and cumin until the onion is translucent and all the liquid has evaporated.

Add the egg white and tofu mixture. Stir well with a wooden spoon and scramble over medium heat until the egg whites are thoroughly cooked. Toss in chives or cilantro. Serve hot.

*Serving size = 1 cup*
*109 calories*
*2.0 grams fat*
*0 milligrams cholesterol*
*702 milligrams sodium*

## RATATOUILLE IN PHYLLO DOUGH

Hubert Keller

*This would be nice served alongside a salad of baby lettuces and fresh herbs dressed with lemon juice and freshly ground pepper.*

SERVES 4

- **Vegetable oil spray for pan coating**
- **2 Japanese eggplants, cut into ¼-inch cubes**
- **2 small green zucchini (1-inch diameter), cut into ¼-inch cubes**
- **2 small yellow zucchini (1-inch diameter), cut into ¼-inch cubes**
- **1 sweet, firm red pepper, cored, seeded, and cut into ¼-inch cubes**
- **1 medium yellow onion, finely chopped**
- **2 garlic cloves, chopped**
- **2 medium tomatoes, peeled, seeded, and diced**
- **Freshly ground pepper**
- **Salt (optional)**
- **½ teaspoon chopped fresh thyme**
- **6 to 8 fresh basil leaves, chopped**

**1 teaspoon mustard seeds (soaked overnight in ⅓ cup white wine, ⅔ cup water, and a dash of vinegar)**
**8 15 × 10-inch sheets oil-free, fat-free phyllo dough**

Spray a nonstick frying pan lightly with pan coating. Over medium heat, sauté the eggplants until soft. Place the eggplants in a mixing bowl. Repeat with the zucchinis and pepper.

Sauté the chopped onions in the same pan until light golden in color. Add the chopped garlic, diced tomatoes, pepper, and salt. Lower the heat and simmer. Add the sautéed vegetables and toss gently over moderate heat for 5 to 8 minutes. Stir in the chopped thyme, basil, and drained mustard seeds. Cool.

Preheat the oven to 325 degrees.

Lay one sheet of phyllo dough on a work surface and spray lightly with the coating. Cover the first layer of phyllo with a second layer and spray again. Divide it, using a sharp, pointed knife, into 4 6 × 7-inch rectangles. Spread 2 tablespoons of the ratatouille in the center of each rectangle. Fold the phyllo over the ratatouille, making sure that everything is completely enclosed, forming a package. Place the package, seam side down, on baker's parchment. Continue, to make 4 packages altogether.

The phyllo packages can be refrigerated a day before baking. Bake until the dough turns golden brown, about 6 to 8 minutes. Serve immediately.

*Serving size = ⅔ cup (one package)*
*194 calories*
*1.8 grams fat*
*0 milligrams cholesterol*
*251 milligrams sodium without added salt*

## ENCHILADAS WITH VEGETARIAN BEAN STEW AND TOMATILLO SAUCE

Jean-Marc Fullsack

*Serve this with Spanish Rice (page 333). You can prepare this 24 hours ahead of time but the tortillas will become quite soft. The Tomatillo Sauce has a fresh and slightly tart flavor with a delicate texture.*

MAKES 12 ENCHILADAS
SERVES 4 TO 6

**1 cup black beans, soaked overnight**
**1 cup red beans, soaked overnight**
**6 cups vegetable stock**
**1 bay leaf**
**2 cups (approximately 1 pound) tomatoes, diced**
**1 large onion, oven roasted (page 133) and chopped**
**1 cup fresh corn kernels**
**1 cup diced green bell pepper**
**½ cup diced red bell pepper**
**2 ounces smoked tofu, diced**
**1 tablespoon minced garlic**
**2 teaspoons ground cumin**
**⅛ teaspoon red chili pepper flakes**
**Freshly ground black pepper**
**Salt**
**12 corn tortillas**
**Fresh chopped cilantro**
**Tomatillo Sauce (recipe follows)**

In a large saucepan, combine the soaked beans, vegetable stock, and bay leaf. Bring to a boil, reduce the heat, and simmer, covered, for 45 minutes, or until the beans are tender. Add the tomatoes, onion, corn, green pepper, red pepper, tofu, garlic, cumin, and chili flakes. Simmer for 15 minutes. Season to taste with pepper and salt.

Preheat the oven to 350 degrees.

Steam the corn tortillas until soft enough to roll without

breaking. Using a slotted spoon, fill each tortilla with a generous ½ cup of beans. Roll and place, seam side down, in a nonstick or lightly oiled baking dish. Pour the beans and their sauce over the stuffed tortillas and bake for 15 minutes, or until bubbling hot. Garnish with the cilantro and serve with tomatillo sauce.

## TOMATILLO SAUCE

MAKES 3 CUPS

**1 pound fresh tomatillos, husked**
**1 cup oven-roasted (page 133) and chopped onion**
**1 cup vegetable stock**
**4 teaspoons minced garlic**
**1 tablespoon minced serrano chili**
**¼ teaspoon cider vinegar**
**Pinch of ground cumin**
**Pinch of sugar**
**½ cup chopped fresh cilantro**
**Salt**

Preheat the oven to 350 degrees.

On a parchment-lined baking sheet, roast the tomatillos for 30 minutes, or until very soft but not split. Coarsely chop them.

In a large saucepan, combine the tomatillos, onion, vegetable stock, garlic, chili, vinegar, cumin, and sugar. Bring to a boil. Reduce the heat and simmer, covered, for 20 minutes. Add the chopped cilantro and transfer to a blender or food processor. Puree until smooth. Season to taste with salt.

*Serving size = 2 enchiladas*
*316 calories*
*3.3 grams fat*
*0 milligrams cholesterol*
*193.1 milligrams sodium without added salt*

## SPINACH AND ROASTED PEPPER TART WITH PICO DE GALLO SALSA

Jean-Marc Fullsack

*For an interesting presentation, roast an additional red pepper and make a lattice work of julienned slices over the tart before baking. This would be very nice with a pasta salad and the Pico de Gallo Salsa (recipe follows).*

MAKES 1 TART
SERVES 6

**1 pound spinach leaves, blanched, squeezed, and chopped**
**2 cups nonfat cottage cheese (16 ounces)**
**1 cup egg whites (approximately 8 eggs)**
**½ cup chopped parsley**
**1 teaspoon salt**
**½ teaspoon black pepper**
**⅛ teaspoon ground nutmeg**
**2 14 × 18-inch sheets fat-free, oil-free phyllo dough**
**2 onions, oven roasted (page 133) and chopped**
**8 ounces smoked tofu, diced**
**1 pound red bell peppers (about 7 peppers), roasted, peeled, and diced (page 133)**

Preheat the oven to 400 degrees.

In a food processor, combine the spinach, cottage cheese, egg whites, parsley, salt, pepper, and nutmeg. Blend well.

Line a 9-inch quiche pan with phyllo dough. Trim the edges with a pair of scissors. Sprinkle the onions and tofu over the bottom of the pan. Pour the spinach mixture over the onions and tofu. Sprinkle the diced red peppers over the top of the tart.

Bake for 30 to 45 minutes, or until a toothpick inserted into the center comes out clean. The center should be barely firm—take care not to overbake. Serve at room temperature.

## PICO DE GALLO SALSA

*This can be prepared up to 3 days ahead of time, though the tomatoes will release some of their juices.*

MAKES 1¼ CUPS

**1 cup tomatoes, peeled, seeded, and diced**
**¼ cup chopped red onion**
**2 tablespoons minced jalapeño pepper**
**1 tablespoon chopped fresh cilantro**
**1 tablespoon fresh lime juice**
**Salt**

In a medium bowl, combine all the ingredients. Mix thoroughly. Season to taste with salt.

*Serving size = ⅙ of tart*
*209 calories*
*1.5 grams fat*
*3.3 milligrams cholesterol*
*805 milligrams sodium*

## CARIBBEAN CURRY

Dennis and Margaret Malone

*This curry is a delightful alternative to the more common East Indian-style curries. Thai green curry paste is a mixture of galanga (a hot ginger), hot green chilies, lemongrass, and Thai basil (a plant similar to the more familiar "sweet" basil but whose leaves have a hotter, more peppery flavor).*

SERVES 4 TO 6

**1½ cups water or vegetable stock**
**1 cup diced onion**
**1 large sweet red pepper, seeded and sliced into ¼-inch strips**

- **2 cups chopped fresh tomatoes**
- **1 tablespoon minced fresh garlic**
- **1 tablespoon minced fresh gingerroot**
- **1 teaspoon Thai green curry paste, or 1 large jalapeño, seeded and finely minced**
- **1 tablespoon ground coriander**
- **1 teaspoon turmeric**
- **1 teaspoon paprika**
- **¼ teaspoon cayenne or to taste**
- **¼ teaspoon ground cardamom**
- **1 cup broccoli florets, cut into ¾-inch pieces and blanched for 3 minutes (page 131)**
- **1½ cups fresh papaya, cut into ½-inch dice**
- **1 cup or 30 sugar snap peas or snow peas, lightly steamed (page 134)**
- **2 tablespoons fresh lime juice**
- **Salt**
- **Freshly ground black pepper**
- **Thin slices of lime (optional)**
- **Sprigs of fresh mint (optional)**

Put the water, onion, and red pepper in a large skillet. Cover and cook over medium heat for about 5 minutes, or until the onion is tender. Add the tomatoes, garlic, gingerroot, green curry paste, and all the spices. Continue to cook, stirring frequently, for about 10 minutes, uncovered, until the sauce thickens.

Add the broccoli, papaya, and the peas, warming them for 1 to 2 minutes. Stir in the lime juice and season to taste with salt and pepper. Serve over Island Rice (page 328) and with the Pear-Jalapeño Raita (page 375). Garnish with slices of lime and sprigs of mint as desired.

*Serving size = 1 cup*
*76 calories*
*0.7 gram fat*
*0 milligrams cholesterol*
*64.3 milligrams sodium without added salt*

## TOFU WITH BLACK BEAN SAUCE

Jean-Marc Fullsack

*This makes a hearty meal for a cold night. Serve it with plain steamed rice.*

MAKES 12 CUPS
SERVES 6

**½ ounce dried shiitake mushrooms**
**1 ounce dried bean curd**
**1 teaspoon Chinese black beans, lightly crushed**
**3 cups carrots, cut in ⅛-inch slices**
**3 cups green bell peppers, cut in ⅛-inch slices**
**2 cups thinly sliced onions**
**1 cup thinly sliced celery**
**2 teaspoons minced garlic**
**1 teaspoon fresh minced gingerroot**
**2 cups vegetable stock**
**½ cup sliced canned bamboo shoots**
**¼ cup low-sodium soy sauce**
**¼ cup sake**
**2 tablespoons ketchup**
**1 tablespoon honey**
**1 pound firm tofu, cut in ½-inch cubes**
**2 cups mung bean sprouts**
**2 tablespoons cornstarch (dissolved in 4 tablespoons cold water)**

In a medium-sized bowl, cover the mushrooms with warm water and soak for 15 to 20 minutes, or until soft. Drain, reserving the liquid, and set aside.

In a large flat dish, soak the dried bean curd in 1 cup of warm water for 5 minutes, or until soft. Drain and set aside.

In a small bowl, soak the black beans in ¼ cup water for 15 to 20 minutes, or until soft. Drain and set aside.

In a large saucepan, sauté the carrots, peppers, onions, celery, garlic, and ginger in ¼ cup vegetable stock for 5 minutes, or until almost tender. Add the remaining vegetable stock, black beans, shiitake mushrooms, and reserved liquid. Add the bean curd, bamboo shoots, ½ cup warm water, soy sauce, sake, ketchup, and honey. Stir well to combine.

Bring to a boil, reduce the heat, and simmer for 10 minutes. Add the tofu and simmer for 10 minutes. Add the bean sprouts and simmer for 2 to 3 minutes more. Add the dissolved cornstarch, stir well, and continue to simmer until the sauce has thickened. Serve in bowls over rice.

*Serving size = 2 cups*
*189 calories*
*2.1 grams fat*
*0 milligrams cholesterol*
*826.3 milligrams sodium*

## MEXICAN SUMMER STEW

Anita and Joseph Cecena

*This is flavorful and makes a hearty meal when served with fresh tortillas and a crunchy green salad.*

MAKES 12 CUPS
SERVES 6 TO 12

**3 cups vegetable stock**
**3 cups texturized vegetable protein chunks (page 120)**
**1 tablespoon ketchup**
**2 onions, sliced ¼ inch thick**
**2 teaspoons minced garlic**
**1 cup white wine**
**6 small zucchini, sliced ½ inch thick**
**4 small yellow crookneck squashes, sliced**
**1 green bell pepper, cut in ½-inch dice**
**2 cups trimmed snow peas**
**3 cups chopped tomatoes**
**3 tablespoons low-sodium soy sauce**
**3 tablespoons chili powder**
**1 tablespoon ground cumin**

**2 cups fresh or frozen corn kernels**
**1 tablespoon cornstarch or arrowroot**
**¼ cup cold water**
**¼ cup chopped fresh cilantro**

In a large saucepan, bring the stock to a boil. Add the vegetable protein and ketchup and remove the pot from the heat. Allow to rest for 10 minutes, or until all the liquid is absorbed. Set aside.

In a large, nonstick sauté pan, braise the onions and garlic in ½ cup white wine for 5 minutes, or until tender. Add the zucchini, squashes, green pepper, snow peas, tomatoes, the rest of the wine, soy sauce, chili powder, and cumin. Simmer for 5 to 10 minutes, or until the vegetables are just al dente. Drain the vegetable protein and add it, along with the corn, and simmer for an additional 10 minutes.

While the stew is simmering during its final minutes, dissolve the cornstarch in ¼ cup cold water and add it to the stew. Stir until thickened. Garnish with cilantro and serve hot.

*Serving size = 1 cup*
*142 calories*
*1.9 grams fat*
*0 milligrams cholesterol*
*205.9 milligrams sodium*

## VEGETABLES BAKED IN PARCHMENT

Paul Bertolli

*This dish is flexible and can serve either as a first or main course. As a main dish, it is complete in itself.*

*Cooking without fats or oils puts greater pressure on the components of a dish to deliver flavor. This recipe will be most successful if you choose vegetables that are at their peak and freshly picked. Cooking vegetables in parchment is certainly one of the best ways to seal in their flavor, as none of the juices can escape. Nor does their combined aroma release until the package is peeled open at the table to the surprised pleasure of your guests.*

*Due to the ever-changing availability of seasonal vegetables, the following recipe is meant as a guideline. You may wish to forgo the peas (for instance, if they are starchy) in favor of asparagus. Or you could substitute artichokes for the fennel. The recipe is forgiving enough to permit these differences. It is advisable, nevertheless, to cut like-textured vegetables, other than those listed here, similarly—for instance, parsnips like carrots, potatoes like beets, celery like fennel, and so on. This will ensure that they cook properly.*

*The simplest way to cook vegetables in parchment is in the oven on a preheated baking sheet. However, you may wish to cook the packages in the coals of the fireplace or grill if you are eating outdoors. If so, wrap the vegetables in an additional layer of heavy-duty foil, lay down a bed of ash over the coals, and allow about 25 minutes for the vegetables to cook.*

SERVES 6

**2 cups thinly sliced fennel bulb**
**¾ cup shelled peas**
**⅔ cup scallions, roots trimmed, cut into 1-inch lengths and split vertically**
**1⅓ cups golden beets, peeled and sliced very thin**
**1 heaping cup yellow or green zucchini, cut into ¼-inch dice**
**1 heaping cup tender string beans, cut into 2-inch lengths**
**1 heaping cup sliced mushrooms**
**1 cup julienned carrots**
**1 cup small turnips, sliced ⅛ inch thick**
**Salt**
**Pepper**
**1 heaping tablespoon chopped fresh tarragon**
**1 tablespoon chopped fresh chives**
**Kitchen parchment paper**
**6 tablespoons water**

Preheat the oven to 400 degrees.

Place 2 standard cookie sheet pans in the oven to warm.

Combine all the vegetables in a large bowl, season them

with salt and pepper, add the fresh tarragon and chives, and mix well. Cut 6 lengths of parchment paper about 18 × 12 inches. Lay the parchment sheets out on a work surface lengthwise. Distribute the vegetables evenly in a mound about a third of the way from the bottom ends. Pour 1 tablespoon of water over each mound of vegetables. Fold the top end over the vegetables to meet the bottom edge. Beginning at either folded corner, make little tight overlapping folds. Proceed all the way around the open side of the parchment until you reach the other corner, then twist the paper to seal the package.

Arrange the packages on the hot pans. Bake for 18 to 20 minutes. The parchment paper will swell and turn a light brown. Serve on warm oval plates immediately and open at the table.

*Serving size = 1 cup*
*94 calories*
*0.6 gram fat*
*0 milligrams cholesterol*
*106.2 milligrams sodium without added salt*

## BEAN BURGERS

Anita Cecena

*This is very easy to prepare and with great results. Serve it with fresh lettuce and tomatoes on a hearty roll. It is also quite satisfying on its own with salsa and nonfat yogurt drizzled over the top.*

MAKES 6 5-INCH BURGERS
SERVES 6

**½ cup minced green onions**
**1½ tablespoons minced garlic**
**2 tablespoons white wine or vegetable stock**
**1 29-ounce can cooked drained pinto beans**
**¾ cup cracker meal**
**2 egg whites**

- ½ **cup chopped fresh parsley**
- 2 **tablespoons seasoned rice vinegar**
- ½ **teaspoon Spike seasoning powder (found in health food stores) or A Little Italian (page 148)**

Preheat the oven to 350 degrees.

In a small nonstick sauté pan, braise the onions and garlic in the white wine until soft.

In a medium bowl, combine the sautéed onions and garlic, beans, cracker meal, egg whites, parsley, vinegar, and seasoning powder. Mash well with a fork or potato masher until blended but not entirely smooth.

On a parchment-lined nonstick baking sheet, drop the mixture by ½-cup amounts and flatten gently with a spoon to form 6 5-inch "burgers." Bake for 25 minutes, or until set and beginning to brown lightly. Serve hot.

*Serving size = 1 5-inch burger*
*179 calories*
*2 grams fat*
*0 milligrams cholesterol*
*738.2 milligrams sodium*

## VEGETABLE STRUDEL

Jean-Marc Fullsack

*This is a very impressive dish to serve, with a delicate flavor that is nicely set off by the Shallot and Mustard Sauce (page 359). Use your favorite combination of vegetables and chop them if you wish. Stir yogurt cheese into the vegetables before wrapping to create a creamy rich filling.*

*This could also be formed into individual portions by starting with 2 sheets of phyllo folded in half to form 4 smaller sheets. The end result will give you more crispy phyllo per portion.*

*When using phyllo, work quickly to prevent it from drying out, for the dough will become brittle and impossible to work with. Keep the phyllo covered with a lightly dampened towel or piece of plastic wrap as you work.*

SERVES 4

**1 large artichoke heart, julienned (heart of a 1-pound artichoke)**
**½ cup julienned and blanched carrot (page 131)**
**1 cup julienned and blanched leek (white part only) (page 131)**
**½ cup 2-inch-length sliced green beans, blanched (page 131)**
**½ cup julienned and blanched fennel bulb**
**½ cup julienned and blanched celery**
**½ cup julienned and blanched mushrooms**
**½ cup peeled, seeded, and julienned apple**
**1 tablespoon chopped fresh parsley**
**1 tablespoon chopped fresh basil**
**1 tablespoon chopped fresh tarragon**
**Freshly ground black pepper**
**Salt**
**4 sheets fat-free, oil-free phyllo dough**
**1 egg white**
**½ teaspoon poppy seeds**
**Parchment paper**
**Shallot and Mustard Sauce (page 359)**

Preheat the oven to 425 degrees.

In a large bowl, combine the artichoke, carrot, leek, green beans, fennel, celery, mushrooms, and apple. Add the parsley, basil, and tarragon. Season to taste with the pepper and salt. Toss well to distribute the herbs and seasonings.

Place the phyllo sheets on a clean dry 15 × 19-inch piece of parchment paper. Quickly spread the vegetable mixture over the center of the sheet, leaving a 2-inch border on each side.

Brush the borders of the phyllo with the egg white and roll the phyllo into a cylinder starting at one of the 18-inch sides. Brush the underside of the 2 ends with egg white and fold the ends under the cylinder to seal. Brush the top of the cylinder with egg white and sprinkle the poppy seeds over it.

Using parchment paper to help lift it, carefully transfer the finished cylinder to a baking sheet. Bake for 20 minutes, or until golden brown. Slice into pieces and serve warm with the Shallot and Mustard Sauce.

*Serving size = ¾ cup*
*153 calories*
*1.4 grams fat*
*0.1 milligram cholesterol*
*385.2 milligrams sodium without added salt*

## TOFU STEW WITH SWEET POTATOES

Jean-Marc Fullsack

*This is a terrific substitute for the kind of meat-based stew that warms a winter meal. It has the same satisfying bold flavors and chunky vegetables but none of the fat.*

MAKES 8 CUPS
SERVES 4 TO 6

**2 cups vegetable stock**
**2 cups sweet potatoes, cut into ½-inch diamond shapes**
**1 cup chopped onions**
**½ cup chopped celery**
**½ cup quartered button mushrooms**
**½ cup turnips, cut into ½-inch diamond shapes**
**½ cup parsnips, cut into ½-inch diamond shapes**
**½ cup sliced carrots**
**½ cup low-sodium soy sauce**
**½ cup mirin**
**¼ cup sake**
**4 garlic cloves, peeled and sliced**
**1 teaspoon minced fresh gingerroot**
**½ cup ¼-inch-sliced yellow squash**
**½ cup ¼-inch-sliced zucchini**
**12 ounces tofu, pressed and cubed**
**Freshly ground black pepper**

**Szechuan peppercorns**
**Salt**
**3 to 4 green onions, chopped**

In a large saucepan, combine the stock, sweet potatoes, onions, celery, mushrooms, turnips, parsnips, carrots, soy sauce, mirin, sake, garlic, and ginger. Bring to a boil. Reduce the heat and simmer for 25 minutes.

Add the zucchini and yellow squash. Simmer for an additional 5 minutes. Add the tofu and simmer 5 minutes more. Season to taste with the pepper, Szechuan peppercorns, and salt. Garnish with chopped green onions and serve.

*Serving size = 1½ cups*
*232 calories*
*3.6 grams fat*
*0 milligrams cholesterol*
*1,589 milligrams sodium*

## TOFU GUMBO

Jean-Marc Fullsack

*This vegetarian gumbo is very high in protein because of the inclusion of the tofu. Serve this rendition of a classic southwestern dish over rice with a slice of corn bread on the side.*

SERVES 6 TO 9

**2 cups diced yellow onions**
**2 cups vegetable stock**
**1½ cups canned crushed Italian tomatoes**
**½ cup ¼-inch sliced carrots**
**1 cup ¼-inch-sliced celery**
**4 cups ¼-inch-sliced okra**
**1 cup diced red bell peppers**
**1 cup diced green bell peppers**
**1 cup sliced yellow squash**
**½ cup fresh corn kernels**

**6 garlic cloves, peeled and sliced**
**1 tablespoon Cajun Spice (page 150)**
**1 teaspoon paprika**
**½ teaspoon fenugreek**
**¼ teaspoon red pepper flakes**
**10 ounces tofu, pressed and cubed**
**Freshly ground black pepper**
**Salt**

In a large saucepan, combine the onions, vegetable stock, tomatoes, carrots, and celery. Bring to a boil and simmer for 10 minutes.

Add the okra, red and green bell peppers, yellow squash, corn, garlic, Cajun Spice, paprika, fenugreek, and red pepper flakes. Continue simmering for another 10 minutes. Add the tofu and simmer an additional 10 minutes. Season to taste with pepper and salt. Serve hot.

*Serving size = 1 cup*
*116 calories*
*2.3 grams fat*
*0 milligrams cholesterol*
*152 milligrams sodium without added salt*

## HALF-HOUR CHILI

*Eating Well* magazine

*You will not miss the beef in this hearty chili. Bulgur adds texture to the spicy mixture of vegetables and beans.*

SERVES 4

**4 tablespoons vegetable stock**
**3 onions, chopped**
**1 carrot, chopped**
**1 tablespoon minced jalapeño pepper (fresh or canned)**
**2 garlic cloves, minced**
**3 to 4 teaspoons chili powder**

**1 teaspoon ground cumin**
**1 28-ounce can plus 1 14-ounce can tomatoes, chopped with their juice**
**1 teaspoon brown sugar**
**2 15-ounce cans red kidney beans, drained and rinsed**
**⅓ cup fine or medium-grain bulgur**
**½ cup nonfat plain yogurt**
**⅓ cup chopped scallions**
**¼ cup chopped fresh cilantro or parsley**

In a Dutch oven or a large saucepan, heat the vegetable stock over medium heat. Add the onions, carrot, jalapeño peppers, garlic, chili powder, and cumin. Braise, covered, for 5 to 7 minutes, or until the onions and carrots are soft.

Add the tomatoes with their juice and the sugar; cook for 5 minutes over high heat. Stir in the beans and bulgur, and reduce heat to low. Simmer the chili, uncovered, for 15 minutes, or until thickened.

Serve with yogurt, scallions, and cilantro or parsley on the side.

*Serving size = 1½ cups*
*119 calories*
*0.9 gram fat*
*0.2 milligram cholesterol*
*489.8 milligrams sodium*

## PEA AND CORN PANCAKES

Jean-Marc Fullsack

*Serve these savory pancakes with an eggplant or roasted bell pepper dish. It would also work well with the Carrot and Ginger Sauce (page 352).*

SERVES 6 (2 PANCAKES EACH)

**1 cup frozen green peas**
**4 egg whites**
**¾ cup nonfat milk**

**1 cup unbleached white flour**
**1 cup fresh or frozen corn kernels, cooked**
**3 tablespoons chopped fresh parsley**
**¾ teaspoon salt**
**¼ teaspoon freshly ground black pepper**

In a blender or food processor, combine the peas, egg whites, and nonfat milk. Add the flour and blend until smooth. Add the corn, parsley, salt, and pepper. Blend just to combine.

Ladle ¼ cup batter onto a hot nonstick griddle or sauté pan. Cook over medium heat until golden brown. Flip and cook the second side. Repeat with the remaining batter. Serve immediately.

*Variation:* Make very small pancakes, using only 1 to 1½ tablespoons batter. Place the pancakes in a serving bowl or individual soup plates and ladle Tomato Consommé (page 204) over.

*Serving size = 2 pancakes*
*139 calories*
*0.4 gram fat*
*0.6 milligram cholesterol*
*370 milligrams sodium*

## SPICY VEGETABLE COUSCOUS

Martha Rose Shulman

***You can vary the vegetables in this filling, piquant couscous according to the seasons.***

SERVES 6 TO 8

**⅓ pound (1 heaping cup) dried chick-peas or white beans, washed, picked over, soaked overnight or for several hours, and drained**
**1 large or 2 small onions, sliced**
**3 to 4 garlic cloves, minced or put through a press**

**2 leeks, white part only, carefully cleaned and sliced**
**1 bay leaf**
**6 cups water**
**1 pound tomatoes, peeled and coarsely chopped, or 1 28-ounce can tomatoes, drained**
**1 fresh jalapeño or other hot green pepper, seeded and sliced**
**½ teaspoon saffron threads**
**¾ pound carrots, thickly sliced**
**¾ pound turnips, peeled and cut into wedges**
**Salt**
**Freshly ground black pepper**
**¾ pound zucchini, thickly sliced**
**Cayenne**
**2 heaping cups couscous**
**½ cup water**
**1 bunch cilantro, chopped**
**Juice of ½ lemon (optional)**
**Whole sprigs of cilantro and harissa sauce, for garnish**

Combine the beans, onion, half the garlic, leeks, bay leaf, and water in a large, heavy-bottomed soup pot or a couscoussier. Bring to a boil, cover, reduce the heat, and simmer 1 hour.

Add the tomatoes, jalapeño, saffron, remaining garlic, carrots, turnips, salt, and pepper to taste. Cover and simmer another hour. Add the zucchini and cayenne to taste. Simmer for another 30 minutes, or until the squash is tender. Adjust the seasonings.

Place the couscous in a large bowl or a casserole. Combine 2 cups broth from the vegetable mixture and ½ cup water. Gradually sprinkle this onto the couscous. Add more water if necessary to cover the couscous. Let the couscous sit for 20 minutes; stir with a wooden spoon or your hands every 5 minutes or more to prevent lumping. The couscous should swell and soften. Add salt to taste.

Heat the cooked couscous through for 15 to 20 minutes in the top part of your couscoussier, or in a strainer or steamer that fits tightly over your soup pot, or in a covered baking dish in a medium oven, or in a microwave for 1 to 2 minutes.

Just before serving, bring the vegetable mixture back to a simmer and stir in the chopped cilantro and optional lemon juice. To serve, spoon the couscous into warmed wide flat soup bowls and ladle on a generous helping of soup. Garnish with sprigs of cilantro and pass the harissa, with a small bowl of broth so that people can dissolve the harissa in a spoonful before adding it to the couscous.

NOTE: Harissa is a fiery hot condiment that is traditional with North African dishes such as couscous. Packed in tubes, it is sold in specialty food stores and Middle Eastern markets.

*Serving size = 2 cups*
*151 calories*
*1.2 grams fat*
*0 milligrams cholesterol*
*126 milligrams sodium without added salt*

## ZUCCHINI STUFFED WITH MUSHROOMS

Alain Rondelli

SERVES 4

**5 large zucchini, about 3 pounds**
**6 garlic cloves, thinly sliced**
**12 ounces medium mushrooms, thinly sliced**
**1 yellow onion, thinly sliced**
**1 cup water**
**½ tablespoon kosher salt**
**2 tablespoons chopped fresh tarragon**
**½ cup peeled, seeded, and diced tomato**
**½ cup chervil leaves**

Cut 4 zucchini in half lengthwise and carefully scoop out the pulp and seeds, taking care not to break the skins (leave ¼ inch of pulp in shell). Chop the pulp and seeds and set aside. Blanch the zucchini in boiling water for 5 minutes and then plunge into ice water. Leave the shells in the water for 10 minutes. Carefully drain and set aside.

Cut the remaining zucchini into quarters lengthwise and then into ¼-inch slices. In a medium-size pan, combine the chopped zucchini, zucchini slices, garlic, mushrooms, onion, water, and salt. Cook over medium-low heat, uncovered, for 35 to 40 minutes, or until the water has evaporated. Remove from the heat and stir in the tarragon.

Stuff the zucchini shells with the vegetable mixture. Place them in a shallow baking dish and bake at 350 degrees for 15 minutes. Finish cooking under the broiler for 3 to 4 minutes, or until the stuffing begins to brown.

To serve, place 2 zucchini halves on each of 4 plates, sprinkle the diced tomato over and around, and sprinkle with the chervil leaves.

*Serving size = 1¾ cups*
*102 calories*
*1 gram fat*
*0 milligrams cholesterol*
*891.7 milligrams sodium*

## BROWN RICE-FILLED CHILIES WITH BLACK BEAN SAUCE

Tracy Pikhart Ritter

SERVES 4

**1½ cups cooked brown rice**
**½ cup diced red bell pepper**
**1 tablespoon roasted ground cumin**
**1 tablespoon roasted ground coriander**
**¼ teaspoon fresh cracked black pepper**
**¼ teaspoon sea salt**
**1 tablespoon chopped fresh cilantro**
**8 whole green chilies, freshly roasted or canned**
**2 ounces nonfat jalapeño Monterey Jack cheese**

**4 ounces vegetable stock plus extra for thinning**
**3 tablespoons minced red onion**
**1 teaspoon minced garlic**
**1 teaspoon ground cumin**
**1 teaspoon ground coriander**
**½ teaspoon chili powder**
**1 tablespoon dry sherry**
**2 tablespoons tomato paste**
**¼ teaspoon minced jalapeño pepper (optional)**
**1½ cups cooked black beans**
**½ cup chopped fresh tomatoes, for garnish**
**1 tablespoon chopped fresh cilantro, for garnish**

Combine the rice with the next 6 ingredients. Fill the chili peppers with the mixture and place them on a lightly sprayed or oiled baking sheet. Grate the cheese and sprinkle it over the peppers.

Preheat the oven to 350 degrees.

Place the stock in a pan. Add the onion, garlic, cumin, coriander, chili powder, and sherry; cook for 3 minutes. Add the tomato paste, pepper, and beans and cook for 5 more minutes.

Reheat the stuffed chilis in the oven for 10 minutes. Place the cooked bean mixture in a blender or food processor and process until smooth and creamy. Add small amounts of stock or water if necessary to thin the mixture.

Place the black bean sauce on a serving platter, set the stuffed chilis on the sauce, and garnish with the tomatoes and cilantro or arrange in individual servings.

*Serving size = 2 stuffed chili peppers*
*270 calories*
*2.5 grams fat*
*1.5 milligrams cholesterol*
*580.8 milligrams sodium without added salt*

## FENNEL AND ONION TART

Alain Rondell

SERVES 4 TO 6

**½ ounce fresh yeast**
**4 cups water**
**2 cups all-purpose flour**
**1 tablespoon kosher salt**
**1 yellow onion**
**5 garlic cloves**
**1 fennel bulb (about 11 ounces), tough outer skin removed**
**1½ tablespoons chopped fresh thyme**
**1 tablespoon plus 1 teaspoon sugar**
**60 pearl onions (12 ounces), peeled**
**⅓ cup balsamic vinegar**
**½ cup chopped fresh chives**

To make the tart shell, mix together the yeast, 1 cup water, flour, and a pinch of salt until well combined. Form the dough into a ball, cover with plastic wrap, and place in the refrigerator for 3 hours.

Mince the yellow onion, garlic, and fennel and place in a medium-sized saucepan. Add 2 cups water, thyme, ½ teaspoon salt, and 1 tablespoon sugar. Cook over medium heat for 25 minutes, or until all the water has been cooked away. Cool to room temperature.

While the fennel-onion marmalade is cooking, place the pearl onions, remaining 1 cup water, ½ teaspoon salt, 1 teaspoon sugar, and balsamic vinegar into a saucepan. Cook over medium-low heat for 20 minutes, or until the water is completely reduced and the onions are tender. Cool to room temperature.

Preheat the oven to 350 degrees.

To assemble the tart, roll the dough out to a circle about 8 inches in diameter and place on a baking sheet. Spread the fennel-onion marmalade over the pastry to within ½ inch of the edge. Top with pearl onions. Bake for 30 to 35 minutes, or until the pastry is golden brown and cooked through. Remove from the oven and garnish with chives. Cut into 4 to 6 wedges and serve warm or at room temperature.

*Serving size = ⅙ of tart*
*217 calories*
*0.8 gram fat*
*0 milligrams cholesterol*
*1,187 milligrams sodium*

## TANDOORI POTATO AND ONION CASSEROLE

Michael Lomonaco

SERVES 8 AS A SIDE DISH

**Spice mixture: 1 tablespoon each of ground cumin, ground coriander seeds, ground cardamom, cinnamon, nutmeg, cayenne, turmeric**
**1 pound small white onions**
**2 pounds Yukon gold or other yellow potatoes**
**1 cup nonfat plain yogurt**
**1 teaspoon fresh hot chili pepper**
**1 tablespoon chopped garlic**
**1 tablespoon grated fresh gingerroot**
**1 cup Vegetable Stock (page 143)**

Blend the spice mixture together and set aside. Peel and slice the onions and potatoes into rounds ¼ inch thick. Combine the yogurt, chili, garlic, ginger, and 1 tablespoon of the spice mix (store the rest to use in other dishes). In a large stainless-steel bowl, toss the sliced onions and potatoes. Add the yogurt mixture and spread the vegetables in an even layer together in a shallow baking dish. Pour the vegetable stock over the top. Bake in a preheated 350-degree oven for 1½ hours, until thoroughly cooked and browned on top. Serve warm.

*Serving size = ¼ cup*
*147 calories*
*1.3 grams fat*
*0.5 milligram cholesterol*
*35.1 milligrams sodium*

## ARMENIAN RAGOUT OF LENTILS, SQUASH, AND APRICOTS

Joyce Goldstein

*This sweet and savory ragout makes a very satisfying and filling dinner when accompanied by steamed basmati rice. It can be prepared ahead of time and reheated, but you will probably need to add more liquid when reheating because the lentils, squash, and apricots absorb much of the pan juices as the dish sits. Fresh green lentils are best, as they hold their shape; however, you can make the ragout with brown soup lentils or red Indian lentils, but they will soften more quickly and become more like a puree.*

SERVES 4

**1½ pounds butternut squash**
**¾ cup green lentils**
**1 cup Vegetable Stock (page 143) plus more as needed for thinning and reheating**
**1 onion, chopped**
**2 garlic cloves, finely minced**
**1 teaspoon ground cumin**
**½ teaspoon ground cinnamon**
**½ cup dried apricots, cut into quarters, soaked in hot water**
**1 cup diced plum tomatoes (optional)**
**2 tablespoons lemon juice**
**Salt and pepper**
**Chopped parsley**

Preheat the oven to 375 degrees.

Bake the butternut squash for 45 to 50 minutes, until tender but firm. When the squash is cool enough to handle, remove the peel, discard the seeds, and cut the flesh into ½-inch chunks. Or you may peel the squash, cut it into ½-inch chunks, and poach them in water or vegetable stock until firm-tender. Drain and set aside.

Cover the lentils with cold water and bring up a boil. Simmer until firm-tender, 20 to 30 minutes. Keep testing, as the cooking time for lentils can vary greatly depending on their age. When the lentils are cooked through, drain them well and set them aside.

Bring the vegetable stock to a boil and add the onion. Reduce the heat and cook, covered, until tender and translucent, about 15 minutes. Add the garlic, cumin, and cinnamon and simmer for a few minutes. Add the dried apricots with some of their soaking liquid, the reserved lentils and squash, and the optional tomatoes; simmer to combine flavors for about 15 minutes. Stir in the lemon juice and season with salt and pepper. If the ragout seems dry, add more apricot liquid or stock. Sprinkle with chopped parsley. Serve with rice.

*Serving size = 1½ cups*
*194 calories*
*0.7 gram fat*
*0 milligrams cholesterol*
*86.7 milligrams sodium without added salt*

## BEETS AND CARROTS WITH WEST INDIAN SPICES

Joyce Goldstein

*These smell so good while they are cooking! Serve them with black beans, rice, and greens for a complete Caribbean experience.*

SERVES 4

**1 pound beets (about 4 medium)**
**1 pound carrots, sliced**
**2 tablespoons grated fresh gingerroot**
**½ cup brown sugar**

**½ cup orange juice**
**¼ cup cider vinegar**
**Grated zest of 1 orange**
**½ teaspoon ground cinnamon**
**½ teaspoon mace**

Wash the beets well and cut off the leaves, leaving an inch or so of stem. Cover with cold water, bring to a boil, and simmer, covered, until tender, about 40 minutes. Drain and cover with cool or lukewarm water. When cool enough to handle, slip off the skins. Cut the beets into slices or chunks.

Peel and cut the carrots into slices or chunks, resembling the beets in size and style. Steam or boil in lightly salted water about 5 minutes or until tender but not soft. Drain.

Combine the ginger, sugar, orange juice, vinegar, orange zest, and spices in a saucepan and bring the mixture to a simmer. Cook until thickened. Simmer the cooked beets and carrots in this sauce for about 5 minutes.

NOTE: Alternatively, you may bake the beets in a foil-covered pan for about an hour. When cool, slip off the skins. Cut the beets into slices or chunks.

*Serving size = 1 cup*
*178 calories*
*0.4 gram fat*
*0 milligrams cholesterol*
*137.1 milligrams sodium*

## COUSCOUS WITH NORTH AFRICAN VEGETABLE TAGINE

Joyce Goldstein

*This vegetable ragout, called a tagine after the covered earthenware dish in which it is cooked, is complex in flavor but not complicated to prepare. The couscous can be steamed at the last minute or hours ahead and revived over steaming water. The seasoned onion and tomato mix-*

*ture also can be prepared ahead of time, and the vegetables added and cooked through just at serving time.*

SERVES 4

COUSCOUS

**2 cups medium-grain couscous**
**3 cups water**
**1 teaspoon salt**
**1 teaspoon ground cinnamon**

Pour the couscous grains into a shallow baking pan or ceramic dish, about 9 inches square and 2 inches high. Bring the water with salt and cinnamon to a boil and pour over the couscous. Cover the pan with foil and let the couscous sit for 5 to 10 minutes. Fluff with a fork. The couscous can be made hours ahead of time and kept warm in a double boiler or over a pan of hot water.

VEGETABLE TAGINE

**1½ cups Vegetable Stock (page 143)**
**1 cup carrot chunks, about 1½ inches in length**
**1 cup green beans, cut in 2-inch lengths**
**1½ cups diced onions**
**3 garlic cloves, finely minced**
**1 tablespoon ground coriander**
**1 tablespoon paprika**
**1 tablespoon ground cumin**
**2 teaspoons freshly ground black pepper**
**¼ teaspoon cayenne**
**6 tablespoons chopped fresh cilantro**
**1 cup diced tomatoes**
**1 cup zucchini, cut in 1-inch slices**
**4 cups Swiss chard, cut into ½-inch-wide strips**
**Salt and pepper**
**2 to 3 tablespoons lemon juice (optional)**

Bring the broth to a boil. Cook the carrots in the broth until tender but not soft. Remove with a slotted spoon and set aside. Drop the green beans into the simmering stock and cook about 5 minutes. Remove the beans with a slotted spoon and immediately refresh them under cold water.

Pour most of the stock into a large sauté pan and bring to a simmer. Cook the onions until tender and translucent, 10 to 15 minutes over moderate heat. Add the garlic, spices, 2 tablespoons of the cilantro, and the tomatoes, and cook 2 minutes longer. (This is the base for the vegetable tagine. You could stop here and add the vegetables just before serving.) Add the zucchini and simmer until the zucchini is tender, about 5 minutes. Add the carrots and Swiss chard and stir well. Simmer until the chard wilts. Add the green beans at the last minute. Season with salt, pepper, and lemon juice. Sprinkle with the rest of the cilantro and serve over couscous.

*Serving size = 2½ cups*
*229 calories*
*1.7 grams fat*
*0 milligrams cholesterol*
*827.4 milligrams sodium*

## SANDWICH WITH SPICED RED PEPPER PUREE, CUCUMBERS, AND GREENS

Joyce Goldstein

*In Greece and Turkey spicy roasted red pepper purees are often served at the start of a meal, accompanied by pita bread. Why not add some sliced cucumbers, greens, and a little minted yogurt for a tasty Middle Eastern sandwich?*

SERVES 4

**2 large red bell peppers**
**1 tablespoon finely minced garlic**
**2 to 3 finely minced jalapeño peppers**
**2 teaspoons ground toasted cumin seed**

**3 tablespoons lemon juice**
**Salt**
**Pepper**
**½ cup nonfat plain yogurt**
**1 teaspoon grated lemon zest**
**3 tablespoons chopped mint**
**1 large or 2 small cucumbers, sliced ⅛ inch thick, peeled and seeded if necessary (English cucumbers won't need peeling)**
**4 large pita breads, or 8 slices whole-grain bread**
**2 bunches of watercress, stems removed**
**16 mint leaves**

Roast the peppers in the broiler, over a grill, or directly on a gas flame. Turn them often until well charred on all sides. Put them in a plastic container to steam for about 15 minutes. Peel, seed, and chop coarsely. Place the peppers, garlic, jalapeño peppers, cumin, and lemon juice in the container of a food processor. Pulse quickly to chop and blend. Season with salt and pepper.

Season the yogurt with lemon zest, mint, salt, and pepper.

Assemble the sandwiches. If using pita breads, cut them in half. Open the pocket and spread the minted yogurt on one side. Top with cucumber slices. Put the pepper puree over the cucumbers and tuck the watercress and mint leaves over the pepper puree.

If using sliced bread, spread yogurt on half the bread and top that side with cucumbers. Put the pepper puree on the other side and top with watercress and mint. Cover with a second slice of bread and cut in half.

*Serving size = 1 sandwich*
*199 calories*
*2.0 grams fat*
*2.2 milligrams cholesterol*
*333 milligrams sodium without added salt*

## MUSHROOMS À LA STROGANOFF

Joyce Goldstein

*Here is the sizzle minus the steak—a traditionally inspired Russian stroganoff of meaty mushrooms. Be sure that the yogurt is at room temperature so that it won't curdle when added to the mushrooms.*

SERVES 2 TO 4

**1 cup Brown Vegetable Stock (page 144)**
**2 cups sliced onions**
**4 cups sliced mushrooms (combination of cultivated and wild if possible)**
**1 tablespoon sweet paprika**
**Pinch of cayenne or hot paprika**
**1 teaspoon grated lemon zest**
**Salt**
**Freshly ground black pepper to taste**
**½ cup nonfat plain yogurt, strained in cheesecloth for 8 hours**
**2 tablespoons chopped fresh dill or parsley**

Heat ½ cup of the stock in a large sauté pan and add the onions. Simmer, covered, until onions are tender, 10 to 15 minutes. Add the mushrooms and simmer for 5 minutes, stirring occasionally. Stir in the paprika, cayenne, lemon zest, and the remaining stock and simmer briskly for about 10 minutes until reduced by one-third. Season to taste with salt and pepper. Remove the pan from the heat, let the mixture rest for about 5 minutes, and then swirl in the yogurt.

Sprinkle with chopped dill or parsley. Serve with slices of baked polenta, steamed brown or wild rice, or noodles.

*Serving size = 1 cup*
*86 calories*
*0.8 gram fat*
*0.4 milligram cholesterol*
*95.8 milligrams sodium without added salt*

## TENDER CORN PANCAKES WITH WATERCRESS SAUCE

Hubert Keller

*This dish has a pretty contrast of colors and a delightful taste that comes from the richness of the roasted bell peppers and corn against the delicate watercress sauce.*

SERVES 4

**1 red bell pepper**
**1 green bell pepper**
**Vegetable oil spray**
**4 ears tender young corn**
**5 egg whites**
**2 tablespoons whole wheat flour**
**Freshly ground black pepper**
**2 bunches of watercress**
**2 tablespoons finely chopped shallots**
**2 tablespoons dry white wine**
**1 cup Vegetable Consommé (page 147)**
**1 tablespoon cooked white rice**
**2 tablespoons finely chopped chives**
**16 asparagus tips, cooked**

Preheat the broiler. Coat the 2 bell peppers very lightly with the pan coating. Place under the broiler and let them roast, turning frequently until the skin is blackened on all sides. When the peppers are charred, cool until comfortable to handle and peel off the blackened skin. Remove the stems, core, and seeds. Slice the peppers into julienned strips 1 inch long and set aside.

Peel the husks and silk from the corn. Bring 5 quarts of water to a boil. Add the corn and boil for 5 minutes, then quickly dip in cold water. Cut the kernels from the cobs. There should be about 1½ cups of cut corn. Place the corn, egg whites, flour, and pepper to taste in a food processor. Blend well. Pour the batter into a small mixing bowl. Wash the watercress and trim off the leaves. Discard the stems. Cook the leaves in boiling water just until tender, about 3 minutes. Drain in a strainer, refresh under cold running water, then squeeze to remove all moisture.

Heat a small saucepan lightly greased with the pan coating. Add the chopped shallots and cook until translucent. Deglaze with the white wine and reduce to almost dry. Add the vegetable consommé, rice, and black pepper to taste. Bring to a boil, lower the heat, and simmer for about 5 minutes. Add the cooked watercress leaves. Blend the mixture in a blender 1 minute; the result will be a light and very tasty watercress sauce.

Combine the sliced bell peppers and chives with the corn batter. Heat a large nonstick sauté pan over medium-high heat. Grease very lightly with the vegetable oil pan coating. Make small pancakes using 1½ tablespoons of batter for each—5 or 6 pancakes can be made at the same time in a good-sized pan. Cook the pancakes until golden brown on one side, flip, and cook until golden brown on the second side. As the pancakes are done, set them aside and keep warm. Repeat with the remaining batter. Coat the center of each of 4 warm plates with watercress sauce. Arrange the pancakes over the sauce and garnish with 4 cooked asparagus tips on each serving.

*Serving size = 8 pancakes with ¼ cup sauce*
*and 4 asparagus tips*
*140 calories*
*1.1 grams fat*
*0 milligrams cholesterol*
*96.5 milligrams sodium*

## GARBANZO STEW

Jean-Marc Fullsack

*This hearty dish would make an excellent accompaniment to the Ratatouille (page 273).*

MAKES 4 CUPS
SERVES 4

**4 cups vegetable stock**
**1 cup dried garbanzo beans, soaked overnight**
**1 cup diced onion**
**1 cup diced tomatoes**
**1 tablespoon minced fresh gingerroot**
**2 teaspoons ground coriander**
**1 teaspoon minced garlic**
**¼ teaspoon ground cumin**
**Freshly ground black pepper**
**Salt**
**1 teaspoon fresh lime juice**
**1 tablespoon chopped fresh parsley**

In a large saucepan, combine the stock and garbanzo beans. Bring to a boil, reduce the heat, and simmer, covered, for 1 hour, or until just tender. Drain, reserving 1 cup of the cooking liquid.

In a large saucepan, combine the cooked garbanzos, reserved liquid, onion, tomato, ginger, coriander, garlic, and cumin. Bring to a boil. Reduce the heat and simmer, covered, for 20 minutes. Season to taste with freshly ground black pepper and salt. Garnish with the lime juice and chopped parsley.

*Serving size = 1 cup*
*134 calories*
*1.9 grams fat*
*0 milligrams cholesterol*
*94.8 milligrams sodium without added salt*

## VEGETARIAN CHILI

Jean-Marc Fullsack

*This is very spicy and flavorful. Try it with fresh corn tortillas and rice with a generous helping of the Mango or Papaya and Beet Salad (page 195) to cool your palate. Or serve it with a green salad for a complete dinner.*

*You can prepare and refrigerate this 2 to 3 days ahead of time. You can also freeze it for up to 3 months, although the corn may darken somewhat.*

MAKES 7 CUPS
SERVES 4 TO 7

**1 cup plus 2 tablespoons vegetable stock**
**¾ cup diced carrots**
**1 cup diced onions**
**1 cup diced green bell peppers**
**1 cup diced red bell peppers**
**1 cup diced celery**
**1 tablespoon minced garlic**
**1 teaspoon dried oregano**
**1 teaspoon dried thyme**
**½ teaspoon ground coriander**
**1 teaspoon ground cumin**
**1½ teaspoons chili powder**
**4 ounces minced canned jalapeño peppers, or to taste**
**2 cups chopped tomatoes**
**3 cups cooked pinto beans**
**1 cup fresh corn kernels**
**1½ tablespoons red miso paste**
**1 tablespoon lemon juice**
**1 teaspoon red wine vinegar**
**1 teaspoon salt**
**Freshly ground black pepper**
**½ cup chopped fresh cilantro**
**Additional chopped cilantro**

In a large nonstick pan in 2 tablespoons vegetable stock, "sweat" the carrots, onions, green and red bell peppers, and celery for 4 to 5 minutes. Add the garlic, oregano, thyme, coriander, cumin, chili powder, jalapeños, tomatoes, pinto beans, and remaining vegetable stock. Bring to a boil, reduce the heat, and simmer for 20 minutes. Add a little extra vegetable or bean liquid if a "saucier" chili is desired. Add the corn kernels and simmer for 7 minutes.

In a small bowl, combine the red miso, lemon juice, and vinegar until dissolved. Stir into the chili with ½ cup of cilantro. Season to taste with the salt and pepper. Serve hot, with the additional chopped cilantro.

*Serving size = 1 cup*
*203 calories*
*1.4 grams fat*
*0 milligrams cholesterol*
*622 milligrams sodium*

## SPRING VEGETABLE STEW

Bradley Ogden

SERVES 6

**2 pounds fresh fava beans, to yield about 1 cup shelled**
**Florets from 1 small bunch of broccoli rabe**
**1 pound fresh black-eyed peas, shelled**
**5 cups Vegetable Stock (page 143)**
**1 fennel bulb, the outside layer peeled away, and cut into 1-inch dice**
**1 pound large asparagus, peeled and cut into 2-inch pieces**
**½ pound sweet garden peas, shelled (won't be much)**
**2 medium tomatoes, peeled, seeded, and cut into 1-inch dice**
**1 small yellow golden squash, sliced into ¼-inch pieces**
**10 ounces curly spinach, washed well**
**Kernels from 2 ears of sweet corn**
**Kosher salt**

**Freshly ground black pepper**
**⅓ cup chervil leaves**
**2 tablespoons tarragon leaves**

Blanch the fava beans in boiling salted water for 2 minutes or until tender. Remove the beans, reserving the cooking water, and plunge them in ice water to cool immediately. Drain and remove the skins from the beans. Bring the water back to a boil, add the broccoli rabe and blanch for 30 seconds, again reserving the water. Remove and cool immediately in the ice water.

Bring the cooking water back to a boil. Blanch the black-eyed peas for 1 minute and cool in the ice water.

In a noncorrosive saucepan, bring the vegetable stock to a boil, add the fennel and asparagus and cook for 30 seconds. Add the blanched vegetables and all the remaining ingredients except the herbs and seasonings and cook for 2 to 3 minutes. Season to taste with salt and pepper, and add the herbs.

NOTE: Fresh black-eyed peas are usually available only in the spring, but vegetables such as string beans could be substituted. Also young bitter greens such as kale or mustard greens can be included.

*Serving size = 2½ cups*
*297 calories*
*1.8 grams fat*
*0 milligrams cholesterol*
*248 milligrams sodium without added salt*

## SPROUTED BREAD WITH SUN-DRIED TOMATO SPREAD

Tracy Pikhart Ritter

*The intense, savory taste of the sun-dried tomato spread used in the bruschetta appetizer adds a delicious kick to this vegetable sandwich.*

MAKES 1 SANDWICH

**2 tablespoons sun-dried tomato spread (page 175)**
**¼ red bell pepper, seeded and sliced**
**¼ green bell pepper, seeded and sliced**
**Few slices of red onion**
**2 tablespoons Vegetable Stock (page 143) or vegetable spray**
**2 slices sprouted or whole wheat bread**
**¼ cup radish sprouts**

Place the spread in a mini food processor or blender and puree slightly to achieve a thinner spread.

Sauté the peppers and onions in vegetable stock for 5 minutes or until soft. Cool.

Toast the bread and spread it with the sun-dried tomato mixture, then layer 1 slice with sautéed peppers and onions and radish sprouts. Cover with the remaining slice of toast.

Serve the sandwich with Corn, Orange, and Tomato Relish (page 371), a tossed green salad, and a legume-based soup.

*Serving size = 1 sandwich*
*148 calories*
*0.8 gram fat*
*0 milligrams cholesterol*
*108.5 milligrams sodium*

## MILD PINTO BEAN CHILI

Jean-Marc Fullsack

*This is a flavorful but much milder variation on the Vegetarian Chili (page 268), suitable for those who prefer to stay clear of peppery "hot" food.*

MAKES 8 CUPS
SERVES 6 TO 8

**5 cups vegetable stock**
**2 cups pinto beans, soaked overnight**
**2 cups diced tomatoes**

**2 medium to large onions, oven roasted (page 133) and chopped**
**1 tablespoon minced garlic**
**2 teaspoons ground cumin**
**1 teaspoon dried oregano**
**½ teaspoon dried thyme**
**¼ teaspoon chili powder**
**⅛ teaspoon red chili pepper flakes**
**1 bay leaf**
**Pinch of sugar**
**1 cup corn kernels**
**½ cup chopped roasted mild green chilis (page 132)**
**2 ounces diced smoked tofu (optional)**
**1 tablespoon red miso paste**
**1½ teaspoons red wine vinegar**
**1½ teaspoons lemon juice**
**1 tablespoon chopped fresh cilantro**
**Cooked rice**
**Corn tortillas**

In a large saucepan, combine the stock, pinto beans, and tomatoes. Bring to a boil, reduce the heat, and simmer, covered, for 45 minutes, or until the beans are tender. Add the onions, garlic, cumin, oregano, thyme, chili powder, chili flakes, and bay leaf. Simmer for 15 minutes. Add the corn kernels, chilis, and optional smoked tofu and simmer for an additional 5 minutes.

In a small bowl, combine the miso, vinegar, and lemon juice. Add to the chili and serve, garnished with the cilantro. Serve with rice and/or corn tortillas.

*Serving size = 1 cup*
*164 calories*
*1.7 grams fat*
*0 milligrams cholesterol*
*45.8 milligrams sodium*

## RATATOUILLE

Jean-Marc Fullsack

*This has a silky texture even though it is untypically made without olive oil. This is delicious with polenta or with French bread and a salad.*

SERVES 4

**1 eggplant (approximately 1¼ pounds)**
**1 onion, roasted and coarsely chopped (to yield 1 cup)**
**1 head of garlic, roasted**
**1 red bell pepper, roasted and diced**
**1 green bell pepper, roasted and diced**
**1 yellow bell pepper, roasted and diced**
**2 tomatoes, peeled, seeded, and cut in ½-inch dice**
**2 zucchini, sliced and quartered**
**2 yellow summer squashes, sliced and quartered**
**¼ fennel bulb, coarsely chopped**
**1 tablespoon chopped fresh basil**
**1 tablespoon chopped fresh parsley**
**1 teaspoon chopped fresh tarragon**
**1 teaspoon dried thyme**
**Freshly ground black pepper**
**Cayenne**
**Salt**

Preheat the oven to 375 degrees.

Cut the eggplant in half and place it, cut side down, on a parchment-lined nonstick baking sheet. Bake for 45 minutes, or until easily pierced with a knife.

When cool enough to handle, scrape out the pulp, roughly chop it, and place in a large nonstick saucepan. (Discard the skin.) Add the onion, garlic, peppers, tomatoes, zucchini, summer squashes, and fennel. Bring to a boil. Reduce the heat and simmer for 30 minutes.

Add the basil, parsley, tarragon, and thyme. Season to taste with pepper, cayenne, and salt. Simmer for an additional 5 minutes and serve hot or at room temperature.

*Serving size = 1¼ cups*
*157 calories*
*1.6 grams fat*
*0 milligrams cholesterol*
*106.2 milligrams sodium without added salt*

## SPICE-DUSTED TOFU "STEAKS" WITH VEGETABLE GRATIN

Tracy Pikhart Ritter

*Soft, spicy tofu seems to melt into the fragrant, sweet, and savory vegetable gratin here for a delectable contrast in texture and flavor. Serve with your favorite potato dish—the Tandoori Potato and Onion Casserole (page 257) or Brown Basmati Lemon Rice (page 341) are wonderful accompaniments.*

SERVES 4

**8 ounces firm tofu**
**4 tablespoons chili powder**
**2 tablespoons ground cumin**
**2 tablepoons ground coriander**
**2 teaspoons paprika**
**½ teaspoon cayenne**
**1 teaspoon salt**

VEGETABLE GRATIN

**¼ cup vegetable stock**
**2 teaspoons balsamic vinegar**
**1 large red onion, sliced thin**
**1 garlic clove, minced**
**Salt**
**Black pepper**
**1 yellow squash, cut into slices**
**1 zucchini, cut into slices**
**2 very ripe tomatoes, sliced**
**2 tablespoons chopped canned green chilis**
**2 tablespoons shredded nonfat jalapeño Monterey Jack cheese**

Drain the tofu well. Slice horizontally to form ½-inch-thick "steaks." Combine the chili, cumin, coriander, paprika, cayenne, and salt. Blend well and coat the tofu on all sides with it. Set aside.

Make the vegetable gratin. In a sauté pan, place the stock, vinegar, onion, garlic, salt, and pepper to taste. Cook slowly for about 8 minutes, or until the onions are soft.

Divide the onion-garlic mixture into 4 parts and arrange into 4 long strips in a 9 × 11-inch baking pan. Lay the squash, zucchini, tomatoes, and chilies on top of the strips. Bake in a 300 degree oven for 10 minutes. Sprinkle with the cheese and bake for 5 minutes, or just until the cheese is melted.

While the vegetables are baking, grill, broil, or bake the tofu steaks on a nonstick baking sheet until soft and heated all the way through, about 15 minutes. (The tofu steaks can be baked while the vegetables are in the oven.) Serve.

*Serving size = 1 cup*
*110 calories*
*2.6 grams fat*
*0.8 milligram cholesterol*
*748.8 milligrams sodium*

## SPRING RAGOUT OF ARTICHOKES, FAVAS, PEAS, AND ASPARAGUS

Joyce Goldstein

*When it comes to vegetables, spring is my favorite season. All of the ones that go into this dish are at their sweetest and most tender in the spring, and they go so well together. Serve the ragout over pasta or stir into risotto for a complete meal.*

SERVES 6

**1 pound fresh fava beans**
**4 globe artichokes**
**1 pound peas**
**1 pound asparagus**

**1 cup Vegetable Stock (page 143)**
**1 onion, chopped (about 1½ cups)**
**2 teaspoons finely minced garlic**
**1 head butter lettuce, cut in ½-inch-wide strips (cut in half, then crosswise)**
**Zest of 1 lemon**
**3 tablespoons finely chopped fresh parsley**
**2 tablespoons chopped fresh basil (or marjoram or mint)**
**Salt and pepper**

Shell the fava beans and simmer them in boiling salted water for 3 to 5 minutes, until tender. Refresh in cold water and peel off the outer skin; you'll have about ½ cup. Set the favas aside.

Cut across the tops of the artichokes and remove the tops, outer leaves, and stems. Drop the artichokes into boiling salted water and cook, covered, for 10 to 15 minutes. Remove the artichokes with a slotted spoon and refresh in cold water. Remove the remaining leaves and scoop out the fuzzy chokes with a spoon. Cut the artichokes into wedges.

Remove the peas from their pods; you should have about 1 cup.

Break off woody stems from asparagus and cut into 2-inch lengths.

Bring the vegetable stock to a simmer in a large sauté pan. Add the onion and garlic and cook until tender and translucent, 10 to 15 minutes. Add the artichoke wedges and cook, covered, until crisp-tender, about 10 minutes. Add the peas and simmer for 5 minutes. Add the asparagus and simmer for 5 minutes. Uncover the pan and stir in the favas, lettuce, and lemon zest and cook until the lettuce is wilted and all the vegetables are tender but not mush. Stir in the parsley and basil. Season with salt and pepper.

*Serving size = 1⅓ cups*
*249 calories*
*1.1 grams fat*
*0 milligrams cholesterol*
*138.1 milligrams sodium without added salt*

## SWEET AND SOUR STUFFED CABBAGE

Joyce Goldstein

*This is a variation on Jewish sweet and sour cabbage. I have substituted a mixture of fresh mushrooms and meaty-tasting dried porcini mushrooms for the traditional ground meat. Stuffed cabbage is best prepared a day or so before serving to give the flavors a chance to come together. Serve with rye bread.*

SERVES 6 TO 8

**½ cup dried porcini mushrooms**
**2 cups rice**
**1 very large or 2 medium green cabbages**
**1 large onion, left whole, and 1 onion, chopped**
**2 egg whites**
**Salt and pepper**
**½ teaspoon grated nutmeg**
**2 cups Brown Vegetable Stock (page 144)**
**1 pound mushrooms, chopped coarsely (about 6 cups)**
**3 cups canned pureed tomatoes**
**½ cup lemon juice**
**1 cup brown sugar**

Soak the porcini in 1 cup of hot water for 30 minutes. Drain and strain the porcini water through a cheesecloth-lined strainer. Reserve the liquid. Chop the porcini medium-fine.

Soak the rice in cold water for 15 minutes. Core the cabbage with a sharp knife. Bring a large kettle of salted water to a boil. Drop in the whole cabbage and cook for 5 to 10 minutes. Remove the cabbage with 2 large spoons and place it in a strainer. When cool enough to handle, remove the largest leaves. (If you are using 2 medium cabbages, save the core and smaller center leaves for another dish.) You will need about 16 to 18 large leaves.

Drain the rice. Quarter the large onion and place it with the egg whites into the container of a food processor and puree. Combine this onion puree with the rice, spices, and soaked and chopped dried mushrooms.

Bring 1 cup of stock and the strained reserved porcini liquids to a boil in a large sauté pan. Add the chopped fresh mushrooms and cook, stirring over high heat until all the liquid is absorbed. Add the mushrooms to the rice mixture.

Place 2 heaping tablespoons of filling on each cabbage leaf and roll up, tucking in the sides. Fasten with toothpicks. In a deep kettle, bring the tomatoes, lemon juice, brown sugar, chopped onion, and 1 cup of stock up to a simmer. Add the cabbage rolls. Cover the kettle and simmer for 1½ to 2 hours, until the rice is cooked. The leaves should be translucent and the porcini should taste like cabbage. Baste the cabbage occasionally. Adjust the sweet and sour ratio and season with salt and pepper.

*Serving size = 1½ cups*
*240 calories*
*0.9 gram fat*
*0 milligrams cholesterol*
*498.0 milligrams sodium without added salt*

## VEGETABLE GUMBO

Michael Lomonaco

SERVES 4

**2 onions, diced**
**4 ribs celery, diced**
**2 red bell peppers, diced**
**2 green bell peppers, diced**
**1 18-ounce can plum tomatoes**
**½ pound okra, sliced**
**10 ounces spinach, chopped**
**1 small head cabbage, shredded**
**3 garlic cloves, crushed**
**3 cloves and 2 bay leaves tied in small cheesecloth sachet**
**6 basil leaves, chopped**
**2 ounces filé powder**

**1 teaspoon black pepper**
**½ teaspoon cayenne**
**1 quart Vegetable Stock (page 143)**
**2 cups cooked brown or white rice**

In a large nonstick casserole, combine all the vegetables and cook over low heat until wilted and the onions become translucent, about 15 minutes. Add the sachet of cloves and bay leaves with the other seasonings; cook for 5 minutes. Warm the vegetable stock and add it; bring to a boil, lower the heat to simmer, and cook for 45 minutes. Discard the bay leaf and clove sachet; stir in the rice, cook for 5 minutes, and serve.

*Serving size = 1½ cups*
*123 calories*
*0.8 gram fat*
*0 milligrams cholesterol*
*165.5 milligrams sodium*

# *Vegetable Side Dishes*

## CRISP BAKED POTATO SKINS WITH CHIVE DIP

Tracy Pikhart Ritter

SERVES 6 AS AN HORS D'OEUVRE

**3 tablespoons paprika**
**3 tablespoons chili powder**
**3 tablespoons roasted ground cumin**
**3 tablespoons ground coriander**
**1 teaspoon garlic powder**
**1 teaspoon onion powder**
**1 teaspoon cayenne pepper**
**½ teaspoon dried thyme leaves**
**½ teaspoon dried oregano leaves**
**½ teaspoon dried rosemary leaves**
**6 baking potatoes, scrubbed clean**

CHIVE DIP

**¼ cup nonfat milk**
**1 cup nonfat cottage cheese**
**1 tablespoon lemon juice**
**1 tablespoon Dijon mustard**
**1 tablespoon prepared horseradish**

- **½ garlic clove, minced**
- **2 teaspoons drained capers**
- **3 tablespoons minced red onion**
- **3 tablespoons chopped fresh chives**
- **½ teaspoon freshly cracked black pepper**
- **Pinch of salt**
- **2 tablespoons chopped fresh herbs, such as parsley, oregano, or thyme (optional)**

Preheat the oven to 375 degrees. Combine the herbs and spices, then set aside.

Slice 4 ¼-inch-thick sides off the potatoes, leaving a potato rectangle. (The potato rectangles can be refrigerated, covered with water, for another use.)

Place the potato skins, cut side up, on a baking sheet and sprinkle with the herb and spice mixture. Bake in the center of the oven for 30 minutes.

Remove the pan from the oven; spray the skins with a fine mist of water and return to the oven for another 15 minutes, or until soft.

While the potatoes are baking, make the chive dip. Combine the milk, cottage cheese, lemon juice, mustard, horseradish, and garlic in this order in a blender or food processor; blend until creamy. Pour into a bowl and add the capers, red onion, chives, black pepper, salt, and the optional chopped herbs. Set aside at room temperature for at least 30 minutes or refrigerate for up to 2 hours. Serve with the potato skins as an appetizer.

*Serving size = 1 skin and 1 tablespoon dip*
*46 calories*
*0.7 gram fat*
*0.2 milligram cholesterol*
*44.9 milligrams sodium without added salt*

## CARCIOFI ALLA ROMANO (ARTICHOKES IN THE ROMAN STYLE)

Donna Nicoletti

*In its traditional preparation, Roman-style artichokes require little oil, so the following adaptation closely resembles the original. The artichokes are excellent served as an appetizer with warm grilled bread.*

SERVES 6

**6 large artichokes**
**1 lemon, halved**
**2 cups good-quality white wine vinegar**
**1 cup lemon juice**
**2 cups water**
**3 teaspoons chopped garlic**
**1 teaspoon salt**
**1 teaspoon freshly ground black pepper**
**1 bunch of mint**
**3 cups bread crumbs**

Cut off the top third of the artichokes. Remove all the outer leaves until you reach the soft light-colored inner leaves. With a spoon, completely remove the choke and the fuzz in the center of the heart. Do not remove the stem, which is one of the tastiest parts. Rub the prepared artichoke hearts all over with a cut lemon as you work to prevent them from turning brown.

Mix the vinegar, lemon juice, water, garlic, salt, and pepper together and bring to a boil in a pot large enough to accommodate all the artichokes (the artichokes must be completely submerged in the liquid). Immerse the prepared artichokes in the boiling liquid and put some weights on top of them (small plates work well) or they will float to the top and not cook evenly. Cook on medium heat for approximately 20 minutes, or until a fork easily pierces the bottoms. Remove from the liquid and cool to room temperature.

While the artichokes are cooking, chop the mint and mix with the bread crumbs. Set aside

When cool, stuff the artichokes with the bread crumb mixture and serve.

*Serving size = 1 artichoke*
*112 calories*
*0.5 gram fat*
*0 milligrams cholesterol*
*448 milligrams sodium*

## BAKED TOMATOES WITH GARLIC

J. E. Hokin

*The tomatoes seem to "ripen" in the oven, their natural flavors combining deliciously with the basil and garlic.*

SERVES 8

**2 cups fresh bread crumbs**
**½ bunch flat-leaf parsley, stems discarded, leaves chopped**
**20 basil leaves, chopped**
**3 garlic cloves, chopped**
**½ teaspoon fine sea salt (optional)**
**½ teaspoon freshly ground pepper**
**1 teaspoon sugar**
**8 tomatoes, tops cut off, seeds and juice removed**

Preheat the oven to 325 degrees.

Mix the bread crumbs, parsley, basil, garlic, optional salt, pepper, and sugar. Stuff the tomatoes with this mixture.

Bake for 45 to 50 minutes, until the tomatoes are soft and the tops are golden brown.

*Serving size = 1 tomato*
*124 calories*
*1.5 grams fat*
*1.2 milligrams cholesterol*
*193.9 milligrams sodium without added salt*

## BRAISED FENNEL

Joyce Goldstein

*To really play up the anise flavor of this celerylike vegetable, add a little Pernod or anise seeds.*

SERVES 6

**2 large or 4 medium fennel bulbs**
**1 cup Brown Vegetable Stock (page 144)**
**1 onion, chopped**
**1 cup diced tomatoes**
**Grated zest of 1 orange**
**1 teaspoon chopped fresh thyme**
**2 tablespoons Pernod or ouzo (optional)**
**Salt and pepper**
**2 teaspoons toasted anise seeds (optional)**

Cut the fennel in half and remove bruised outer layers. Cut it into quarters, remove the tough core and cut in ¼-inch slices; you should have about 6 cups. Cook the fennel in boiling salted water for 3 to 5 minutes until al dente; do not overcook. Drain.

Bring the vegetable stock to a simmer in a large saucepan. Add the onion and cook, covered, until tender, about 10 minutes. Add the fennel, tomatoes, orange zest, and thyme and simmer, covered, until very tender, about 15 minutes. Uncover the pan, raise the heat, and reduce liquids rapidly.

Add the optional Pernod or ouzo, and season with salt and pepper. Top with the toasted anise seeds if desired. This may be served hot or at room temperature.

*Serving size = 1¼ cups*
*62 calories*
*0.7 gram fat*
*0 milligrams cholesterol*
*15.5 milligrams sodium without added salt*

## BRUSSELS SPROUTS WITH GARLIC AND GINGER

Joyce Goldstein

*Brussels sprouts are rarely a popular vegetable because they are most often cooked until they are gray and soggy and smell like tired cabbage. Here's a recipe that treats brussels sprouts as a crisp, fragrant, and green vegetable.*

SERVES 2 TO 3

**1 pound brussels sprouts, ends trimmed**
**1½ cups vegetable stock or water**
**1 tablespoon finely minced garlic**
**1 tablespoon grated fresh gingerroot**
**1 teaspoon grated lemon zest**
**1½ teaspoon anise seed**
**Salt**
**Pepper**

Cut the brussels sprouts in half. Place, flat side down, on a cutting board and cut the sprouts into very thin strips; you'll have about 3 cups. Bring 1 cup stock or water to a simmer in a large sauté pan. Add the sprouts, garlic, ginger, and lemon zest. Cook, uncovered, over high heat, stirring often, until the sprouts are tender-crisp, 5 to 7 minutes. Add more broth or water as needed. Stir in anise seed and season with salt and pepper. Serve with steamed rice.

NOTE: Snow peas or sugar snap peas can be similarly prepared. Remove the strings and tops. Cook snow peas 3 to 5 minutes, sugar snaps a little longer.

*Serving size = 1⅓ cups*
*86 calories*
*1.1 grams fat*
*0 milligrams cholesterol*
*39.8 milligrams sodium without added salt*

## MOROCCAN SPICE CARROTS

Joyce Goldstein

*This dish is sweet and subtly hot. It's best served with couscous and some braised greens, along with a legume-based salad or soup, for a complete dinner.*

SERVES 4

**1½ pounds carrots (8 to 10)**
**1 cup vegetable stock**
**3 tablespoons brown sugar**
**1 teaspoon ground cinnamon**
**½ teaspoon ground cumin**
**¼ teaspoon cayenne**
**½ cup fresh orange juice**
**Grated zest of 1 orange**
**⅓ cup currants or brown raisins, plumped in hot water (optional)**
**Salt**
**Freshly ground black pepper**
**3 tablespoons chopped fresh mint**

Peel and slice the carrots about ¼ inch thick. You should have about 3½ cups.

Bring the stock to a boil in a sauté pan over moderate heat and drop in the sliced carrots.

Add the sugar and spices and stir well. Reduce the heat and simmer until the carrots are crisp-tender. Stir in the orange juice and orange zest and optional currants or raisins and simmer a few minutes longer. Season with salt and pepper and additional cayenne to taste. Sprinkle with chopped mint and serve at once.

NOTE: Beets or a combination of carrots and beets can be used. First boil the beets until tender, then peel and cut into chunks. If combining with carrots, add the beets when you add the orange juice.

*Serving size = 1 cup*
*130 calories*
*0.6 gram fat*
*0 milligrams cholesterol*
*193.1 milligrams sodium without added salt*

## GREEK-STYLE GREEN BEANS
Joyce Goldstein

*The Greeks are not of the al dente vegetable school and this ragout of tender green beans braised with onion, tomatoes, and oregano may convince you that not all vegetables have to be crunchy and firm to be toothsome.*

SERVES 4

**1 pound green beans (Blue Lakes preferred), trimmed and cut in 2-inch lengths**
**½ cup vegetable stock**
**1 onion, chopped or thinly sliced**
**1 garlic clove, finely minced**
**1½ teaspoons dried oregano**
**¾ cup peeled, seeded, and diced tomato**
**1 tablespoon tomato puree (optional)**
**Salt**
**Pepper**
**Lemon wedges, for garnish**

Drop green beans into a large pot of salted water and cook until firm-tender or al dente. Drain and refresh in ice water. Drain again and set aside.

Bring the vegetable stock to a boil in a large sauté pan. Add the onion and simmer, covered, until tender and translucent, about 10 minutes. Add the garlic, oregano, tomato, and optional tomato puree and simmer about 5 minutes. Add the green beans and simmer until tender and some of the sauce is absorbed, 5 to 7 minutes. Season with salt and pepper. Serve with lemon wedges.

*Serving size = ¼ pound*
*66 calories*
*0.7 gram fat*
*0 milligrams cholesterol*
*150.9 milligrams sodium without added salt*

## CITRUS BRAISED ARTICHOKES

Joyce Goldstein

*This recipe is of Sicilian inspiration. The combination of citrus and a little hot pepper is an interesting contrast for the meaty artichokes.*

SERVES 6

**6 large globe artichokes**
**¼ cup lemon juice**
**½ cup orange juice**
**½ cup tangerine juice or additional orange juice**
**1 cup water**
**1 teaspoon red pepper flakes**
**6 garlic cloves**
**Bay leaf**
**Zest of 1 orange**
**Zest of 1 lemon**
**3 tablespoons chopped parsley**

Cut the stems and tops of the leaves off the artichokes. Drop into boiling salted water and cook for 8 to 10 minutes. Remove the artichokes with a slotted spoon and rinse with cold water. When cool enough to handle, remove the leaves and scoop out the fuzzy choke, leaving the trimmed hearts.

Bring the citrus juices, water, red pepper flakes, garlic cloves, bay leaf, and zests to a simmer in a wide saucepan. Drop in the artichoke hearts and simmer until firm-tender, 15 to 20 minutes longer. Remove the artichoke hearts with a slotted spoon. Garnish with the chopped parsley. Serve with a lemon or orange wedge, if desired. These are good served warm or at room temperature.

*Serving size = 1 artichoke*
*55 calories*
*0.3 gram fat*
*0 milligrams cholesterol*
*49.8 milligrams sodium*

## TURKISH EGGPLANT WITH CHILIES AND YOGURT

Joyce Goldstein

*Traditionally, this tangy puree is accented with chopped walnuts. If you want crunch, add the chopped celery instead. Simmering the garlic takes the harshness away while it leaves the great flavor.*

SERVES 4

**2 large eggplants**
**¼ cup Brown Vegetable Stock (page 144)**
**3 garlic cloves, finely minced**
**1 cup nonfat plain yogurt**
**2 to 3 tablespoons fresh lemon juice**
**3 tablespoons chopped dill**
**3 tablespoons chopped Italian parsley**
**2 to 3 jalapeño peppers, very finely minced**
**Salt**
**Freshly ground black pepper**
**½ cup chopped celery (optional)**

Broil or grill the eggplants, turning often for even cooking. When charred all over and very soft, 15 to 20 minutes, place them in a drainer tray until cool enough to handle. Carefully remove skin and put the eggplant pulp in a strainer so the bitter juices will drain away; drain for about 12 to 15 minutes. Put the vegetable stock and garlic in a small sauté pan and simmer over low heat for a few minutes. Put the drained eggplant pulp in a food processor and pulse just enough to achieve a rough puree. Add the garlic and the rest of the ingredients except the celery. Pulse quickly to combine. Adjust seasoning. If you are using the celery, fold it in at the end. Serve warm accompanied by steamed rice or at room temperature as a dip with bread or lavosh.

*Serving size = 1 cup*
*80 calories*
*0.5 gram fat*
*1 milligram cholesterol*
*124.5 milligrams sodium without added salt*

## BRAISED OKRA WITH TOMATOES

Natalie Ornish

*Try this with the Vegetarian Red Beans and Seven-Grain Dirty Rice (page 342) and/or corn bread and chipotle chilies for a southwestern treat. To make things easier, you could omit the chili peppers, lemon juice, and zest with very good results.*

SERVES 4

**½ pound fresh or frozen okra**
**1 cup diced onion**
**2 teaspoons minced garlic**
**¼ cup white wine**
**1 7-ounce can chopped tomatoes**
**1 teaspoon Chinese chili sauce, or 1 to 2 teaspoons canned chipotle chilies in adobo sauce**
**2 tablespoons lemon juice**
**1 teaspoon lemon zest**
**Freshly ground black pepper**
**Salt**

If using fresh okra, rinse in cold water and dry with a towel. Trim off the stalk end. Cut into ¼-inch slices and set aside.

In a large, nonstick sauté pan, braise the onion and garlic in the white wine until tender. Add the okra, tomatoes, and chili sauce and stir well. Bring to a boil, reduce the heat, and simmer, covered, for 8 to 10 minutes, or until the okra is just tender. (If using frozen okra, just cook until heated through.) Add the lemon juice and zest. Season to taste with pepper and salt.

*Serving size = ¾ cup*
*68 calories*
*0.4 gram fat*
*0 milligrams cholesterol*
*166.3 milligrams sodium without added salt*

## STUFFED BAKED POTATOES

J. E. Hokin

*For variety, substitute cabbage or chard for the spinach.*

SERVES 6

**6 large potatoes (about 6 ounces each), baked**
**2 small garlic cloves, chopped**
**2 tablespoons vegetable stock**
**1 cup nonfat milk, warmed**
**1½ cups Nonfat Yogurt Cheese (page 148)**
**1 teaspoon fine sea salt (optional)**
**½ teaspoon freshly ground pepper**
**½ teaspoon Hungarian paprika**
**1 pound spinach, cleaned, cooked, drained, and chopped**

Preheat the oven to 350 degrees. Slice off the tops of the potatoes, scoop out the flesh and transfer to a mixing bowl. Reserve the skins.

Simmer the garlic in the stock until softened, about 3 minutes. In a large bowl, mash the potato with the warmed milk, yogurt cheese, sautéed garlic, salt, pepper, paprika, and spinach. Stuff the potato mixture into the reserved potato skins.

Place the potatoes in a baking dish, and bake them until heated through, about 20 minutes.

*Serving size = 1 potato*
*286 calories*
*0.6 gram fat*
*1.8 milligrams cholesterol*
*134.1 milligrams sodium without added salt*

## GREEN VEGETABLES WITH ROASTED PEPPER PUREE

J. E. Hokin

*You will not miss the mayonnaise or cream sauce usually served with the vegetables since the roasted pepper puree creates a thick and very tasty but fat-free sauce.*

SERVES 6

**½ cup vegetable stock**
**2 red or yellow bell peppers, roasted, seeded, and chopped (page 133)**
**½ small onion, chopped**
**1 garlic clove, coarsely chopped**
**1 tablespoon red wine vinegar**
**1 teaspoon lemon juice**
**2 pounds cooked green vegetables, such as green beans, broccoli, asparagus, and snow peas**

Add the stock to a saucepan and, over a medium to high flame, cook until the stock has been reduced to 1 tablespoon.

Combine this concentrated vegetable stock with the roasted peppers, onion, garlic, vinegar, and lemon juice in a saucepan. Bring to a boil, cover, and lower the heat to a simmer. Cook for 30 minutes. Let cool to room temperature.

Puree the pepper mixture until smooth. Reheat the sauce, and spoon onto serving plates. Arrange the vegetables on top of the puree.

*Serving size = 1 cup vegetables and 3 tablespoons sauce*
*55 calories*
*0.5 gram fat*
*0 milligrams cholesterol*
*25.2 milligrams salt*

## OLD-FASHIONED MASHED POTATOES

J. E. Hokin

SERVES 8

**2 pounds baking potatoes, scrubbed but not peeled**
**½ cup nonfat milk**
**1 cup Nonfat Yogurt Cheese (page 148)**
**3 tablespoons butter substitute**
**1 teaspoon fine sea salt (optional)**
**1 teaspoon Hungarian paprika**
**½ teaspoon freshly ground white pepper**

Bring a large pan of water to a boil. Cut potatoes into large pieces and cook in the water about 30 minutes or until tender. Drain the potatoes. Use a potato ricer or sieve and return them to the saucepan. Or mash them in the saucepan.

Add the remaining ingredients and mash or beat the potatoes until smooth and well mixed. Taste and correct seasoning. Reheat when ready to serve.

*Serving size = 1 cup*
*168 calories*
*2.1 grams fat*
*1.0 milligram cholesterol*
*87.7 milligrams sodium without added salt*

## RED ONIONS SIMMERED WITH SHERRY VINEGAR

J. E. Hokin

*The long, slow cooking intensifies the natural sweetness of the onions.*

SERVES 8

**2 tablespoons vegetable stock**
**1½ pounds red onions, peeled and sliced**
**2 teaspoons sugar**
**1 teaspoon coarse sea salt (optional)**
**½ teaspoon freshly ground pepper**
**3 tablespoons sherry wine vinegar or to taste**

Heat the stock in a large saucepan, add the onions, sugar, salt, and pepper. Cook over a low heat, covered, for 35 minutes, until the onions color slightly.

Add the vinegar and cook for 30 minutes, covered, over a low heat; the onions should be very soft. Adjust the seasoning and serve.

*Serving size = ¼ cup*
*34 calories*
*0.4 gram fat*
*0 milligrams cholesterol*
*14.8 milligrams sodium without added salt*

## SAUTÉED ZUCCHINI WITH MUSTARD DILL SAUCE

Tracy Pikhart Ritter

*This creamy, herb-spiked vegetable dish is satisfying and rich. The combination of both Dijon and grainy mustard adds flavor and also helps to thicken and emulsify the sauce.*

SERVES 6

**3 whole zucchini**
**2 egg whites**
**¼ teaspoon cayenne**
**½ cup all-purpose flour**
**Pinch of salt**
**Pinch of freshly ground pepper**
**Vegetable oil spray**
**½ cup diced shallots or white onion**
**2 cups vegetable stock**
**4 tablespoons chopped fresh dill**
**2 ounces nonfat milk**
**2 tablespoons grainy-style mustard**
**2 tablespoons Dijon mustard**
**½ teaspoon salt**
**½ teaspoon freshly ground black pepper**
**1 tablespoon chopped fresh dill**

Wash and lightly scrub the zucchini. Cut the ends off and slice lengthwise into ¼- to ½-inch slices.

Lightly beat the egg whites and cayenne pepper together, then set aside. Season the flour with salt and pepper and set aside as well.

Heat a large skillet and lightly spray it with vegetable oil pan coating. Dip the zucchini into the beaten egg whites and then dredge in the seasoned flour. Shake off any excess. Brown the zucchini on one side for 1 minute, drain off any excess oil, and turn over.

Add all the remaining ingredients, except the dill for garnish, to the pan. Blend ingredients, bring to a boil, and reduce to a simmer. Cover and cook zucchini and sauce for 20 more minutes, until the sauce is thickened and the zucchini is still slightly soft to the touch.

If a thicker sauce is desired, remove the zucchini to a serving platter or plates and return saucepan with sauce to heat. Bring to a boil and reduce until desired thickness is reached.

Serve with roasted rosemary potatoes, pasta, or rice. Garnish with fresh chopped dill.

*Serving size = ½ zucchini with sauce*
*78 calories*
*0.8 gram fat*
*0.2 milligram cholesterol*
*351.6 milligrams sodium*

## ARTICHOKE HEARTS WITH SWEET PEPPERS, SAFFRON, AND BASIL

Alain Rondelli

*This can be prepared up to 24 hours in advance.*

SERVES 4

**8 artichokes (about 4½ pounds)**
**2 red bell peppers, seeded and diced**
**2 yellow bell peppers, seeded and diced**
**1 yellow onion, diced**
**4 garlic cloves, finely sliced**
**⅛ teaspoon saffron**
**½ teaspoon kosher salt**
**Juice of one lemon**
**1 tablespoon tomato paste**
**1 quart water**
**20 small whole basil leaves**

Remove all the leaves and stems from the artichokes. Peel the stems and bases of any tough skin. Discard the leaves. Put the artichoke hearts and stems into a large saucepan along with the peppers, onion, garlic, saffron, salt, lemon juice, tomato paste, and water. Bring the mixture to a boil, then reduce the heat to medium. Continue cooking for about 35 minutes, or until the artichokes are tender but not mushy. Remove the artichoke hearts and stems and continue cooking the other vegetables until the liquid is reduced to 1 cup. Remove the chokes from the artichoke hearts, cut into quarters, and return to the sauce. Cool to room temperature; refrigerate for 1½ to 2 hours.

To serve, divide the artichokes and sauce evenly among 4 plates and sprinkle attractively with the basil leaves.

*Serving size = 2 artichokes with sauce*
*86 calories*
*0.4 gram fat*
*0 milligrams cholesterol*
*1,005 milligrams sodium*

## OVEN-ROASTED POTATOES WITH FRESH HERBS

Tracy Pikhart Ritter

*Oil and butter are not necessary to create delicious oven-roasted vegetables. Here, fresh herbs and vegetable stock are used to coat small red potatoes before they are baked. Add carrots and turnips for variety.*

SERVES 4 TO 6

**2 pounds small red potatoes**
**2 tablespoons vegetable stock**
**1 teaspoon chopped fresh rosemary or ¼ teaspoon dried**
**2 teaspoons chopped fresh parsley or 1 teaspoon dried**
**⅛ teaspoon dried sage leaves**
**2 teaspoons paprika**
**2 teaspoons freshly ground black pepper**
**1 teaspoon salt (optional)**
**Vegetable oil spray**

Preheat the oven to 375 degrees.

Clean and quarter the potatoes. Toss with the remaining ingredients until well coated.

Lightly wipe or spray a baking pan with vegetable oil. Place the potatoes in a single layer on the pan and bake for 30 minutes, until the potatoes are soft and brown.

*Serving size = 1 cup*
*163 calories*

*0.4 gram fat*
*0 milligrams cholesterol*
*33.6 milligrams sodium without added salt*

## POTATO AND TOMATO GRATIN

Joyce Goldstein

*You'll need a nonstick baking dish for this gratin if you want to unmold it. If not, simply serve it from the baking dish.*

SERVES 3 TO 4

**1 cup vegetable stock**
**1 medium onion, chopped (about 1 cup)**
**2 garlic cloves, finely minced**
**2 cups plum tomatoes, seeded and diced**
**2 teaspoons chopped fresh thyme or 4 tablespoons chopped fresh basil**
**2 large baking potatoes, peeled and cut into ⅛-inch-thick slices**
**Salt**
**Pepper**
**Chopped parsley (optional)**

Bring the vegetable stock to a boil in a medium sauté pan. Add the onion and cook, covered, until soft and translucent, about 15 minutes. Add the garlic and cook for a minute or two, then add the tomatoes and herbs. Simmer, uncovered, for about 10 minutes, stirring occasionally, until thickened.

Preheat the oven to 350 degrees.

Place about one-third of the tomato sauce on the bottom of an 8- or 10-inch baking dish or pie pan. Top with potato slices sprinkled with a little salt and pepper, then more sauce, then potatoes, salt and pepper, then tomato sauce, then potatoes, then salt and pepper. Bake for 40 to 45 minutes, covered, until potatoes are cooked through. Sprinkle with chopped parsley, if desired. Cut into wedges and serve.

*Serving size = 1 cup*
*147 calories*
*0.8 gram fat*
*0 milligrams cholesterol*
*94.4 milligrams sodium without added salt*

## ROASTED JAPANESE EGGPLANT WITH GREEN HERB SAUCE

Catherine Pantsios

*If you have a garden or a good greengrocer, you can experiment with other combinations of herbs. Chervil, tarragon, and chives all work well.*

SERVES 6 AS AN APPETIZER, 3 AS A SIDE DISH

**6 Japanese eggplants, 6 to 8 inches long**
**1 cup fresh cilantro leaves**
**1 cup fresh Italian parsley leaves**
**1 teaspoon roasted ground cumin seeds**
**Zest of 2 lemons**
**½ cup lemon juice**
**Black pepper**
**Salt**

Over a grill or gas flame, roast the eggplant until the skin blackens and the flesh is soft. Allow to cool and peel carefully with a small sharp knife to remove all the skin, being careful that the eggplants keep their shape.

Puree the remaining ingredients in a blender or food processor. Pour the sauce over the eggplants and allow them to marinate in the sauce for at least an hour.

*Serving size = 1 eggplant with sauce*
*46 calories*
*0.4 gram fat*
*0 milligrams cholesterol*
*59.1 milligrams sodium without added salt*

## MARINATED BUTTERNUT SQUASH

Donna Nicoletti

Agrodolce, *or sweet and sour flavors, is classic Sicilian. The sweetness of the squash and the tanginess of the balsamic vinegar combine to make a side dish that will complement any savory main course.*

SERVES 6 TO 8

**1 medium butternut squash**
**¼ cup balsamic vinegar**
**2 tablespoons water**
**½ teaspoon salt**
**½ teaspoon freshly ground pepper**
**2 tablespoons mint, chopped**

Peel the skin from the squash and cut it in half. Carefully remove the seeds and stringy matter. Cut the squash into medium dice from the center.

In a sauté pan, put the balsamic vinegar and water, salt and pepper, and heat. Add the squash and cook for just a few minutes; it should remain firm. Remove the squash and liquid from the heat and put into a separate bowl. Cool completely. Add the chopped mint and serve as a garnish or side dish.

*Serving size = ½ cup*
*52 calories*
*0.1 gram fat*
*0 milligrams cholesterol*
*170 milligrams sodium*

## ROASTED AND RUSTIC SWEET PEPPERS

Michael McDermott

*The stunning colors make for a wonderful presentation and the fresh taste will complement a variety of dishes—especially grains, pastas, or beans. This can be prepared and refrigerated for up to 2 days.*

MAKES 3 CUPS
SERVES 3 TO 6

**3 roasted red bell peppers (page 133), sliced ¼-inch thick**
**3 roasted green bell peppers (page 133), sliced ¼-inch thick**
**3 tablespoons red wine vinegar**
**2 teaspoons minced garlic**
**¼ teaspoon dried basil**
**¼ teaspoon dried thyme**
**¼ teaspoon dried rosemary**
**¼ teaspoon dried marjoram**
**¼ teaspoon dried oregano**

In a large bowl, combine the peppers with the remaining ingredients. Toss well and marinate for at least 30 minutes. Serve at room temperature.

*Serving size = ½ cup*
*52 calories*
*0.1 gram fat*
*0 milligrams cholesterol*
*170.3 milligrams sodium*

## SICILIAN SWEET AND SOUR PUMPKIN SQUASH

Joyce Goldstein

*A specialty of Palermo, this dish is known as* Fegato ai Sette Cannoli, *or "Liver from the Seven Fountains." Sicilians think cooked squash has the meaty texture of liver, though there is no taste comparison.* Sette cannoli *refers to a seven-spouted fountain in the Vucceria market.*

*Instead of frying the pumpkin squash in the traditional style, bake it, then cut it into cubes. The onions are cooked in a sweet and sour sauce that is then tossed with the cooked pumpkin, and the mixture is topped with fresh mint. This dish keeps for a few days in the refrigerator.*

SERVES 4

**2 pounds pumpkin or butternut squash**
**Salt and pepper**
**1½ cups Brown Vegetable Stock (page 144)**
**2 onions, thinly sliced**
**6 tablespoons sugar**
**⅔ cup red wine vinegar**
**½ cup chopped fresh mint**

Preheat the oven to 375 degrees. Cut the pumpkin in half and remove the seeds. Place the pumpkin cut side down on a baking sheet. Bake about 45 minutes or until tender but not mush. The pumpkin flesh should be firm enough to cut into ½-inch cubes or slices. Sprinkle with salt and pepper.

Bring 1 cup of the stock to a boil in a saucepan and cook the onions in it, uncovered, over moderate heat until tender. When most of the liquid has evaporated, sprinkle the onions with sugar and cook until the onions begin to caramelize. Add the vinegar and the remaining stock and continue to cook until deep golden brown but not burned. Add water if the mixture seems dry; the onions should end up in a sweet and sour syrup. Toss the pumpkin cubes with the onion mixture and stir well to coat. Sprinkle with coarsely chopped mint.

NOTE: If you can't find a nice pumpkin, butternut or banana squash will do and can be prepared the same way.

*Serving size = 1¼ cups*
*166 calories*
*0.3 gram fat*
*0 milligrams cholesterol*
*80.1 milligrams sodium without added salt*

# *Pasta / Pizza / Polenta / Bread Dishes*

## LINGUINE WITH GREENS, POTATOES, GARLIC, HOT PEPPER, AND TOMATOES

Joyce Goldstein

*This pasta is wonderful when little new potatoes are at their sweetest. While most of us can find little red potatoes (known in the trade as "creamers") at our market, try to keep your eyes open for butter-tasting yellow Finnish potatoes, the nutty bintjis, and sweet ruby crescents as well. The richness of the potato provides a nice contrast for the tart and pungent greens.*

SERVES 4

**6 to 8 little new potatoes**
**½ cup cooked green beans (optional)**
**½ pound pasta (shells, penne, linguine, farfalle)**
**½ cup vegetable stock**
**½ cup diced onions**
**2 teaspoons finely minced garlic**
**2 teaspoons hot red pepper flakes (optional)**
**1½ cups diced, peeled plum tomatoes**
**½ cup juice from the tomatoes or tomato juice**

**4 cups assorted greens (escarole, arugula, dandelion, chard)**
**Salt and pepper**

Bake the potatoes in a 350-degree oven for 35 to 40 minutes, until tender but firm. Or steam them in water or vegetable stock to cover. If you steam them in vegetable stock, reserve it for the pasta sauce. When cool enough to handle, cut the potatoes into 1-inch chunks. If you are including green beans, cook them in vegetable stock and immediately refresh in cold water. Drop the pasta into a large kettle of boiling salted water. Stir.

Heat the ½ cup stock in a sauté pan over moderate heat. Add the onions and cook, covered, until tender, about 10 minutes. Add the garlic and optional hot red pepper flakes and cook 2 minutes longer. Add the tomatoes, tomato liquid, potatoes, and greens and optional beans and cook until the greens are wilted and the potatoes are heated through. Season with salt and pepper. When the pasta is al dente, drain it and toss with the sauce in a warmed bowl.

NOTE: Canned tomatoes can be substituted for fresh.

*Serving size = 2 cups*
*307 calories*
*1.4 grams fat*
*0 milligrams cholesterol*
*271.0 milligrams sodium without added salt*

## PASTA WITH RED PEPPERS, GREENS, WHITE BEANS, GARLIC, AND LEMON ZEST

Joyce Goldstein

*The fleshy peppers play nicely off the rich white beans, accented by the tart greens and lemon.*

SERVES 2

**½ cup white beans, soaked in water overnight**
**1 bay leaf**
**4 garlic cloves**
**⅓ cup vegetable stock**
**2 red bell peppers, cut in ½-inch strips**
**4 cups Swiss chard or escarole, washed well and cut into ½-inch strips**
**1 tablespoon grated lemon zest**
**Salt**
**Freshly ground pepper**
**2 tablespoons lemon juice**
**½ pound penne and farfalle pasta**

Rinse the beans, put them in a saucepan, and cover with 2 cups cold water. Add the bay leaf and 2 cloves of garlic and bring to a boil over high heat. Reduce the heat and simmer until tender, 45 to 60 minutes. Remove the pot from the heat.

Bring the vegetable stock to a simmer in a sauté pan over moderate heat. Add the pepper strips and simmer for 5 to 8 minutes, then add the greens, 2 cloves of garlic that have been minced, and lemon zest and stir well, until the greens are wilted, 3 to 4 minutes. Drain the beans (most of the liquid will have been absorbed) from the cooking liquid with a slotted spoon and add them to the peppers and greens. Warm through. Season to taste with salt, pepper, and lemon juice.

Meantime, cook the pasta according to directions. Drain and toss with the beans and vegetables.

NOTE: This can be made with roasted peppers, in which case steam the greens, as above, in the stock and add the peppers with the beans. Also, any remaining bean liquid could be used as a pasta sauce; you will have enough for ½ pound.

*Serving size = 1⅔ cups vegetables and 2 ounces pasta*
*195 calories*
*1.2 grams fat*
*0 milligrams cholesterol*
*394.7 milligrams sodium without added salt*

## PASTA WITH ROASTED EGGPLANT AND TOMATO SAUCE

Joyce Goldstein

*Most eggplant pastas have a tendency to be rather oily because eggplant is so porous that it absorbs every drop of oil that touches it. To cook the eggplant without oil you could peel and boil it, but then it would taste like old socks. By baking the eggplant, you eliminate the problem: The eggplant steams in its skin and remains very moist and flavorful. Just add tomato sauce, garlic, capers, and the herb of your choice for a very satisfying dish.*

MAKES 2 MAIN DISHES OR 4 FIRST COURSES

**1 medium eggplant**
**½ pound penne, rigatoni, or pasta shells**
**1½ cups tomato sauce**
**4 garlic cloves, finely minced**
**2 tablespoons capers, rinsed and coarsely chopped**
**Pinch of hot red pepper flakes**
**2 teaspoons dried oregano, or 4 tablespoons chopped fresh basil**
**Salt**
**Freshly ground black pepper**

Preheat the oven to 450 degrees.

Prick the eggplant in a few places with a knife. Place on a baking sheet and roast for about 40 minutes, turning occasionally for even cooking, until the eggplant is tender but not falling apart. When the eggplant is cool enough to handle, peel it and dice the pulp. Place the pulp in a colander to drain away any bitter juices. Discard the skin.

Bring a large pot of salted water to a boil. Drop in the pasta and stir.

Warm the tomato sauce in a large sauté pan over moderate heat. Add the eggplant and the rest of the ingredients and warm through. Season to taste. Adjust salt, pepper, and hot red pepper. If the tomatoes are tart, add a pinch of sugar to compensate. When the pasta is al dente, drain and toss with the sauce. Serve at once.

NOTE: Two roasted and peeled red or green peppers, cut and diced, can be added to the dish.

*Serving size = 2⅓ cups*
*129 calories*
*0.8 gram fat*
*0 milligrams cholesterol*
*630 milligrams sodium without added salt*

## SPAGHETTI WITH SICILIAN GREENS

Joyce Goldstein

*The Arabic influence on Sicilian cuisine makes itself felt in this pasta with the addition of currants to the confit of greens and saffron to the onions.*

SERVES 3

**¼ teaspoon crushed saffron filaments**
**2 tablespoons white wine**
**½ cup sun-dried tomatoes (not in oil), cut into ¼-inch strips**
**1 cup vegetable stock**
**¼ cup currants**
**½ pound spaghetti**
**2 cups yellow onions, sliced ¼-inch thick**
**1 cup fennel, sliced ⅛ inch thick**
**1 tablespoon minced garlic**
**6 cups greens cut into ½-inch strips (escarole, chard, dandelion, and so on)**
**Salt and pepper**

Combine the saffron and white wine in a small pan. Simmer a minute or two over low heat. Set aside to steep.

Soak the sun-dried tomatoes in vegetable stock for 30 minutes. Plump the currants in hot water.

Bring a large pot of salted water to a boil. Drop in the spaghetti and stir.

Drain the tomatoes and set aside; reserve the soaking liquid. Bring the tomato liquid to a simmer in a large sauté pan. Simmer the onions until they are tender and translucent, 10 to 15 minutes. Add the saffron and wine and simmer 1 minute longer. Add the fennel, garlic, and sun-dried tomatoes and simmer 3 to 4 minutes. Drain the currants but reserve the water. Add the greens and currants to the onion mixture and cook until greens are wilted. Season with salt and pepper. Add currant liquid if needed for texture and balance of flavor. Cook the spaghetti until al dente. Toss all together.

*Serving size = 1⅔ cups*
*296 calories*
*2.1 grams fat*
*0 milligrams cholesterol*
*244.3 milligrams sodium without added salt*

## SPINACH RAVIOLI

Jean-Marc Fullsack

*The pot-sticker skins make this very easy to prepare. Look for them in the Asian foods department of your local supermarket or in a Chinese food market.*

*Try these with the Tomato and Roasted Bell Pepper Sauce (page 354), the sauce from the Pasta with Tomato, Basil, and Garlic Sauce (page 312), or almost any sauce you choose. They would also be delicious with the Tomato Consommé (page 204) ladled over them. Prepare and refrigerate the ravioli on a parchment-lined cookie sheet in single layers up to 6 hours ahead of time.*

MAKES 48 RAVIOLI
SERVES 6 TO 8

**1 cup tomatoes, peeled, seeded, and diced**
**1 small onion, oven roasted (page 133) and chopped**
**1 cup minced mushrooms**
**2 teaspoons minced garlic**
**½ pound spinach leaves, blanched (page 131) and chopped**
**½ cup nonfat cottage cheese**
**2 tablespoons minced fresh basil**
**Freshly ground black pepper**
**Salt**
**48 eggless pot-sticker skins**

In a large saucepan, combine the tomatoes, onion, mushrooms, and garlic. Cook over medium heat until the liquid from the mushrooms completely evaporates and the mixture is somewhat dry. Be careful not to burn it. Set aside to cool.

In a large bowl, combine the tomato mixture, spinach, cottage cheese, and basil. Season to taste with pepper and salt.

On a cutting board, lay out a single layer of pot-sticker skins. Using a pastry brush, moisten the edges with water. Place 1 tablespoon of the spinach mixture onto the center of each skin. Cover with a second potsticker skin and press the edges together with the tines of a fork to seal.

Cook the ravioli in boiling water or vegetable stock for 3 minutes, or until the potsticker skin is al dente. Serve hot.

*Serving size = 6 ravioli*
*107 calories*
*0.9 gram fat*
*0.6 milligram cholesterol*
*140.3 milligrams sodium without added salt*

## MUSHROOM LASAGNE

Tina Salter and Christine Swett

*When the porcini mushrooms have reopened their "gills" during the soaking is when the flavor has increased. Any variety of mushrooms can be used. You can save some time by chopping the mushrooms in a food processor. Be sure to use the pulse function. You want the mushrooms to be chopped but not pureed.*

MAKES 1 9 × 13-INCH LASAGNE
SERVES 9

**1 eggplant (approximately 1¼ pounds)**
**2 ounces dried porcini mushrooms, soaked 20 minutes in 1 cup water**
**2 pounds fresh domestic mushrooms**
**3 onions, finely minced**
**1 cup red wine**
**1 28-ounce can crushed tomatoes with puree**
**¼ cup chopped fresh parsley**
**2 teaspoons chopped fresh thyme or 1 teaspoon dried**
**1 teaspoon ground nutmeg**
**½ teaspoon red hot pepper flakes**
**1 pound nonfat cottage cheese**
**1 cup Nonfat Yogurt Cheese (page 148)**
**1 pound soft tofu**
**1 pound lasagne noodles**
**4 large ripe tomatoes, thinly sliced**

Preheat the oven to 350 degrees.

On a nonstick baking sheet roast the eggplant for 1 hour. Peel and finely chop the pulp. Set aside.

Drain the porcini mushrooms and preserve their soaking liquid. Chop the fresh and soaked mushrooms coarsely and set aside.

In a large sauté pan, put the mushroom soaking liquid and the onions. Sauté until just translucent. Add the mushrooms and red wine, then sauté over medium heat for 15 minutes, or until all the liquid has evaporated. At this point stir in the eggplant and add the crushed tomatoes, then continue cooking until very soft and the liquid has evaporated again. Add the parsley, thyme, ground nutmeg, and red pepper flakes, then set aside.

In a food processor, combine the cottage cheese, yogurt cheese, and tofu. Pulse to just combine. Set aside.

Cook the pasta according to the package directions. Drain and set aside.

To assemble the lasagne, spread ½ cup of the mushroom mixture over the bottom of a lasagne pan. Cover with ½ cup of the cheese mixture. Cover the cheese mixture with a layer of noodles.

Repeat with the remaining ingredients, using one-third of the remaining ingredients for each layer, ending with the noodles. Layer the sliced tomatoes over the top layer of noodles and bake for 40 minutes. Remove from the oven and let rest 15 minutes before serving.

*Serving size = 2 cups*
*191 calories*
*1.8 grams fat*
*2.3 milligrams cholesterol*
*160 milligrams sodium*

## PASTA CARDOZO

John Cardozo

*The sauce is filled with the meatlike texture of the vegetable protein. It makes a filling and satisfyingly delicious meal.*

SERVES 6

**1 cup water or vegetable stock**
**3 tablespoons ketchup**
**1 cup texturized vegetable protein chunks (page 120)**
**1 cup chopped onion**
**3 tablespoons minced garlic**
**½ cup vegetable stock or white wine**
**1 cup diced celery**
**1 cup diced carrots**
**1 28-ounce can chopped tomatoes**
**2 tablespoons tomato paste**

**2 tablespoons soy sauce**
**¼ teaspoon dried red chili flakes**
**1 teaspoon dried oregano**
**Freshly ground black pepper**
**Salt**
**1 pound dried pasta**
**¼ cup chopped fresh basil**

In a medium saucepan, bring the water or stock to a boil. Remove from the heat and add the ketchup. Add the vegetable protein chunks, cover, and let soak for 5 minutes. Drain well, chop into ¼-inch bits, and set aside.

In a large saucepan, braise the onion and garlic in the ½ cup of stock or wine for 5 minutes, or until tender. Add the celery and carrots and braise an additional 5 minutes. Add the chopped tomatoes, vegetable protein, tomato paste, soy sauce, chili flakes, and oregano. Simmer over low heat for 30 minutes. Season to taste with pepper and salt. Let the sauce rest while the pasta cooks, according to package directions. Ladle the sauce over the pasta, garnish with the basil, and serve immediately.

*Serving size = 1 cup pasta and 1 cup sauce*
*226 calories*
*1.4 grams fat*
*0 milligrams cholesterol*
*794.4 milligrams sodium without added salt*

## PASTA WITH TOMATO, BASIL, AND GARLIC SAUCE

Conrad and Marsha Knudsen

*This is exceptionally easy to prepare and a good sauce to keep on hand in your refrigerator. It will keep well for up to 3 days in the refrigerator or frozen for up to 2 months.*

MAKES 6 CUPS SAUCE
SERVES 6

**12 cups canned chopped tomatoes (2 28-ounce cans)**
**3 tablespoons chopped garlic**
**1 cup chopped fresh basil**
**1 teaspoon sugar**
**Freshly ground black pepper**
**Salt**
**10 ounces angel hair pasta**
**¼ cup chiffonaded fresh basil**

In a large, nonstick saucepan, combine the tomatoes, garlic, basil, and sugar. Bring to a boil and simmer, uncovered, over low heat for 30 minutes. Season to taste with pepper and salt.

Prepare the pasta according to the package directions. Drain the pasta well and divide into 6 servings. Ladle sauce over each serving and garnish with the chiffonaded basil.

*Serving size = 1 cup sauce and 1 cup pasta*
*242 calories*
*1.4 grams fat*
*0 milligrams cholesterol*
*484.7 milligrams sodium without added salt*

## ITALIAN-STYLE VEGETABLES WITH PASTA

Tracy Pikhart Ritter

*Fresh, seasonal vegetables are sautéed in vegetable stock instead of oil to release their flavors. Fresh herbs and reconstituted sun-dried tomatoes add authentic Italian taste to this savory tomato-based pasta sauce.*

SERVES 4

**2 tablespoons vegetable stock**
**1 red bell pepper, seeded and coarsely chopped**
**1 yellow bell pepper, seeded and coarsely chopped**
**1 green bell pepper, seeded and coarsely chopped**
**2 small zucchini, cut into ½-inch slices**

- **½ red onion, chopped**
- **1 garlic clove, minced**
- **1 14-ounce can whole peeled tomatoes in sauce**
- **4 large sun-dried tomatoes, softened and chopped**
- **2 tablespoons chopped fresh oregano or ½ teaspoon dried**
- **2 tablespoons chopped fresh basil or 1 teaspoon dried**
- **½ teaspoon sea salt**
- **½ teaspoon freshly ground black pepper**
- **4 2½-ounce servings of your favorite pasta**

Heat a large skillet. Add the stock and all the ingredients except the pasta. Cover and cook over medium-low heat for 15 to 20 minutes, or until al dente.

Cook the pasta according to the package directions. Drain well and serve with the vegetable sauce.

*Serving size = 1 cup pasta and 1 cup sauce*
*280 calories*
*1.9 grams fat*
*0 milligrams cholesterol*
*481.2 milligrams sodium*

## ORZO WITH LEMON AND HERBS

Martha Rose Shulman

*Orzo is a rice-shaped pasta, as popular in Greece, where it is called* kritharaki *or* orza, *as it is in Italy, where it is called* manestra *or* riso. *Part of its appeal for a cook is that it is very difficult to overcook. This is a lightened but wonderful version of a traditional Greek dish to serve as a side dish or a main course.*

Makes 6 cups
Serves 4 to 6

- **2 quarts vegetable stock**
- **2 cups medium orzo**
- **¾ cup chopped fresh herbs (parsley, basil, or tarragon)**

**¼ cup fresh lemon juice**
**Freshly ground black pepper**
**Salt**

In a large saucepan, bring the vegetable stock to a boil. Add the orzo and cook for 10 to 15 minutes, or until just tender. Drain well and toss with herbs and lemon juice. Season to taste with pepper and salt. Serve hot, at room temperature, or chilled.

NOTE: You can prepare this up to 6 hours in advance. Serve at room temperature or reheat in a 350-degree oven for 15 to 20 minutes.

*Serving size = 1 cup*
*237 calories*
*1.2 grams fat*
*0 milligrams cholesterol*
*91 milligrams sodium without added salt*

## INDONESIAN "FRIED" NOODLES

Conrad and Marsha Knudsen

MAKES 8 CUPS
SERVES 4 TO 8

**1 pound soba noodles**
**3 tablespoons low-sodium soy sauce**
**1½ tablespoons brown sugar**
**1 to 3 teaspoons crushed red chili peppers**
**1 cup finely chopped onion**
**3 teaspoons minced garlic**
**1 tablespoon peeled and grated gingerroot**
**1 cup snow peas**
**6 green onions, chopped**
**1 teaspoon lime zest**
**1 cup bean sprouts**

**½ pound tofu, cut into ½-inch cubes**
**Fresh lime juice**
**Chopped fresh cilantro**

Prepare the noodles according to the package directions, drain well, and set aside.

In a large, nonstick sauté pan combine the soy sauce, brown sugar, and crushed red peppers. Stir to dissolve the sugar. Add the onions, garlic, and ginger and cook for 1 to 2 minutes. At this point add the snow peas, green onions, and lime zest. Toss, then cook for 1 to 2 minutes, or until the peas are tender and bright-colored. Add the bean sprouts and tofu. Continue cooking and toss just until the bean sprouts are slightly wilted.

Add the soba noodles and toss well. Add lime juice to taste and garnish with the cilantro.

*Serving size = 1½ cups*
*186 calories*
*1.1 grams fat*
*0 milligrams cholesterol*
*640.5 milligrams sodium*

## PIZZA

Jean-Marc Fullsack

*Top this pizza with your favorite vegetables, such as peppers and mushrooms. The dough can be prepared and frozen up to 2 months. Allow it to return to room temperature before assembling. The pizza sauce can be kept refrigerated for up to 3 days.*

1 16-INCH PIZZA
SERVES 8

**1½ cups warm water**
**1 tablespoon active dry yeast**
**1 teaspoon honey**
**4 cups unbleached flour**

**½ teaspoon salt**
**1 onion, roasted and sliced (page 133)**
**1 cup canned or fresh tomato puree**
**1 teaspoon dried thyme**
**1 teaspoon chopped fresh basil**
**1 teaspoon chopped fresh parsley**
**1 teaspoon dried oregano**
**1 teaspoon minced garlic**
**1 teaspoon black pepper**
**Pinch of salt**
**Pinch of sugar**
**1 eggplant, oven roasted (page 132)**
**1 zucchini, sliced ⅛ inch thick and blanched (page 131)**
**1 yellow squash, sliced ⅛ inch thick and blanched (page 131)**
**4 plum tomatoes, sliced ⅛ inch thick**
**1 teaspoon chopped fresh basil**

In a large bowl, combine the water, yeast, honey, and 4 teaspoons flour. Stir gently to combine. Cover the bowl with a damp towel and let stand for 30 minutes in a warm place until foamy.

Add the remaining flour and salt, then knead for about 10 minutes, until the dough is well combined and smooth; add small amounts of additional flour if the dough is sticky. Transfer the dough to a large bowl, cover with a damp towel, and let rise in a warm place for about 45 minutes, or until doubled in volume. Punch the dough down and roll to fit into a 16-inch pizza pan. Set aside.

Preheat the oven to 450 degrees. In a large bowl, combine the onions, tomato puree, thyme, basil, parsley, oregano, garlic, pepper, salt, and sugar and stir to combine. Spread the mixture over the dough.

Chop the flesh of the roasted eggplant and spread over the sauce. Layer the zucchini, yellow squash, plum tomatoes, and basil over the eggplant.

Bake the pizza for 15 to 20 minutes, or until the dough is golden brown. Serve hot.

*Serving size = 1/8 of a 16-inch pizza*
*267 calories*
*0.8 gram fat*
*0 milligrams cholesterol*
*279.2 milligrams sodium without added salt*

## POLENTA ALLA VENEZIANA

Joyce Goldstein

SERVES 4

*This is a dinner divine. The creamy polenta is a fine support player to a rich ragout of mushrooms, asparagus, and tomato.*

**4 cups cold water or vegetable stock or more as needed**
**1 cup coarse cornmeal for polenta**
**Salt**
**Freshly ground black pepper**
**1 cup Brown Vegetable Stock (page 144) or water**
**1 cup diced yellow onions**
**2½ cups asparagus, cut into 1-inch lengths**
**4 cups thickly sliced mushrooms**
**1½ cups diced plum tomatoes (optional)**
**2 tablespoons finely chopped fresh parsley**
**2 teaspoons finely minced garlic**
**1 tablespoon grated lemon zest**

Stir the water or stock and cornmeal together in a large heavy saucepan. Cook over low heat, stirring often and scraping the bottom of the pot, until the mixture is thick and no longer feels grainy on the tongue, about 30 minutes. If it still feels grainy and all the liquid has been absorbed, add more, stirring it in well. Season to taste with salt and pepper. Keep warm over hot water.

Keep the polenta in a soft state by adding water or stock from time to time. Or pour it into a sheet pan lined with baker's parchment. Refrigerate. When firm, turn out onto a work surface and cut into triangles or finger lengths; warm in the oven or broiler.

Bring the vegetable stock to a simmer in a sauté pan. Add the onions and cook, covered, over moderate heat, until the onions are tender and translucent, about 15 minutes. Add the asparagus and mushrooms and stir well, simmering uncovered for 5 to 7 minutes until tender. Add the optional diced tomatoes, season with salt and pepper, and stir in the parsley, garlic, and lemon zest. Warm through. Spoon this mixture over either soft or baked polenta and serve at once.

NOTE: White mushrooms can almost always be found at the supermarket. If you can find brown mushrooms, chanterelles, or other wild mushrooms they will add a greater depth of flavor to this dish. Dried mushrooms soaked in hot water and drained also can intensify the flavor: strain the soaking liquids through cheesecloth and add them to the sauce for an even richer ragout. When asparagus is not available, increase the mushroom quantity to 5 to 6 cups. This sauce can also be used over pasta or rice or stirred into a basic risotto.

*Serving size = 2 cups*
*339 calories*
*2.1 grams fat*
*0 milligrams cholesterol*
*90.0 milligrams salt without added salt*

## BLACK PEPPER POLENTA WITH BELL PEPPER SAUCE AND SHIITAKE MUSHROOMS

Hubert Keller

SERVES 4

**3 red bell peppers**
**Vegetable oil spray**
**1 small onion, diced**
**2 small garlic cloves, chopped**

- **3 large tomatoes, peeled, seeded, and chopped**
- **Pinch of chopped thyme**
- **5 fresh basil leaves**
- **1 teaspoon honey**
- **Freshly ground black pepper**
- **8 to 10 medium shiitake mushrooms**
- **3½ cups Vegetable Consommé (page 147)**
- **1 cup coarse cornmeal**
- **⅓ cup grated nonfat Parmesan**
- **½ teaspoon coarsely ground black pepper**
- **4 pinches of fresh chervil (keep whole for garnishing)**

Preheat the broiler. Coat the peppers very lightly with the vegetable oil spray. Place under the broiler and roast, turning frequently, until the skin is blackened on all sides. When the peppers are completely charred, cool them until they can be handled comfortably and peel off the skin. Remove the stems, core, and seeds. Chop the peppers and set them aside.

Lightly spray the bottom of a saucepan with the vegetable oil. Add the diced onion and simmer over medium heat, stirring until translucent, about 1½ minutes. Add the garlic, tomatoes, bell peppers, thyme, basil, honey, and freshly ground pepper.

Cook over low heat for 15 to 20 minutes, until the bell peppers and tomato mixture start to thicken; if the mixture seems to be reducing too fast, add 1 or 2 tablespoons of water. Transfer to a blender or food processor and puree until completely smooth. Transfer to a small saucepan and keep warm.

Remove and discard the stems of the shiitake mushrooms. Mince the mushrooms. Lightly spray a nonstick frying pan with the vegetable oil and set over medium heat. Sauté the mushrooms, add freshly ground pepper, and keep warm.

Bring the vegetable consommé to a boil in a heavy saucepan. Pour in the cornmeal in a thin stream while whisking constantly until it begins to thicken, about 20 minutes. Stir in the Parmesan and the coarsely ground black pepper. Divide the polenta among 4 warmed soup plates. Spoon the red pepper sauce gently all around the polenta. Top the polenta with the sautéed shiitake mushrooms and sprinkle with chervil.

*Serving size = 1½ cups*
*226 calories*
*1.4 grams fat*
*1.2 milligrams cholesterol*
*120.2 milligrams sodium*

## POLENTA WITH SUN-DRIED TOMATOES AND BLACK BEANS

Tracy Pikhart Ritter

SERVES 6

**4 cups water or vegetable stock**
**1 cup polenta or finely ground cornmeal**
**1 tablespoon ground cumin**
**1 teaspoon freshly ground black pepper**
**1 teaspoon ground basil or oregano**
**3 tablespoons chopped scallions**

SUN-DRIED TOMATO PESTO

**½ cup softened sun-dried tomatoes**
**2 garlic cloves, minced**
**¼ cup balsamic vinegar**
**½ cup chopped fresh basil**
**¼ cup chopped fresh Italian parsley**
**1 teaspoon capers**
**1 teaspoon balsamic vinegar**
**1 large fresh tomato, seeded**

BLACK BEANS

**2 cups cooked black beans**
**4 garlic cloves, minced**
**1 jalapeño pepper, seeded and minced**
**½ red onion, minced**
**1 tablespoon black pepper**
**1 teaspoon black pepper**
**1 teaspoon ground cumin**
**½ cup dry sherry**

Bring the water or stock to a boil; slowly add the polenta, stirring constantly to avoid lumps. Add the cumin and pepper. Reduce to a simmer and cook, stirring often, for 20 minutes, until the polenta is thick and begins to pull away from the sides of the pot. Add the basil and scallions. Set aside.

Add all the ingredients for the Sun-Dried Tomato Pesto to the blender and process at high speed until well blended and smooth. Pour into a bowl and set aside.

In a large saucepan or skillet, cook the garlic, jalapeño, onion, pepper, and cumin in the sherry for 3 minutes until soft. Add the cooked black beans and continue to heat until hot. Add vegetable stock if moister beans are desired.

Serve the polenta with the black beans spooned over. Garnish with the tomato pesto.

*Serving size = 1½ cups*
*265 calories*
*1.9 grams fat*
*0 milligrams cholesterol*
*33.4 milligrams sodium*

## POLENTA AND MUSHROOMS

Michael Lomonaco

SERVES 6

**1 cup polenta or finely ground cornmeal**
**½ teaspoon dried thyme leaves**
**2 tablespoons chopped fresh parsley**
**½ teaspoon dried oregano leaves**
**Pepper to taste**
**1 cup sliced mushrooms, steamed for 3 minutes or sautéed in vegetable stock**
**½ cup nonfat plain yogurt**

In a nonstick pot, bring 2 cups water to boil. Using a whisk, slowly stir in the cornmeal, taking care to avoid lumps. Return the mixture to the boil, lower the heat, and simmer for about 10 minutes. After the polenta has cooked, stir in the herbs, seasoning, mushrooms, and yogurt. Cook for 5 minutes. Using a nonstick baking pan, pour the polenta in and set aside to cool. When the polenta is cool and firm, cut it into pieces about 2 inches by 2 inches. Broil, toast, or grill the pieces and serve with the tomato sauce of your choice or as a side dish with vegetables, stew, or chili.

NOTE: Any type of mushrooms, or a combination, will work here.

*Serving size = ½ cup*
*100 calories*
*0.5 gram fat*
*0.3 milligram cholesterol*
*16 milligrams sodium*

## BASIC BREAD DOUGH FOR FOCACCIA OR LOAVES

Donna Nicoletti

MAKES 1 LOAF (30 SLICES)

**4 cups bread flour**
**1½ teaspoons salt**
**3 tablespoons active dry yeast**
**1⅓ cups lukewarm water (100 degrees maximum)**
**Spray bottle of water**

Put the flour, salt, and yeast in an electric mixer that has a dough hook attachment. With the mixer on low speed, slowly add the warm water. When the dough forms a ball, turn up the speed to medium to knead for 7 minutes. The dough is completely kneaded if you press your finger into it and it bounces back.

Put the dough into a large bowl and cover tightly with

plastic wrap. Keep in a warm—but not hot—spot in the kitchen until it doubles in volume. Punch the dough down, cover again with plastic, and let rise a second time.

At this point the dough is ready to be used in various recipes. Directions follow for focaccia or a simple loaf.

*For focaccia:* Preheat the oven to 350 degrees. Lay the dough on a cookie sheet with sides or a jelly roll pan. A pizza pan or baking tile can also be used. Press the dough out to the corners of the pan. If it resists, don't worry. The dough must rise again and then it will fill the pan. After it has doubled and covers the whole pan, press your fingers into the surface to give it its traditional indentations. The dough is now ready for a choice of toppings such as tomato sauce or dried or fresh herbs (rosemary is a favorite) and coarse grain salt. Put the pan in the oven, lightly spray the top with water, and bake for 25 to 30 minutes, or until it is lightly brown on the bottom. Slip out immediately and cool on a rack.

*For bread loaf:* Preheat the oven to 475 degrees. Put the dough in a 12 × 17-inch bread loaf pan, and let it rise until it is doubled. Slash the top of the bread in three places with a knife and, if you wish, sprinkle with flour. Put in the oven and spray the oven with water to help form a good crust. After 10 minutes, reduce the temperature to 400 degrees and spray the oven once again. Bake the bread for approximately 30 to 40 minutes. To check for doneness, turn the bread out of the pan and tap on the bottom. If it sounds hollow, it is ready to come out of the oven. Cool on a rack.

NOTE: Alternatively, before the final rising you can halve the dough and form two cylinders to yield two baguettes after allowing the dough to double in the rising. Bake as above.

*Serving size = 1 slice*
*67 calories*
*0.3 gram fat*
*0 milligrams cholesterol*
*117.6 milligrams salt*

## PASTA WITH TOFU, CORN, AND SAFFRON

Tracy Pikhart Ritter

*The combination of tofu, sweet peppers, and corn in a spicy vegetable broth with pasta creates a nicely textured dish. The saffron gives it a delicate flavor and pale peach color.*

SERVES 6

**½ red onion, minced**
**¼ bay leaf**
**½ teaspoon saffron threads**
**1 teaspoon orange zest**
**1 quart vegetable stock**
**1 8-ounce brick firm tofu, cut into cubes**
**2 teaspoons chili powder**
**2 teaspoons ground cumin**
**2 teaspoons ground coriander**
**½ teaspoon salt, or to taste**
**1 pound pasta**
**Vegetable oil cooking spray**
**2 red bell peppers, roasted (page 133), peeled, and cut into julienne strips**
**Kernels from 2 large ears of corn or 1 cup frozen, rinsed**
**1 bunch basil, cut in chiffonade**

Place the onion, bay leaf, saffron, zest, and stock in a sauté pan. Bring to a boil, reduce to a simmer, and reduce by half. Strain to clear the liquid of solids and set aside. Meanwhile, put the water for the pasta on to boil.

Combine the tofu, chili, cumin, coriander, and salt, if desired. Cook the pasta according to the manufacturer's instructions. Five minutes before the pasta is done, heat a skillet, spray with vegetable oil cooking spray, and add the tofu, peppers, and corn. Cook for 1 minute. Add the strained vegetable sauce and bring to a simmer.

Drain the pasta well and add to the tofu mixture. Toss the

pasta with the sauce and continue to cook for 1 to 2 minutes, until thickened. Garnish with the basil.

*Serving size = 2 cups*
*377 calories*
*2.9 grams fat*
*0 milligrams cholesterol*
*228.3 milligrams sodium*

## SPAGHETTI WITH BEANS AND PISTOU SAUCE

Tina Salter and Christine Swett

*The various beans and vegetables make this a very colorful dish. An interesting combination might be yellow split peas, black beans, garbanzo beans, navy beans, red beans, and pinto beans—probably there are dozens more. If you want to, you could start with 2½ cups of various types of canned beans that you have rinsed well and drained.*

MAKES 8 CUPS
SERVES 4 TO 6

**1 cup mixed beans, soaked overnight**
**⅛ cup lentils**
**3 cups Vegetable Stock (page 143)**
**1 cup white wine**
**1 cup roasted and sliced onion (page 133)**
**¼ cup julienned carrots**
**¼ cup julienned celery**
**¼ cup julienned fennel**
**¼ cup julienned leeks, white part only**
**¼ cup julienned turnip**
**¼ cup julienned green bell pepper**
**¼ cup green beans, cut into 2-inch lengths**
**8 ounces dried fettuccine or spaghetti**
**1½ cups Pistou Sauce (page 361)**
**Chopped fresh basil**
**Freshly ground black pepper**
**Salt**

In a medium saucepan, combine the beans, lentils, stock, and wine. Simmer for 45 minutes, or until tender. Drain well and set aside.

In a large nonstick sauté pan, sweat the onions, carrots, celery, fennel, leeks, turnip, pepper, and green beans for 5 minutes, or until just tender. Set aside.

Cook the pasta according to the package directions. Drain well. In a large serving bowl, combine the beans, vegetables, and pasta with 1 cup Pistou Sauce and toss well. Season to taste with salt and pepper. Garnish with the remaining pistou and basil.

*Serving size = 1½ cups*
*314 calories*
*1.5 grams fat*
*0 milligrams cholesterol*
*256 milligrams sodium without added salt*

# Rice and Other Grains

## ISLAND RICE

Dennis and Margaret Malone

*This rice dish is subtly aromatic and has a light flavor. Prepare it up to 2 days in advance and reheat in a microwave oven or steamer.*

SERVES 4

**3 cups water**
**1½ cups medium-grain brown rice**
**2 tablespoons finely sliced fresh lemongrass**
**2 teaspoons finely minced lime zest**
**1 teaspoon salt**

In a medium saucepan, combine all the ingredients. Simmer over very low heat 50 minutes, or until the water is absorbed and the rice is al dente, cooked but still firm. Fluff the rice with a fork and serve hot.

*Serving size = ¾ cup*
*83 calories*
*0.6 gram fat*
*0 milligrams cholesterol*
*586.2 milligrams sodium*

## RICE PILAF WITH CARROTS, RAISINS, AND ORANGE ZEST

Joyce Goldstein

*This pilaf could be Persian, Afghani, or from a Russian province in the Caucasus.*

SERVES 4

**1 cup Basmati rice**
**3 cups hot vegetable stock**
**1 onion, chopped (about 1 cup)**
**½ teaspoon ground cinnamon**
**½ teaspoon ground cumin**
**5 large carrots, peeled and coarsely grated (2½ to 3 cups)**
**Grated zest of 1 orange**
**⅓ cup raisins and/or apricots, plumped in hot water, coarsely chopped**

Cover the rice with cold water and soak for an hour. Drain. Bring the stock to a boil in a medium saucepan. Keep warm. Ladle 1 cup of the stock into a sauté pan and add the chopped onion. Cook until the onion is tender and translucent, about 15 minutes. Add the spices and cook for a few minutes longer. Add the carrots, orange zest, and rice and cook for a minute or two. Add the rest of the stock and the drained fruit and cover the pan. Reduce heat and cook until the rice has absorbed the liquid, about 20 minutes. Let stand, covered, for 10 minutes longer. Fluff with a fork. Serve with steamed spinach topped with a dollop of nonfat yogurt.

*Serving size = 1¾ cups*
*244 calories*
*1.1 grams fat*
*0 milligrams cholesterol*
*94.9 milligrams sodium*

## RICE, LENTIL, AND SPINACH PILAF

Joyce Goldstein

*This combination of lentils, greens, and rice is typical of the Middle East. Instead of serving the greens and lentils over rice they are combined before serving. Accompany this with a dollop of yogurt or mint chutney or a spiced fruit chutney. You can substitute cooked chick-peas for the lentils.*

SERVES 4

**½ cup green lentils**
**1 cup Basmati rice**
**2 cups water**
**¾ cup vegetable stock**
**2 onions, chopped**
**2 garlic cloves, minced**
**4 celery stalks, chopped**
**2 teaspoons ground cumin**
**½ teaspoon ground cinnamon**
**Grated zest of 1 lemon**
**1 cup diced peeled tomatoes (optional)**
**3 to 4 cups well-washed fresh spinach or Swiss chard, cut in ½-inch strips**
**Salt**
**Pepper**

Wash the lentils, place them in a saucepan, and cover with cold water. Bring to a boil, reduce the heat, and cover the pan. Simmer for 25 to 40 minutes, until tender but still al dente. Drain.

Bring the rice and 2 cups of water to a boil. Reduce heat and simmer about 20 minutes, covered, until the rice has absorbed all of the liquid. Set aside.

Bring the vegetable stock to a boil in a saucepan. Add the onions and simmer until tender and translucent, about 10 minutes. Add the garlic, celery, cumin, and cinnamon and simmer for 5 minutes longer. Add the lentils and lemon zest and optional tomatoes to the pan. Heat through and then stir in the greens. When the greens are tender, fold the lentil and greens mixture into the rice. Season with salt and pepper.

NOTE: You may make this ahead of time and place in a baking pan, cover with foil, and warm in the oven for 15 to 20 minutes. Cooked cubes of carrots or butternut squash may also be added to this mixture.

*Serving size = 2 cups*
*169 calories*
*1.2 grams fat*
*0 milligrams cholesterol*
*162.3 milligrams sodium*

## RISOTTO WITH BUTTERNUT SQUASH, GREENS, AND TOMATOES

Joyce Goldstein

*This risotto would be at home in northern Italy or Portugal, where similar ingredients are combined with rice, but here the mixture is baked in a casserole rather than cooked over a flame. The sweetness of the squash and the onion provide a wonderful contrast with the greens and tomatoes.*

SERVES 6

**6 to 7 cups vegetable stock**
**2 cups diced yellow onion**
**1½ cups butternut squash, cut into ½-inch cubes**
**2 cups Arborio rice**
**¾ cup canned plum tomatoes, drained, cut in ½-inch dice, juices reserved**
**½ teaspoon ground nutmeg (optional)**
**1 teaspoon grated orange zest (optional)**
**3 cups Swiss chard, cut into ½-inch strips**
**Salt**
**Pepper**

Bring 1 cup stock to a simmer in a large sauté pan. Add the onions and simmer for 10 to 15 minutes, or until they are tender and translucent.

While the onions are cooking, bring the rest of the stock to a boil in a large saucepan. Drop the butternut squash into the boiling stock, reduce the heat, and simmer until the squash is cooked but still firm. Remove the squash with a slotted spoon and set aside. Keep the stock at a simmer.

Add the rice to the cooked onions and cook 3 to 5 minutes, until the rice is opaque. Ladle 1 cup of the simmering stock into the rice and stir until the stock is absorbed. Add another cup of stock and cook over low heat, stirring occasionally. Repeat the process with 1 more cup of stock; the rice will absorb the stock more slowly now but you can't rush it. When the rice is almost al dente, stir in the cooked squash and the tomatoes, the optional nutmeg and orange zest, and cook for a few minutes. Add 1½ cups more simmering stock and cook again until nearly absorbed, then add the greens and stir until they are wilted. Season to taste with salt and pepper. Serve at once. The mixture should be a little soupy in the bowl and the rice should be al dente, soft on the outside and firm in the center.

*Serving size = 2 cups*
*308 calories*
*0.8 gram fat*
*0 milligrams cholesterol*
*212.2 milligrams sodium without added salt*

## BASMATI RICE WITH PEAS

J. E. Hokin

*Try serving this elegant rice dish with Red Onions Simmered with Sherry Vinegar (page 294) for a satisfying light supper.*

SERVES 6

- **2 cups and 2 tablespoons vegetable stock**
- **½ small onion, finely chopped**
- **1 garlic clove, minced**
- **½ teaspoon dried basil**
- **1 cup Basmati rice**
- **1 teaspoon fine sea salt**
- **½ teaspoon freshly ground pepper**
- **1 pound peas, shelled, or 10-ounce package frozen tiny peas**

Heat the 2 tablespoons vegetable stock in a 4-quart saucepan, and add the onion, garlic, and basil. Cook 2 minutes over low heat. Add the 2 cups of stock, rice, salt, and pepper. Cover and cook over low heat for 20 minutes. Stir in the peas and cook until done, about 5 minutes more.

*Serving size = ¾ cup*
*75 calories*
*0.3 gram fat*
*0 milligrams cholesterol*
*407.1 milligrams sodium*

## SPANISH RICE

Paul Paulsen

*This is a great combination of fresh flavors. Serve it with a spinach salad with a cilantro-based dressing.*

MAKES 9 CUPS
SERVES 6 TO 9

- **1 cup chopped onion**
- **4 teaspoons minced garlic**
- **6 tablespoons white wine**
- **1 28-ounce can stewed tomatoes**
- **1 cup diced green bell pepper**
- **1 cup diced red or yellow bell pepper**

**1 cup sliced mushrooms**
**1 15-ounce can drained or vacuum-sealed corn kernels**
**4 to 6 tablespoons medium or hot salsa**
**1 teaspoon dried basil**
**1 teaspoon Italian seasoning (A Little Italian, page 148)**
**4 cups cooked brown rice**
**Black pepper**
**Salt**
**Chopped fresh cilantro, for garnish**

In a large, nonstick pan, braise the onion and garlic in the wine until tender. Add the stewed tomatoes, peppers, mushrooms, corn, salsa, basil, and Italian seasoning. Bring to a boil and simmer for 8 to 10 minutes.

In a large serving bowl, combine the hot cooked rice with the sauce and toss well to combine. Season to taste with pepper and salt. Garnish with chopped fresh cilantro and serve.

*Serving size = 1½ cups*
*289 calories*
*2.1 grams fat*
*0 milligrams cholesterol*
*788.8 milligrams sodium without added salt*

## KASHE

Natalie Ornish

*For centuries kashe was considered peasant food in Russia. While this recipe calls for buckwheat, a grain indigenous to Russia, kashe can also be made from wheat, barley, and millet. Whatever grain is used, it is usually browned in a pan to produce a nutty flavor.*

MAKES 3 CUPS
SERVES 6

**2 cups chopped onion**
**½ cup white wine**
**1 teaspoon dried thyme**

**1 teaspoon celery seeds**
**½ teaspoon sugar**
**¼ teaspoon ground cinnamon**
**1 cup kashe**
**1 raw egg white**
**2½ cups boiling water**

In a large nonstick sauté pan, sauté the onions in the white wine until translucent. Add the thyme, celery seeds, sugar, and cinnamon. Stir to combine well. Transfer to a medium bowl and set aside.

In another bowl combine the kashe and the egg white. Mix thoroughly to coat the kashe. Transfer the kashe to a large nonstick sauté pan and toast it, stirring frequently, until the grains are dry and light brown.

Add the boiling water and onion mixture. Reduce the heat, cover, and simmer for 12 to 15 minutes. Serve warm.

*Serving size = ½ cup*
*150 calories*
*1 gram fat*
*0 milligrams cholesterol*
*16.2 milligrams sodium*

## WILD RICE PANCAKES

Jean-Marc Fullsack

*Serve these very tasty and colorful savory pancakes over a puddle of the Carrot and Ginger Sauce (page 352) and lightly garnished with some chopped fresh herbs.*

MAKES 12 PANCAKES
SERVES 4 TO 6

**2 cups wild rice, cooked**
**½ cup flour**
**2 large egg whites (approximately ½ cup)**
**½ cup nonfat milk**

**¼ cup frozen peas**
**¼ cup fresh corn kernels**
**¼ cup red bell peppers, seeded and cut in ⅛-inch dice**
**¼ cup chopped green onions**
**2 tablespoons chopped fresh parsley**
**¼ teaspoon salt**
**⅛ teaspoon pepper**

Cook the wild rice according to the package directions and allow to cool.

In a large bowl, blend together the flour, egg whites, and milk until smooth. Add the cooked wild rice, peas, corn, red bell peppers, green onions, parsley, salt, and pepper. Stir to combine.

Ladle ¼ cup batter onto a hot nonstick griddle or sauté pan. Cook over medium heat until golden brown. Flip and repeat. Serve immediately.

*Serving size = 3 pancakes*
*187 calories*
*0.6 gram fat*
*0.6 milligram cholesterol*
*202.6 milligrams sodium*

## WARM SAFFRONED RICE SALAD WITH ASPARAGUS AND CREOJA SAUCE

Hubert Keller

SERVES 4

**1 cup long-grain white rice**
**2½ cups water**
**12 threads saffron**
**Freshly ground pepper**
**2 tablespoons finely chopped chives**
**¼ pound mixed baby lettuces, washed and dried**
**1 head endive, leaves separated**
**24 medium asparagus tips**

**4 tablespoons lemon juice**
**16 freshly toasted baguette slices**
**1 cup Creoja Sauce (page 350)**
**1 ripe tomato, peeled, seeded, and chopped**

Preheat the oven to 325 degrees. Place the rice and water in a flame-proof casserole. Add the saffron and pepper. Bring to a boil, stirring once or twice. Cover and bake in the oven for 20 minutes; the rice should be perfectly cooked and all the liquid absorbed. Mix in the chopped chives and keep warm.

Season the lettuces, endive, and asparagus tips with the lemon juice and freshly ground pepper. Place the lettuce in the center of each of 4 dinner plates. Arrange the asparagus tips attractively to one side. Garnish with the endive leaves.

Top the lettuces with the warm rice. Set the baguette slices on the side opposite from the asparagus, and top with Creoja Sauce on the side or spooned over the rice. Garnish each serving with a little of the chopped tomato.

*Serving size = 3 cups*
*199 calories*
*1.2 grams fat*
*0.1 milligram cholesterol*
*74.6 milligrams sodium*

## VEGETABLE RISOTTO WITH SAFFRON

Hubert Keller

SERVES 4

**Vegetable oil spray**
**½ cup finely chopped onion**
**½ teaspoon black mustard seeds**
**1 cup long-grain white rice**
**2 to 2½ cups Vegetable Consommé (page 147)**
**Zest of 4 limes**
**½ teaspoon saffron threads**

**2 garlic cloves, finely chopped**
**6 shiitake mushrooms, diced (optional)**
**4 tablespoons fresh shelled or frozen green peas**
**Freshly ground black pepper**
**8 basil leaves, chopped**
**2 tablespoons finely chopped chives**
**½ teaspoon finely chopped thyme**
**2 tomatoes, peeled, seeded, and diced**

Heat a nonstick saucepan over moderately low heat. Spray lightly with pan coating. Add the onion and cook slowly until translucent. Add the mustard seeds and cook until they turn gray, sputter, and pop. Pour in the rice and cook very gently over low heat, stirring, for 2 to 3 minutes.

Add the vegetable consommé, the lime zest, saffron, garlic, shiitake mushrooms, green peas, and pepper to taste. Bring to a boil over high heat, lower the heat, and keep stirring gently. Simmer for 20 to 25 minutes, until the rice is tender and fluffy. Add water or vegetable consommé as necessary. Add the basil, chives, thyme, and diced tomatoes and combine carefully. Cook for 2 more minutes and serve immediately.

*Serving size = 1⅓ cups*
*226 calories*
*0.9 gram fat*
*0 milligrams cholesterol*
*15.7 milligrams sodium*

## HOT RICE WITH FRESH VEGETABLES

Deborah Madison

*The heat of the rice brings out the flavors of the herbs and vegetables. Thickened bean broth provides an oil-less dressing to moisten the rice and carry the flavors. (If you haven't any bean broth, add an extra tomato for moistness.) The vegetables and herbs listed below are mainly suggestions. Feel free to use others that are appealing to you and in season and omit those you don't care for.*

SERVES 4 TO 6

**½ teaspoon salt**
**2 cups long-grain brown rice**
**1 cup bean broth, preferably from white beans (page 346)**
**3 to 4 ripe tomatoes, halved, seeded, and chopped, with their juice**
**1 bunch scallions, trimmed and finely chopped**
**½ jalapeño pepper, seeded and minced**
**1 firm zucchini, cleaned, trimmed, and cut into small cubes**
**3 celery ribs, trimmed, cleaned, and finely diced**
**1 large cooked artichoke heart, diced**
**4 baby carrots, finely diced**
**1 small green bell pepper, seeded and diced**
**2 garlic cloves, minced**
**½ cup finely chopped Italian parsley**
**½ cup chopped basil**
**2 tablespoons chopped celery or lovage leaves**
**Salt**
**Freshly ground black pepper**
**Fresh lemon juice or vinegar to taste**

Bring 2 quarts of water to a boil, add ½ teaspoon salt, then the rice. Lower the heat to a simmer and cook for approximately 45 minutes, or until the rice is done.

While the rice is cooking, boil the bean broth in a small pan until reduced to ⅓ cup. Pour into the bottom of a serving bowl large enough to contain the rice and the vegetables. Set aside and cool to room temperature.

Add all the vegetables and herbs to the bowl. When the rice is ready, drain off any excess water and add it, while steaming hot, to the vegetables. Toss well and season with salt to taste, plenty of black pepper, and a squeeze of fresh lemon juice.

*Serving size = ¼ cup*
*201 calories*

*1.7 grams fat*
*0 milligrams cholesterol*
*381.3 milligrams sodium without added salt*

## WILD RICE PILAF WITH DRIED FRUIT

Bradley Ogden

MAKES 3½ CUPS

- **¾ cup diced onion**
- **½ cup wild rice**
- **3 sprigs of fresh thyme**
- **1 teaspoon kosher salt**
- **½ teaspoon freshly cracked black pepper**
- **2 cups water**
- **2 cups apple cider**
- **¼ cup dry sour cherries**
- **¼ cup dry currants (or raisins)**

Combine all the ingredients, except the cherries and currants, in a medium-sized heavy-bottomed saucepan and cook slowly, covered, over medium heat for approximately 35 minutes. Add the dried fruit and cook for another 15 minutes, or until the rice is tender but not mushy. Cool, drain off any excess liquid, and serve.

NOTE: Other dried berries can be substituted for the cherries and currants.

*Serving size = 1 cup*
*169 calories*
*0.3 gram fat*
*0 milligrams cholesterol*
*790.6 milligrams sodium*

## BROWN BASMATI LEMON RICE

Tracy Pikhart Ritter

*The subtle, nutty taste of Basmati rice is enhanced with the addition of fresh lemon zest and sweet spices. Rinsing the rice before cooking washes away the excess starch, yielding rice that is very light and fluffy.*

SERVES 6

**1 cup brown Basmati rice**
**2 cups water or Vegetable Stock (page 143)**
**Grated zest of 1 lemon**
**¼ teaspoon ground nutmeg**
**¼ teaspoon ground cloves**
**½ teaspoon ground cinnamon**
**½ teaspoon ground cumin**
**½ teaspoon ground coriander**
**Pinch of saffron (optional)**
**1 tablespoon chopped fresh parsley, for garnish**

Rinse the rice and soak it for 20 minutes in cold water.

Add all the ingredients except for the parsley to a 2-quart pot. Bring to a boil, lower the heat, stir, and simmer, covered, for 20 minutes, or until the water is absorbed and the rice is cooked. Garnish with the chopped parsley.

NOTE: This can also be made with white Basmati rice.

*Variation:* To ½ cup of the rice add ¼ cup cooked lentils, ½ teaspoon chopped fresh parsley, and lemon juice to taste.

*Serving size = ½ cup*
*118 calories*
*1 gram fat*
*0 milligrams cholesterol*
*3.7 milligrams sodium*

## VEGETARIAN RED BEANS AND SEVEN-GRAIN DIRTY RICE

Tracy Pikhart Ritter

*The lusty flavors of Cajun cooking transform this vegetarian dish into something special.*

MAKES 8 CUPS
SERVES 6 TO 8

**2 cups brown rice**
**1½ cups chopped red onion**
**3 garlic cloves, minced**
**1 cup finely diced carrots**
**½ cup chopped celery**
**1 jalapeño pepper, seeded and minced**
**1 tablespoon ground cumin**
**1 tablespoon ground coriander**
**2 teaspoons chili powder**
**3¾ cups vegetable stock**
**1 bay leaf**
**1½ cups cooked red beans (page 124)**
**1½ cups chopped tomatoes**
**½ cup fresh or frozen corn kernels**
**½ teaspoon sea salt**
**3 tablespoons chopped fresh parsley**
**3 tablespoons chopped fresh cilantro**

Place a medium-sized pot over medium heat. Add the first 9 ingredients and heat for 3 to 5 minutes, stirring almost constantly, until lightly browned. In another pot, bring the stock and bay leaf to a boil and add to the rice mixture. Cover the pan, lower the heat, and simmer for 15 minutes.

Add the beans, tomatoes, corn, and salt. Stir, cover, and simmer for 15 more minutes, or until the liquid is absorbed. Remove from the heat and add the parsley and cilantro. Serve.

*Serving size = 1 cup*
*308 calories*
*2.7 grams fat*
*0 milligrams cholesterol*
*281.2 milligrams sodium*

## QUINOA TABOULI

Martha Rose Shulman

*This is much like the traditional bulgur tabouli but with quinoa. Serve this brightly flavored salad in the traditional manner, with hummus and pita bread.*

MAKES 6 CUPS
SERVES 6 TO 8

**½ cup quinoa**
**1 cup water**
**2 cups chopped tomatoes (approximately 1 pound)**
**2 cups chopped fresh parsley**
**1 cup chopped fresh mint**
**½ cup chopped green onions**
**½ cup lemon juice**
**½ teaspoon ground cumin**
**Freshly ground black pepper**
**Salt**
**1 head romaine lettuce, broken into leaves**
**½ pint cherry tomatoes**

In a medium-sized bowl, soak the quinoa in cold water for 5 minutes. Drain and rinse under cold running water.

In a medium saucepan, combine the soaked quinoa and water and bring to a boil.

Reduce the heat and simmer, covered, for 15 to 20 minutes, or until just tender. Drain, reserving the cooking liquid.

In a large bowl, toss the quinoa with the tomatoes, parsley, mint, green onions, lemon juice, and cumin. Season to taste with pepper and salt. Chill and serve on a large serving platter with the romaine lettuce leaves and garnished with the tomatoes. If you can get them, yellow "cherry" tomatoes make a very striking contrast here.

If you like a salad with a little more moisture, add some of the reserved quinoa cooking liquid when you combine the quinoa with the vegetables and cumin.

*Serving size = 1 cup*
*151 calories*
*2.1 grams fat*
*0 milligrams cholesterol*
*129.8 milligrams sodium without added salt*

## RICE PILAF

Anita Cecena

*Home gardeners who raise large zucchini should try this as a stuffing for baked zucchini. For variation, fresh chopped herbs such as rosemary, thyme, and savory can be stirred into the rice just before it is layered into the casserole and prior to microwaving. Leftovers can be cut into squares, wrapped in plastic, and frozen.*

Makes 8 cups
Serves 6 to 8

**Vegetable oil spray**
**1 cup brown rice**
**½ cup wild rice**
**3 cups Vegetable Stock (page 143)**
**¾ pound fresh mushrooms, sliced**
**1 10-ounce package frozen spinach, thawed and chopped**
**1 cup nonfat plain yogurt**
**Freshly ground black pepper**
**Salt**

Lightly spray a large nonstick sauté pan with a thin coating of the vegetable oil spray. Sauté the brown and wild rice until brown. Add the vegetable stock. Bring to a boil, reduce the heat, and cover. Simmer for 45 minutes, or until tender. Set aside.

Lightly spray a second large, nonstick sauté pan with the spray. Add the mushrooms and sauté until tender. Set aside.

In a medium bowl, combine the spinach and yogurt. Beat until fluffy with a wire whisk. Set aside.

Lightly coat a 9 × 13-inch glass casserole dish with pan spray. Cover the bottom of the casserole with half the rice. Cover the rice with half the spinach mixture. Cover the spinach with half the mushrooms. Repeat the layers, ending with the mushrooms.

Cover tightly with plastic wrap and cook in a microwave oven for 10 to 15 minutes, or until hot. Alternatively, bake at 350 degrees for 50 minutes in a conventional oven. Season to taste with pepper and salt.

*Serving size = 1 cup*
*82 calories*
*0.6 gram fat*
*0.5 milligram cholesterol*
*95.1 milligrams sodium without added salt*

# *Dressings and Sauces*

## REDUCED BEAN BROTH TO REPLACE OIL

Deborah Madison

*If the beans haven't been cooked in an excessive amount of water, the resulting broth—especially where aromatic seasonings have been used—is often quite flavorful. When further reduced, it becomes viscous and thick, with lots of body. While it doesn't replace oil in terms of flavor, it can act as a medium to hold and take on the flavors of garlic, shallots, herbs, mustard, and spices—in other words, the seasonings used in many salad dressings. Similarly, the cooking liquid from boiled grains like rice and quinoa are somewhat thick and can be used.*

To reduce the bean broth, pour it into a saucepan and boil slowly until it is reduced by roughly half or until it is somewhat thickened. Pick up a spoonful and slowly pour it back into the pan to see if it looks viscous. Precise amounts and times are impossible to give because they depend on the quality of broth you start with and the type of beans used. If very watery and thin, it will take longer to reduce.

If your beans have been cooked with sage, peppercorns, and aromatic herbs like parsley, bay leaf, and thyme, then your broth is off to a good start. If it hasn't been so endowed and is weakly flavored, reduce it with a bay leaf, pinch of thyme, some parsley, a few garlic cloves, and any other aromatics that will echo the final use of the broth—fennel seeds if it's going to be used on a fennel salad, for example. When it has achieved some body, cool, then strain. Substitute wherever salad oil is called for.

## HORSERADISH YOGURT DRESSING

Joyce Goldstein

*This dressing is very versatile. It can be a dip for raw vegetables such as carrots, peppers, and cucumbers. It is excellent spooned over cooked leeks, beets, potatoes, or carrots. And it can be thinned a bit with water or vinegar and used as a salad dressing for romaine, cucumbers, radishes, and green onions.*

MAKES 1¾ CUPS

**2 tablespoons finely minced onion**
**5 to 6 tablespoons grated horseradish (see note)**
**4 tablespoons white vinegar**
**1½ cups nonfat plain yogurt**
**3 tablespoons finely chopped fresh dill**
**Salt and black pepper**

Combine all of the ingredients in a mixing bowl.

NOTE: This is a good method for grating horseradish: Peel a piece weighing about ½ pound. Slice it across the grain and then chop coarsely. Put the slices in a blender or food processor with the vinegar. You will need about ¾ cup of sliced horseradish to get 5 to 6 tablespoons grated.

*Serving size = 2 tablespoons*
*23 calories*
*0.1 gram fat*
*0.4 milligram cholesterol*
*41.5 milligrams sodium without added salt*

## TOMATO HONEY VINAIGRETTE

Joyce Goldstein

*This is good on cold poached leeks, cooked carrots, and beets.*

MAKES 1¼ CUPS

**1 cup canned plum tomatoes, drained, juices reserved, pureed in food processor**
**2 tablespoons tomato puree**
**1 tablespoon honey**
**2 tablespoons balsamic vinegar**
**1 tablespoon red wine vinegar**
**Salt and pepper**
**Pinch of ground cinnamon (optional)**
**Grated orange zest (optional)**

Combine all the ingredients in a bowl and whisk together well. If the sauce is too thick, thin it with a bit of tomato juice.

*Serving size = 2 tablespoons*
*13 calories*
*0.1 gram fat*
*0 milligrams cholesterol*
*69.1 milligrams sodium without added salt*

## TOMATO YOGURT RUSSIAN DRESSING

Joyce Goldstein

*The ideal dressing for a summer tomato, cucumber, and red onion salad, it would also be nice on just lettuce, even a wedge of iceberg. And it gives you yet another potato salad option.*

MAKES ABOUT 1¼ CUPS

**1 teaspoon dry mustard**
**2 teaspoons sugar**
**2 tablespoons lemon juice**
**1 tablespoon red wine vinegar**

**4 tablespoons tomato puree**
**1 cup nonfat plain yogurt**
**Salt**
**Pepper**

Combine all the ingredients in a bowl and whisk together well.

*Serving size = 2 tablespoons*
*21 calories*
*0.2 gram fat*
*0.4 milligram cholesterol*
*72 milligrams sodium without added salt*

## HONEY CUMIN CHIQUITA BANANA VINAIGRETTE

Tracy Pikhart Ritter

*The banana imitates the texture and viscosity of oil, and creates a flavorful dressing that is delicious on mixed greens or cold steamed vegetables.*

MAKES 1 CUP

**1 ripe medium banana**
**½ cup water**
**2 tablespoons sherry wine vinegar**
**1 tablespoon grainy mustard**
**1 tablespoon honey**
**1 tablespoon roasted ground cumin**
**¼ teaspoon sea salt**
**⅛ teaspoon fresh cracked black pepper**

Place the ingredients in the order given in a blender. Blend on high speed for 1 minute until creamy and smooth. Refrigerate for 1 hour before using.

*Serving size = 2 tablespoons*
*27 calories*
*0.4 gram fat*

*0 milligrams cholesterol*
*101.4 milligrams salt*

## CREOJA SAUCE

Hubert Keller

*This delicious dressing is one of my favorites. Use it on any kind of salad, such as mixed greens, pasta salad, cucumber salad, or green bean salad.*

SERVES 4

**2 to 3 medium carrots, peeled**
**1 peeled garlic clove**
**1 tablespoon nonfat plain yogurt**
**1 tablespoon balsamic vinegar**
**Juice of ½ lemon**
**Freshly ground black pepper**
**1 tablespoon finely chopped red onion**
**1 tablespoon finely chopped celery**
**1 tablespoon finely chopped carrot**
**1 tablespoon finely chopped green bell pepper**
**1 tablespoon finely chopped chives**
**1 tablespoon finely chopped cilantro**
**6 fresh basil leaves, chopped**

Put the carrots and garlic through an electric juicer. Pour the mixture into a bowl and whisk in the nonfat yogurt, vinegar, lemon juice, and ground pepper. Add the red onion, celery, chopped carrot, bell pepper, chives, cilantro, and basil. Mix gently and set aside at room temperature for 15 minutes before serving.

*Serving size = 2 tablespoons*
*27 calories*
*0.1 gram fat*
*0.1 milligram cholesterol*
*32.9 milligrams sodium*

## GREEN CHILI SAUCE WITH CUMIN AND CARDAMOM

Deborah Madison

*The cardamom reveals the origins of this Yemenite-based sauce. Its sweetness is barely detectable as such, but it gives an added dimension to the chilies. This is delicious with yams and sweet potatoes, with corn dishes, stirred into soups, or spread on crackers. Any fresh green chili can be used: serranos, jalapeños, Anaheims. Even a green bell pepper, mixed with a small amount of hot chili, can be used by those who have a low tolerance for heat.*

MAKES ½ CUP

**4 ounces fresh green chilies, roughly chopped**
**4 large garlic cloves, peeled and diced**
**½ cup roughly chopped parsley**
**½ cup roughly chopped cilantro**
**Fresh lemon juice or water**
**1 teaspoon black pepper**
**1 teaspoon ground cumin**
**¼ to ½ teaspoon ground cardamom**
**Pinch of salt**

Puree the chilies with the garlic and fresh herbs in a small food processor. Add a little lemon juice or water to help blend the mixture, if necessary, then add the spices and blend again. Dilute with additional water or lemon juice, as needed.

Store in the refrigerator in a covered glass jar. This will keep a week or more. If you want a very hot sauce, do not remove the seeds and veins from the chilies before you chop them.

*Serving size = 2 tablespoons*
*18 calories*
*0.2 gram fat*
*0 milligrams cholesterol*
*64 milligrams sodium without added salt*

## CARROT AND GINGER SAUCE

Jean-Marc Fullsack

*Try this with grilled eggplant or other vegetables. It can be prepared and refrigerated up to 24 hours in advance.*

MAKES 1½ CUPS
SERVES 6

**1 cup peeled and diced carrots**
**⅓ cup chopped onion**
**1½ cups vegetable stock**
**¼ cup orange juice concentrate**
**1 teaspoon peeled and minced fresh gingerroot**
**2 tablespoons nonfat plain yogurt**
**Freshly ground black pepper**
**Salt**

In a nonstick sauté pan, sweat the carrots and onion over medium heat in 2 tablespoons vegetable stock until the onions are translucent. Add the remaining vegetable stock and simmer, covered, for 15 minutes. Add the orange juice concentrate and ginger. Cook for 1 minute.

In a blender, puree the vegetables and yogurt until smooth. Season to taste with pepper and salt. Serve warm.

*Serving size = ¼ cup*
*46 calories*
*0.2 gram fat*
*0.1 milligram cholesterol*
*73.2 milligrams sodium without added salt*

## WHITE BEAN SAUCE

Jean-Marc Fullsack

*If you like your sauces creamier, feel free to add this to a food processor and puree until smooth. Use the sauce as a bed for the Stuffed Tomatoes with French Lentils (page 230) or unpureed as a substitute for the lentil stuffing.*

MAKES 2 CUPS
SERVES 4

**½ cup dry white navy beans**
**1 cup vegetable stock**
**2 cups tomatoes, peeled, seeded, and chopped**
**¼ cup minced carrots**
**¼ cup minced celery**
**¼ cup minced leeks**
**¼ cup minced onions**
**2 garlic cloves, minced**
**½ teaspoon dry savory**
**¼ teaspoon dry thyme**
**1 bay leaf**
**Freshly ground black pepper**
**Salt**

Place the dried beans in a large bowl and cover with 4 cups of cold water. Soak overnight or for 1 hour in water which has been boiled for 2 to 3 minutes.

Drain the beans and place in a large saucepan. Add the vegetable stock, tomatoes, carrots, celery, leeks, onions, garlic, savory, thyme, and bay leaf. Bring to a boil and reduce the heat. Simmer for 1 hour, or until the beans are tender. Season to taste with the pepper and salt.

*Serving size = ½ cup*
*130 calories*
*0.9 gram fat*
*0 milligrams cholesterol*
*340 milligrams sodium without added salt*

## TOMATO AND ROASTED BELL PEPPER SAUCE

Jean-Marc Fullsack

*This very flavorful sauce is an easy way to dress up a platter of grilled vegetables. This is also great on blanched vegetables or pasta. It can be prepared and refrigerated up to 4 days in advance and will keep frozen for up to 2 months.*

MAKES 3 CUPS

**1 large roasted onion (page 133), sliced**
**2 roasted garlic cloves (page 132), peeled**
**2 large tomatoes, peeled, seeded, and chopped**
**2 red bell peppers, roasted (page 133), peeled, and chopped**
**½ cup vegetable stock**
**2 tablespoons chiffonaded basil**
**½ teaspoon balsamic vinegar**
**⅛ teaspoon Tabasco**
**Freshly ground black pepper**
**Salt**

In the bowl of a food processor, combine all the ingredients and process until smooth. Season to taste with pepper and salt. Warm and serve.

*Serving size = ⅓ cup*
*18 calories*
*0.2 gram fat*
*0 milligrams cholesterol*
*70 milligrams sodium without added salt*

## MANCHURIAN SAUCE

Michael McDermott

*This sauce can be used in many ways: as a marinade, a dip for crepes or vegetables, or as a base for salad dressings, sauces, soups, stir-fried veg-*

*etables, cooked grains, and noodles. It will last in the refri to 10 days, although the green onions will lose some of thei color.*

MAKES 1 CUP

**½ cup soy sauce**
**½ cup vegetable stock**
**½ cup thinly sliced green onions**
**1 teaspoon minced fresh gingerroot**
**1 teaspoon minced garlic**
**½ teaspoon wasabi (or ½ teaspoon minced jalapeño pepper)**

In a medium-sized bowl, combine all the ingredients and whisk until well blended. Refrigerate for at least 30 minutes before serving.

NOTE: If you are watching your sodium intake, substitute one of the low-sodium varieties of soy sauce, but keep in mind that these may still be quite high in salt.

*Serving size = 1 tablespoon*
*6 calories*
*0 grams fat*
*0 milligrams cholesterol*
*514 milligrams sodium without added salt*

## TOMATO AND BASIL PESTO

Bradley Ogden

MAKES ⅔ CUP

**1 medium vine-ripened tomato**
**½ cup loosely packed basil leaves**
**2 tablespoons chopped Italian parsley**
**½ teaspoon minced garlic**

**1 tablespoon balsamic vinegar**
**1 teaspoon lemon juice**
**Salt**
**Freshly ground black pepper**

Core the tomato and cut it in half. Grill over very hot coals for only a few minutes to take on some color and flavor. Remove from the grill and set aside to cool.

Place the basil, parsley, and garlic in a food processor. Process until smooth. Add the tomato, vinegar, and lemon juice and process. Season with the salt and pepper to taste.

*Serving size = 2 tablespoons*
*11 calories*
*0.1 gram fat*
*0 milligrams cholesterol*
*6.1 milligrams sodium without added salt*

## YOGURT GARLIC SAUCE

Joyce Goldstein

*This classic Middle Eastern sauce is usually spooned over rice, cracked wheat, steamed spinach, or mushrooms. It also will work well on root vegetables such as beets, leeks, celery root, and carrots.*

*For a Greek mezze or appetizer salad/dip called Tzatziki, hang the yogurt in cheesecloth for 3 days (page 148), omit the paprika, and add ½ cup chopped or grated cucumber to this mixture.*

MAKES ABOUT 1 CUP

**1 cup nonfat plain yogurt**
**1 large garlic clove, minced fine**
**2 tablespoons chopped mint or dill**
**1 green onion, finely minced**
**Grated lemon zest (optional)**
**1 teaspoon paprika**
**½ teaspoon salt**

Combine all the ingredients in a bowl with a whisk.

*Serving size = ¼ cup*
*36 calories*
*0.2 gram fat*
*1 milligram cholesterol*
*338 milligrams sodium*

## YOGURT "TARTAR" SAUCE

Joyce Goldstein

*If you were wondering what to spoon onto your baked potato, I think you'll find this the perfect topping. This familiar American sauce is actually a variation on the classic French rémoulade. To accentuate the tartness, add the vinegar from the cornichons. The amount of chopped onion is up to you.*

*This will keep for a few days in the refrigerator.*

MAKES ABOUT 1¼ CUPS

**1 cup nonfat plain yogurt**
**2 tablespoons finely minced white onion**
**2 tablespoons chopped cornichons**
**2 tablespoons vinegar from the cornichons or more to taste**
**1 tablespoon chopped capers**
**1 tablespoon chopped parsley**
**1 tablespoon Dijon mustard**
**½ teaspoon freshly ground black pepper**
**Salt**

Combine all the ingredients in a bowl with a whisk. Serve with baked potatoes, steamed carrots, leeks, beets, green beans, or the Celery Root, Orange, Grapefruit, and Spinach Salad on page 183.

*Serving size = 2 tablespoons*
*15 calories*

*0.1 gram fat*
*0.4 milligram cholesterol*
*170 milligrams sodium without added salt*

## MANGO SALSA
Jean-Marc Fullsack

*This is very summery and light, very nice with the Spiced Lentil and Fava Bean Salad with Fennel (page 191) and tomato-based dishes. It can be prepared and refrigerated up to 4 hours before serving.*

MAKES 2½ CUPS

**1 diced fresh mango**
**½ cup diced red bell pepper**
**½ cup diced red onion**
**½ cup peeled, seeded, and diced tomatoes**
**1 tablespoon minced jalapeño pepper**
**1 tablespoon minced fresh mint**
**1 tablespoon seasoned rice vinegar**
**1 tablespoon fresh lime juice**

In a large serving bowl, combine all the ingredients. Toss well and serve.

*Serving size = 2 tablespoons*
*13 calories*
*0.1 gram fat*
*0 milligrams cholesterol*
*7.4 milligrams sodium*

## TOMATO SALSA
Tracy Pikhart Ritter

*No fat-free pantry should be without a spicy salsa. More or fewer chilies can be added according to your taste. Serve this salsa with Vegetarian Red Beans and Seven-Grain Dirty Rice (page 342), Brown Rice-Filled*

*Chilies with Black Bean Sauce (page 254), or with fat-fr… chips.*

MAKES 2 CUPS

**2 large ripe beefsteak or similar tomatoes, seeded and cut into ½-inch cubes**
**¼ small red onion, minced**
**¼ serrano or jalapeño pepper, seeds and membrane removed, minced, or 1 teaspoon red pepper flakes**
**1 tablespoon fresh chopped cilantro or to taste**
**1 teaspoon fresh chopped oregano, or a pinch of dried oregano leaves**
**½ teaspoon fresh cracked black pepper**
**Salt to taste**
**Lime juice to taste (optional)**

Combine all ingredients. Set aside for 1 hour or more before using. This keeps well refrigerated for 2 to 3 days.

*Serving size = ¼ cup*
*11 calories*
*0.2 gram fat*
*0 milligrams cholesterol*
*56.9 milligrams sodium without added salt*

## SHALLOT AND MUSTARD SAUCE

Jean-Marc Fullsack

*Serve with the Vegetable Strudel (page 245), with steamed vegetables, or over rice.*

MAKES 1 CUP

**4 shallots**
**2 cups vegetable stock**
**½ cup chopped fennel**
**1 teaspoon nonfat milk powder**

**2 teaspoons Dijon mustard**
**1 teaspoon chopped fresh tarragon**
**Freshly ground black pepper**
**Salt**

Preheat the oven to 350 degrees.

Bake the unpeeled shallots on a nonstick baking sheet for 35 minutes, or until soft and tender. Peel and chop roughly.

In a medium saucepan, combine the vegetable stock, fennel, shallots, and milk powder. Bring to a boil, reduce the heat, and simmer for 30 minutes.

Transfer to a food processor and puree until smooth. Whisk in the mustard and tarragon. Season to taste with pepper and salt. Serve.

*Serving size = ¼ cup*
*27 calories*
*0.4 gram fat*
*0 milligrams cholesterol*
*51 milligrams sodium without added salt*

## TINA'S PASTA PRIMAVERA SAUCE

Tina Salter

MAKES 3 CUPS

**3 garlic cloves, peeled and minced**
**2 tablespoons vegetable stock**
**2 cups button mushrooms or any fresh mushrooms, quartered**
**1 basket cherry tomatoes, halved**
**1 red bell pepper, julienned**
**Salt (optional)**

In a large nonstick sauté pan, sauté the garlic in 2 tablespoons of vegetable stock. Add the mushrooms and cook for 3 to 5 minutes, until the juices begin to run. Add the cherry tomatoes and red bell pepper. Continue to cook for 2 to 3 minutes to warm all thoroughly. Add salt to taste and serve.

*Serving size = ¾ cup*
*60 calories*
*1.0 gram fat*
*0 milligrams cholesterol*
*14.8 milligrams sodium without added salt*

## PISTOU SAUCE

Jean-Marc Fullsack

*This intensely garlicky sauce is wonderful with vegetables, pasta, or simply for bread.*

MAKES 1½ CUPS

**Approximately 1 pound tomatoes (2 large)**
**1 large onion, unpeeled**
**6 garlic cloves, unpeeled**
**1 cup chopped fresh basil**
**1 teaspoon minced garlic**
**Salt**

Preheat the oven to 350 degrees.

Slice the tomatoes into ¼-inch slices. Bake on a parchment-lined baking sheet for 30 to 45 minutes, or until the tomatoes lose their sheen and begin to shrivel. Bake the whole unpeeled onion on a nonstick baking sheet at the same time about 45 minutes, or until the onion is tender to a knife. Add the garlic cloves to the baking pan with the onion after 10 minutes.

Peel the baked onion and chop roughly with the baked tomatoes. In a medium nonstick sauté pan, combine the onions and tomatoes. Squeeze the garlic pulp from each clove into the onion-tomato mix and simmer, uncovered, for 10 minutes. Add the basil and raw minced garlic and blend. Add salt to taste and serve warm or at room temperature.

*Serving size = 2 tablespoons*
*17 calories*
*0.1 gram fat*
*0 milligrams cholesterol*
*29.3 milligrams sodium without added salt*

## TOFU AND MISO DRESSING

Jean-Marc Fullsack

*This is a delightful dressing for mixed greens. It can be kept refrigerated for up to 1 week.*

Makes 1½ cups

**1 cup soft tofu**
**3 tablespoons fresh lemon juice**
**1 tablespoon Dijon mustard**
**1 tablespoon mellow white miso (page 117)**
**1 tablespoon sake**
**1 tablespoon honey**
**1 tablespoon poppy seeds (optional)**

In a blender, combine the tofu, lemon juice, mustard, miso, sake, and honey and puree until smooth. Add the optional poppy seeds and stir to combine.

*Serving size = 2 tablespoons*
*23 calories*
*0.7 gram fat*
*0 milligrams cholesterol*
*70.5 milligrams sodium*

## TOMATO SWEET PEPPER KETCHUP

Tracy Pikhart Ritter

MAKES 2½ CUPS
SERVES 10

**2 tablespoons water or vegetable stock**
**5 garlic cloves, minced**
**½ red onion, minced**
**¼ teaspoon dried oregano**
**2 pounds fresh or canned tomatoes, peeled and seeded**
**2 roasted red bell peppers (page 133), peeled, seeded, and chopped**
**2 to 3 tablespoons balsamic vinegar**
**¼ teaspoon cayenne**
**¼ teaspoon salt**
**Pinch of ground cinnamon**
**Pinch of ground cloves**
**Pinch of ground allspice**

In a large saucepan, put the water or stock, garlic, onion, and oregano. Cook for 2 to 3 minutes. Be careful not to burn the garlic. Add the remaining ingredients and cook over medium-low heat for 20 to 30 minutes until thickened.

Place all ingredients in a food processor and process until smooth.

To thicken further, return to a pot and cook over medium-low heat for 10 more minutes, or until reduced to desired thickness. Take care that the ketchup does not scorch on the bottom of the pan.

This will keep well for 2 weeks in the refrigerator or longer frozen.

*Serving size = ¼ cup*
*140 calories*
*1.9 grams fat*
*0 milligrams cholesterol*
*341.9 milligrams sodium*

## SPICY CINNAMON-CHILI PASTE
Wolfgang Puck

*Use this paste to perk up marinades or sauces. One or 2 tablespoons in tomato sauce will perk it up.*

MAKES ABOUT 1½ CUPS

**1 pound (2 or 3) red bell peppers, cored, cut in half, and seeded**
**2 jalapeño peppers, cored**
**1 bunch cilantro**
**12 garlic cloves**
**1 tablespoon ground cinnamon**
**1 teaspoon ground coriander**
**About ½ teaspoon salt**

Preheat the oven to 500 degrees.

Place all of the ingredients, except the salt, in a large piece of heavy aluminum foil. Wrap securely and airtight, place on a baking tray, and bake for 45 minutes, until the peppers are tender.

Unwrap the package, being careful that the steam does not burn you, and puree the ingredients in a food processor or blender. Season with salt to taste and cool. Use as needed.

NOTE: The paste, tightly covered, can be refrigerated for up to 1 month and frozen for up to 3 months.

*Serving size = 2 tablespoons*
*20 calories*
*0.2 gram fat*
*0 milligrams cholesterol*
*99.8 milligrams sodium*

## TOMATO KETCHUP

Wolfgang Puck

*The length of time it takes for the ketchup to thicken depends upon the water content of the tomatoes. So be patient—it really is worth the wait. Try this only when you can get flavorful, vine-ripened tomatoes.*

MAKES 2 CUPS

**2 pounds ripe (about 5 or 6 medium) tomatoes, rinsed and diced**
**2 large garlic cloves, smashed**
**½ small onion, diced**
**¼ large (1-ounce) red bell pepper, diced**
**½ cup plus 2 tablespoons light corn syrup**
**½ cup plus 2 tablespoons cider vinegar**
**1 tablespoon salt**
**2 teaspoons pickling spices**
**¼ cup tomato paste**

In a medium stainless-steel or enamel saucepan, over a low flame, cook the tomatoes and garlic until the sauce begins to bubble. Add the onion and red pepper and cook 1 or 2 minutes. Stir in the corn syrup, vinegar, salt, and pickling spices and continue to simmer over the low flame until the sauce reduces and thickens, about 1½ hours, stirring occasionally. (The sauce will reduce by about one-half). Do not rush. Cook over a low flame to prevent scorching.

Strain through a food mill and stir in the tomato paste. Correct seasoning to taste, cool, and refrigerate in a covered container until needed. The ketchup will thicken slightly as it cools, but it is not the consistency of store-bought ketchup.

NOTE: The ketchup will keep up to three weeks.

*Serving size = 2 tablespoons*
*52 calories*
*0.3 gram fat*
*0 milligrams cholesterol*
*448.4 milligrams sodium*

# *Chutneys, Relishes, Raitas, and Pickles*

## PEACH AND APRICOT CHUTNEY

Jean-Marc Fullsack

*Try this with any curried or highly spiced dish.*

MAKES 2 CUPS
SERVES 6 TO 8

**2 ounces (approximately ½ cup) dried apricots, diced**
**1 cup pitted and diced fresh ripe peaches**
**1 cup peeled, seeded, and diced tomatoes**
**1 cup diced onion**
**¼ cup seasoned rice vinegar**
**1 tablespoon minced red jalapeño pepper**
**1 tablespoon minced green jalapeño pepper**
**1 tablespoon minced fresh gingerroot**
**Pinch of ground cloves**
**Pinch of turmeric**
**Pinch of cayenne**
**¼ cup chopped fresh cilantro**

In a small bowl, cover the apricots with warm water. Soak for 20 minutes. Drain and transfer to a nonreactive saucepan.

Add the peaches, tomatoes, onion, vinegar, jalapeños, ginger, cloves, turmeric, and cayenne. Stir, bring to a boil, reduce the heat, and simmer, covered, for 20 minutes. Cool before adding the cilantro. Store, refrigerated, in a sterilized jar for up to 1 week.

*Serving size = ¼ cup*
*62 calories*
*0.3 gram fat*
*0 milligrams cholesterol*
*6.3 milligrams sodium*

## FRESH CORIANDER OR MINT CHUTNEY

Joyce Goldstein

*This is a spicy and refreshing chutney that works well with almost any vegetable curry—and of course, saffron rice. This keeps well for about a day, after which the color begins to fade, though the taste is still good.*

MAKES ABOUT 1½ CUPS

**3 to 4 bunches fresh cilantro**
**3 to 4 bunches fresh mint leaves (about 2 tightly packed cups)**
**1 onion, diced (about ¾ cup)**
**2 to 3 walnut-sized pieces of fresh gingerroot, peeled**
**3 to 4 jalapeño peppers, diced**
**½ cup lemon juice**
**¼ cup water**
**½ teaspoon salt**
**1 teaspoon sugar**

Put all the ingredients in the container of a blender or food processor. Puree to a fine consistency. Keep refrigerated until serving time.

*Serving size = 2 tablespoons*
*12 calories*

*0.1 gram fat*
*0 milligrams cholesterol*
*242.3 milligrams sodium*

## PINEAPPLE CHUTNEY

Jean-Marc Fullsack

*This very beautiful and tasty dish would be a wonderful accompaniment to many dishes, especially Indian ones such as curries. This can be prepared and refrigerated in sterilized jars for up to 2 weeks.*

MAKES 3 CUPS

**2 cups diced fresh pineapple**
**½ cup rice wine vinegar**
**½ cup small-diced red onion**
**½ cup small-diced red bell pepper**
**2 tablespoons honey**
**1½ tablespoons minced jalapeño pepper**
**1½ tablespoons minced fresh gingerroot**
**1 tablespoon lime juice**
**1 teaspoon minced garlic**
**1 teaspoon turmeric**
**⅛ teaspoon ground cloves**
**½ cinnamon stick**

In a large nonstick, nonreactive saucepan, combine all the ingredients. Bring to a boil, reduce the heat, and simmer, covered, for 1 hour. Cool to room temperature before serving or storing in the refrigerator.

*Serving size = 2 tablespoons*
*27 calories*
*0.2 gram fat*
*0 milligrams cholesterol*
*0.8 milligram sodium*

## LEMON-FIG CHUTNEY

Catherine Pantsios

*This excellent sweet-and-sour chutney makes a good candiment in an Indian meal. Black Mission figs are essential here.*

MAKES 1 QUART

**1 cup fresh figs (Black Mission), halved**
**2 cups lemon slices (cut in half lengthwise, then cut across into ¼-inch slices, seeds removed)**
**1 cup chopped yellow onions**
**1 cup raisins**
**½ cup mild honey, such as orange blossom**
**1 teaspoon salt**
**1 cup white wine vinegar or apple cider vinegar**
**2 teaspoons peeled and freshly grated gingerroot**
**¼ teaspoon ground cloves**
**¼ teaspoon ground cinnamon**
**¼ teaspoon ground nutmeg**

Combine all the ingredients in a heavy saucepan and bring to a boil. Reduce the heat and simmer, covered, for 1 hour. Simmer, uncovered, for another ½ hour. This keeps for 2 weeks in the refrigerator.

*Serving size = 2 tablespoons*
*42 calories*
*0.1 gram fat*
*0 milligrams cholesterol*
*79.3 milligrams sodium*

## PEAR CARDAMOM RELISH

Tracy Pikhart Ritter

MAKES 2 CUPS

**10 firm, ripe pears, peeled, cored, and coarsely chopped**
**2 tablespoons poppy seeds**
**½ teaspoon ground cardamom**
**½ teaspoon ground cinnamon**
**1 teaspoon minced fresh gingerroot**
**½ cup white wine vinegar**
**¼ cup sugar**
**1 cup pear nectar**
**½ teaspoon sea salt**

Combine all the ingredients in a nonreactive pan. Bring to a boil, reduce the heat to low, and simmer for about 25 minutes, until thickened. Cool. Serve with grilled or roasted vegetables.

*Serving size = 2 tablespoons*
*42 calories*
*0.1 gram fat*
*0 milligrams cholesterol*
*79.3 milligrams sodium*

## TOMATO MINT RELISH

Tracy Pikhart Ritter

*Serve with the Bean Burgers (page 244).*

MAKES 1½ CUPS

**4 cups peeled whole tomatoes**
**½ cup minced red onion**
**1 cup red wine vinegar**
**½ cup light brown sugar**

- 2 teaspoons chopped fresh mint
- 1 teaspoon ground cumin
- 1 teaspoon ground coriander
- 1 teaspoon black mustard seeds
- 1 teaspoon peeled and minced fresh gingerroot
- 2 garlic cloves, minced
- ½ teaspoon cayenne
- ½ teaspoon sea salt

Place all ingredients in a nonreactive saucepan. Bring to a boil, reduce to a simmer, and cook for 30 minutes over low heat. Cool before serving.

*Serving size = 2 tablespoons*
*18 calories*
*0.2 gram fat*
*0 milligrams cholesterol*
*40 milligrams sodium*

## CORN, ORANGE, AND TOMATO RELISH

Jean-Marc Fullsack

*This very pretty relish can be prepared and refrigerated up to 6 hours in advance.*

MAKES 2 CUPS

- 1 cup fresh corn kernels (1 large ear)
- 1 large orange
- ¾ cup diced tomatoes
- ¼ cup diced red bell pepper
- 1 tablespoon chopped fresh cilantro
- 1 small jalapeño pepper, finely minced
- 1 tablespoon seasoned rice vinegar
- 1 tablespoon fresh lime juice
- Freshly ground black pepper
- Salt

Bring 6 quarts of water to a boil. Add the corn. Allow the water to return to a boil and blanch the corn for 1 minute, or just until tender. Drain and refresh under cold running water. Drain well and set aside.

Peel the orange including the white pith and the membrane between segments. Cut each segment into quarters.

In a large bowl, combine the corn, orange pieces, tomato, red bell pepper, cilantro, and jalapeño. Pour the vinegar and lime juice over the vegetables and toss well. Season to taste with pepper and salt. Serve at room temperature.

*Serving size = ¼ cup*
*38 calories*
*0.3 gram fat*
*0 milligrams cholesterol*
*39.6 milligrams sodium without added salt*

## CHICK-PEA AND VEGETABLE PICKLES

Deborah Madison

*You can't make a meal of spicy pickles, but they can make a wholesome nibble before, if not with, dinner.*

MAKES ABOUT 3 CUPS

**½ cup dried chick-peas, soaked overnight, or 1 can, drained**
**Salt**
**1 small rutabaga**
**1 small turnip**
**2 medium carrots**
**8 garlic cloves**
**2 serrano chilis**
**10 black peppercorns**
**1 cup white wine or apple cider vinegar**
**3 tablespoons sugar or to taste**
**Several sprigs of mint**

If using dried chick-peas, cover with fresh water; cook until tender but not mushy, about 1 hour 15 minutes. Season to taste with salt. If using canned chick-peas, rinse them well and set aside.

Peel the vegetables if the skins look old or scarred, then cut them into quarters. Cut the quarters into triangular pieces about ¼ inch thick. Peel the garlic and slice in half lengthwise.

Put the vegetables in a nonreactive pan with the garlic, chilis, peppercorns, ½ teaspoon salt, vinegar, and sugar. Add water to cover, bring to a boil, then lower the heat and simmer 15 minutes. When finished, transfer the contents to a bowl, add the chick-peas, and submerge the mint sprigs in the liquid. The vinegar will turn them gray-green, but the heat will release their aroma. Cover and refrigerate until well chilled. Serve garnished with fresh mint leaves.

*Serving size = ¼ cup*
*52 calories*
*0.2 gram fat*
*0 milligrams cholesterol*
*177.9 milligrams sodium without added salt*

## MIKE'S KOREAN-STYLE PICKLED VEGETABLES

Catherine Pantsios

*These are good for snacking or as a small salad or side dish.*

MAKES ABOUT 2 QUARTS

**4 large carrots**
**6 unwaxed Japanese or English cucumbers**
**1 6-inch piece of daikon root**
**15 garlic cloves, thinly sliced**
**1 tablespoon salt**
**2 cups rice vinegar**
**4 tablespoons sugar**

Peel the carrots and slice at a slight angle into ⅛-inch-thick slices using a mandoline, a Japanese Benriner-type slicer, or a sharp knife. Repeat this process with the cucumbers. Peel the daikon and cut in half lengthwise, then slice across, also on an angle, into slightly thinner slices than the carrots and cucumbers.

Blanch the carrots and garlic in boiling water for 20 seconds, then cool quickly in cold water.

Place the cucumbers and daikon in a bowl and toss with the salt. Allow them to drain in a sieve for 10 minutes, then pat dry. Heat the vinegar with the sugar until it boils and the sugar dissolves. Combine all the vegetables and pour the vinegar-sugar mixture over them. Allow the vegetables to steep for at least 10 minutes before serving. These keep well for up to 1 week in the refrigerator.

*Serving size = ¼ cup*
*28 calories*
*0.1 gram fat*
*0 milligrams cholesterol*
*234.2 milligrams sodium*

## COOKED TOMATO CHUTNEY

Tracy Pikhart Ritter

MAKES 1 CUP

- **4 cups peeled and seeded chopped fresh or canned tomatoes**
- **3 tablespoons finely chopped red onion**
- **2 garlic cloves, minced**
- **1 teaspoon peeled and minced fresh gingerroot**
- **2 teaspoons black mustard seeds**
- **¼ cup sherry wine vinegar**
- **½ cup light brown sugar**
- **¼ teaspoon salt**
- **¼ teaspoon cracked black pepper**

Combine all the ingredients in a nonreactive pan. Bring to a boil, reduce the flame to low, and simmer for about 40 minutes, or until thickened. Cool before serving. Serve this chutney with quesadillas or grilled vegetables. It will keep for up to 2 weeks in the refrigerator.

*Serving size = 2 tablespoons*
*68 calories*
*0.7 gram fat*
*0 milligrams cholesterol*
*87.5 milligrams sodium*

## PEAR-JALAPEÑO RAITA

Dennis and Margaret Malone

*This is a wonderful nondairy alternative to the classic yogurt-based raita and the flavor is delightful. Serve as a cooling contrast to spicy Indian dishes.*

Makes 3 cups

**10 ounces extra-firm tofu**
**½ cup roughly chopped onion**
**¼ cup lime juice**
**1 jalapeño pepper, roughly chopped**
**3 cups fresh pears (approximately 1½ pounds), peeled, seeded, and cut in ½-inch dice**
**¼ cup chopped fresh mint**
**½ teaspoon salt**

In a blender or food processor, combine the tofu, onion, lime juice, and minced jalapeño. Process until very smooth and then transfer to a large bowl. Add the pears, mint, and salt. Gently toss to combine thoroughly. Cover with plastic wrap and refrigerate for at least 1 hour. Serve chilled or at room temperature.

*Serving size = ¼ cup*
*42 calories*
*0.6 gram fat*
*0 milligrams cholesterol*
*100.2 milligrams sodium*

## SPICED SPINACH WITH YOGURT
Jean-Marc Fullsack

*Serve this wonderful condiment with Vegetable Brochettes (page 231) and rice. The recipe doubles easily if you want to use it as a full side dish for more people. It can be prepared and refrigerated up to 2 hours ahead of serving.*

MAKES 1½ CUPS
SERVES 3 TO 6 AS A SIDE DISH OR CONDIMENT

**1 pound fresh spinach**
**2 teaspoons ground cumin**
**2 teaspoons ground coriander**
**1 teaspoon minced garlic**
**1 cup nonfat plain yogurt**
**⅛ teaspoon ground nutmeg**
**Freshly ground black pepper**
**Salt**

Wash the spinach well and shake gently to remove the excess water.

In a dry large pan or skillet, toast the ground cumin and coriander, taking care not to let the spices turn dark brown and burn.

Add the damp spinach and garlic, then stir continuously to wilt the spinach leaves. Transfer to a serving bowl, stir in the yogurt and nutmeg, and season to taste with pepper and salt. Serve at room temperature or chilled.

*Serving size = ¼ cup*
*45 calories*
*0.6 gram fat*
*0.7 milligram cholesterol*
*132.3 milligrams sodium*

## PERSIMMON RELISH

Wolfgang Puck

*Persimmons must be very ripe for the best flavor. If persimmons are not in season, mango or papaya can be substituted.*

SERVES 6

**1 cup diced (about 2 medium) very ripe persimmons**
**½ cup diced onion**
**½ jalapeño pepper, cored, seeded, and diced**
**2 tablespoons lime juice**
**3 teaspoons chopped cilantro**
**Pinch of cayenne pepper**
**Salt**

In a small bowl, combine all the ingredients and season with salt to taste.

*Serving size = 2 tablespoons*
*9 calories*
*0 grams fat*
*0 milligrams cholesterol*
*0.4 milligram sodium*

# Desserts

All of these desserts are delicious and very low in fat. However, some are high in sugar, so please consume them in moderation if you want to lose weight.

## APPLE PANCAKES WITH CINNAMON NONFAT YOGURT

Michael Lomonaco

SERVES 4

**1 cup all-purpose flour**
**3 tablespoons nonfat egg substitute**
**1½ cups nonfat plain yogurt**
**½ teaspoon baking powder**
**3 tablespoons orange juice**
**3 tablespoons maple syrup**
**4 Granny Smith or other tart apples, peeled, cored, and sliced**
**¼ teaspoon ground cinnamon**
**Mint leaves**

Combine the flour, egg substitute, 1 cup yogurt, baking powder, orange juice, and 2 tablespoons maple syrup into a batter. If you like thinner pancakes, add 2 to 4 tablespoons of water at this point. Let rest for ½ hour. Meanwhile, in a nonstick skillet, sauté the sliced apples with 1 tablespoon water until the slices are tender and caramelized. Combine the remaining yogurt and maple syrup with the cinnamon. Using a nonstick omelette pan, make thin crepes by pouring 3 tablespoons of the batter into the preheated pan and rolling it around to uniformly cover the surface of the pan. Cook over medium heat about 1 minute, flip with a spatula and cook the other side for about 10 seconds. Continue until all the batter has been used. For each serving, roll each of two crepes around 2 tablespoons of the apples. Garnish with a dollop of flavored yogurt and a mint leaf.

*Serving size = 3 (4- to 5-inch) pancakes with filling*
*278 calories*
*1.2 grams fat*
*1.6 milligrams cholesterol*
*138.3 milligrams sodium*

## PERSIMMON SPICE MUFFINS

Paul Bertolli

*Persimmons are an excellent moisture retainer in baked goods, making them ideal to use with oat bran, which tends to absorb a lot of moisture. They are available in the late fall. Choose fruit that is as soft as possible. (Hachiya is the variety to look for; the smaller, more compressed varieties with lighter skin are intended to be eaten while the fruit is still firm.) The flesh should look translucent and have a jellylike texture. Slice the persimmon in half and scrape the pulp from the peel. To make a puree, put it through a strainer or blend it in a food processor.*

MAKES 16 MUFFINS

**3 cups oat bran**
**3 teaspoons baking powder**
**½ teaspoon ground cloves**
**1 teaspoon ground cinnamon**
**½ teaspoon ground ginger**

- **1 teaspoon salt**
- **5/8 cup persimmon puree**
- **½ cup honey**
- **5/8 cup nonfat milk**
- **2 egg whites (from 2 large eggs)**
- **1 cup grated McIntosh apple**
- **¼ cup dried currants**

Preheat the oven to 375 degrees.

Place paper liners in 16 muffin tin openings. Combine the oat bran, baking powder, spices, and salt in a mixing bowl and blend well. Combine the remaining ingredients in a separate bowl, blend them, stir them into the dry ingredients, and mix well.

Spoon the mixture into the muffin pans, filling each opening to the top (the muffins won't rise much), and smooth them over with the back of a spoon. Bake for 30 minutes or until brown on top and set in the center.

Cool the muffins thoroughly before serving.

*Serving size = 1 muffin*
*90 calories*
*0.5 gram fat*
*0.2 milligram cholesterol*
*235.0 milligrams sodium*

## APPLE BREAD PUDDING

Jean-Marc Fullsack

*This is a comforting dessert or a satisfying breakfast dish on a blustery winter day. Baking it in a shallow dish yields a pudding with lots of crusty topping.*

MAKES 6 CUPS
SERVES 6 TO 12

- **2 cups nonfat milk**
- **¾ cup maple syrup**
- **1 tablespoon ground cinnamon**

**1 cup egg whites (6 to 8 eggs)**
**4 cups diced bread**
**2 cups apple, peeled, cored, and diced**
**1 cup raisins**

Preheat the oven to 350 degrees. In a large bowl, combine the milk, maple syrup, and cinnamon. In another bowl, beat the egg whites until frothy. Add the egg whites to the milk mixture and stir to combine thoroughly. Add the bread and toss well. Set aside to soak for 30 minutes.

Fold in the diced apples and raisins and pour into a nonstick or lightly oiled 8 × 12 × 2-inch baking dish. Bake for 45 to 50 minutes, or until the top is very brown and crisp. A knife inserted into the middle should come out clean at this point. Serve warm or at room temperature.

*Serving size = ½ cup*
*192 calories*
*0.4 gram fat*
*0.7 milligram cholesterol*
*61.1 milligrams sodium*

## ANGEL FOOD CAKE

Joyce Goldstein

*This simple cake is especially nice with berries.*

SERVES 8 TO 10

**1 cup cake flour**
**1½ cups sugar**
**2 cups egg whites (6 to 8 eggs)**
**1 teaspoon pure vanilla extract**
**¼ teaspoon almond extract**
**¼ teaspoon salt**

Preheat the oven to 350 degrees.

Sift the cake flour and ¾ cup sugar together three times. Set aside. Whip the egg whites until foamy with the whisk attachment of an electric mixer. Gradually beat in the rest of the sugar. Add the extracts and salt. Beat just until stiff peaks form. Do not overbeat. Remove the bowl from the mixer.

With a whisk or spatula fold the flour and sugar mixture by thirds into the egg whites. Place the batter in an ungreased 10-inch tube pan. Bake for 40 to 45 minutes, or until the cake is golden brown and springs back to the touch. Invert the cake until cool. Remove it from the pan and serve.

*Serving size = 1/10 cake*
*168 calories*
*0.1 gram fat*
*0 milligrams cholesterol*
*97.4 milligrams sodium*

## BAKED FIGS WITH GRAND MARNIER CREAM AND RASPBERRIES

Joyce Goldstein

*Fresh figs are the treat of late summer and are wonderful paired with raspberries. The Grand Marnier cream adds a level of complexity that makes this a voluptuous dessert.*

SERVES 4

**12 ripe fresh purple figs**
**1 teaspoon mixed ground cinnamon and cloves or Chinese Five Spices**
**½ cup brown sugar**
**½ cup water**
**1 cup nonfat plain yogurt, drained in cheesecloth in a strainer for 2 days in refrigerator**
**2 tablespoons sugar**
**¼ cup Grand Marnier**
**½ cup raspberries**

Preheat the oven to 350 degrees.

Prick the figs with a fork in a few places and place them

in a baking dish. Combine the spices and brown sugar. Sprinkle over the figs and then add the water to the dish. Bake, uncovered, for ½ hour, basting often. Combine the thickened yogurt with the sugar and Grand Marnier. Place the figs in serving dishes. Top with a dollop of yogurt and a few raspberries.

NOTE: To make a fig and berry gratin, spoon the flavored yogurt over the cooked figs, add the raspberries, and place under the broiler for about 5 minutes, until lightly browned.

*Serving size = 3 figs and 3 tablespoons yogurt and 2 tablespoons raspberries*
*276 calories*
*0.7 gram fat*
*1 milligram cholesterol*
*51.2 milligrams sodium*

## BLUEBERRY COMPOTE

Joyce Goldstein

*This is good spooned over lemon or melon sorbet or chunks of melon.*

MAKES APPROXIMATELY 4 CUPS
SERVES 4 TO 8

**3 cups blueberries**
**1 tablespoon lemon juice**
**½ teaspoon finely chopped lemon peel**
**½ teaspoon ground cinnamon**
**⅓ cup port**
**¾ cup sugar**

Simmer 2 cups of the blueberries with the lemon juice, peel, cinnamon, port, and sugar for about 5 minutes. Stir in the remaining cup of blueberries and serve warm or at room temperature.

*Serving size = ½ cup*
*110 calories*
*0.2 gram fat*
*0 milligrams cholesterol*
*4.7 milligrams sodium*

## BROILED PINEAPPLE WITH CINNAMON AND RUM

Joyce Goldstein

*A tropical treat, simple to prepare and even easier to eat.*

SERVES 4 TO 8

**1 medium ripe pineapple, peeled, cored, and sliced about 1 inch thick**
**1 cup brown sugar**
**1 teaspoon ground cinnamon**
**Pinch of ground cloves or nutmeg**
**½ teaspoon pure vanilla extract**
**½ cup Meyers dark rum**

Place the pineapple slices in a baking pan that will fit under the broiler. Combine the sugar, cinnamon, and cloves and sprinkle over the pineapple. Broil until tender and somewhat caramelized. Remove the pineapple to a serving platter. Combine the vanilla and rum and pour into the pan over low heat, on top of the stove, loosening any brown bits with a spoon. Pour the rum syrup over the pineapple. Serve warm.

*Serving size = ½ cup*
*123 calories*
*0.2 gram fat*
*0 milligrams cholesterol*
*6.4 milligrams sodium*

## STRAWBERRY SORBET

Joyce Goldstein

MAKES 1 QUART

**5 pints ripe strawberries**
**1 cup sugar**
**½ cup water**
**Pinch of salt**
**1 tablespoon lemon juice**
**2 tablespoons cassis liqueur or kirsch**

Puree the berries in the container of a food processor and strain to remove the seeds; you should have about 4 cups of puree. Heat the sugar, water, and salt in a saucepan over medium heat until the sugar is dissolved. Stir into the berry puree and refrigerate until cold. Stir in the lemon juice and cassis or kirsch. Freeze in an ice cream maker according to the manufacturer's instructions.

*Serving size = ½ cup*
*132 calories*
*0.3 gram fat*
*0 milligrams cholesterol*
*4.7 milligrams sodium*

## COEUR À LA CRÈME

J. E. Hokin

*Until now, this was the richest dessert one could eat. I have substituted nonfat yogurt cheese to create a fat-free replacement for this classic.*

*You will need a heart-shaped porcelain cheese mold with draining holes and some cheesecloth for this.*

SERVES 8 TO 10

**1 pound Nonfat Yogurt Cheese (page 148)**
**1 tablespoon pure vanilla extract**
**2 tablespoons confectioners' sugar (optional)**
**1 pint strawberries, cleaned and sliced**

Place the yogurt cheese in a medium-sized bowl. Add the vanilla and sugar and stir until well blended. Line the mold with cheesecloth. Spoon the cheese mixture into the mold, smooth the top, and set on a plate. Refrigerate for 24 hours to allow the cheese to drain and produce a firm heart shape.

Unmold onto a serving plate. Remove the cheesecloth and serve with strawberries.

*Serving size = ¼ cup*
*55 calories*
*0.2 gram fat*
*1 milligram cholesterol*
*43.8 milligrams sodium*

## ALMOND CAKE WITH STRAWBERRIES AND KIRSCH

Paul Bertolli

*This light cake, like a soufflé, relies upon beaten egg whites for its airy structure. Ripe raw strawberries, sliced and lightly sugared, peaches, or any other juicy fruit may be substituted for the cherries with equal success.*

*You may also wish to alter the flavor of the cake with anise, which is particularly harmonious with strawberries or vanilla extract. Or if you prefer the flavor of lemon, add a teaspoon of zest to the beaten egg whites before folding in the flour and sugar.*

SERVES 16 TO 20

**1½ cups egg whites (about 10 large eggs)**
**1 teaspoon almond extract**
**1¼ cups superfine sugar**
**1 cup cake flour**
**1 cup confectioners' sugar**
**2½ cups fresh pitted Bing or Burlatt cherries**
**2 tablespoons water**
**2 tablespoons kirsch**

Have ready a 9 × 3-inch springform pan fitted with a "collar": Cut a piece of baking parchment about 5 inches wide and 30 inches long. Fold it twice vertically. Fit the strip inside the edges of the pan so that it rises above the top about 2 inches. The collar will contain the cake as it rises up and sets.

Preheat the oven to 350 degrees.

Combine the egg whites, almond extract, and half the superfine sugar in an electric mixer. Using the whisk attachment, beat the mixture until the whites hold stiff peaks when the whisk is lifted. Add the remaining superfine sugar a small amount at a time and continue to beat the whites after each addition only enough to incorporate the sugar. Transfer the whites to a large bowl. Combine the cake flour and confectioners' sugar and sift them into another bowl. Using a spatula, fold the flour mixture into the whites about ¼ cup at a time. Work fast and do not overmix. Keep the mixture as light and airy as possible.

Pour the mixture into the cake pan and carefully even the surface with a spatula. Bake the cake for 45 minutes, or until uniformly light brown and slightly springy to the touch at the center.

Cool on a rack before removing from the pan.

In the meantime, combine the cherries, water, and kirsch in a skillet. Bring to a boil and simmer for 5 minutes. If your cherries are tart, you may wish to add a bit of sugar to taste. Keep in mind, however, that the cake is sweet. The cherries should be quite juicy. Transfer to a bowl and let them cool.

Serve a wedge of the cake with several spoonfuls of the cherries and some of the kirsch-flavored syrup.

*Serving size = 1⁄16 of the cake*
*157 calories*
*0.4 gram fat*
*0 milligrams cholesterol*
*34.8 milligrams sodium*

## WARM CREPES WITH PEARS AND CARAMEL-RED WINE SAUCE

Paul Bertolli

*The combination of pears and red wine, fruits of the autumn harvest, is a natural one. It is not only the evocative flavors of this dessert but also its tawny colors that make it so appropriate to serve in the fall season. The choice of the Bartlett pear is not arbitrary; it is one of the best cooking pears, for its musky perfume doesn't fade with heat (as is the case with the more fragile Comice) and it holds its texture well. What's more, cooked Bartletts have a smooth, buttery quality that requires no enrichment.*

*There are several simple steps to this recipe that can all be done in advance. First, assemble the batter, then precook the pears, and finally, make the caramel-red wine sauce. Just before serving, roll up the pears in the crepes, warm them in the oven, and spoon the sauce over.*

SERVES 8

**½ cup all-purpose unbleached flour**
**1½ teaspoons granulated sugar**
**¼ teaspoon salt**
**2 egg whites**
**⅓ cup nonfat milk**
**⅓ cup plus ¾ cup water**
**5 ripe Bartlett pears (2 pounds)**
**½ fresh vanilla bean**
**½ cup sugar**
**2 cups dry red wine (preferably Zinfandel)**
**½ cup Dannon nonfat plain yogurt**
**2 teaspoons confectioners' sugar**

Place the flour, sugar, and salt in a medium-sized bowl. Add the egg whites and the milk, and whisk until the mixture is smooth. Add the ⅓ cup water and continue to whisk until the ingredients are well blended. If there are any lumps in the batter, pass it through a fine sieve.

Heat a 6-inch Silverstone or other nonstick pan. Pour about 2 tablespoons of batter into the pan and quickly tilt the pan to cover the entire bottom. The faster you spread the batter, the thinner your crepe will be. Let the crepe cook for about 30 seconds, or until the edges are brown.

Use a blunt knife tip to lift the edge and turn the crepe over by hand. Let it cook an additional 30 seconds on the second side. Remove and cool the crepes one on top of another on a plate. You should have 8 crepes.

Peel, quarter, and core the pears, reserving the peels, and cut them into rough 1-inch chunks. Place the pears in a saucepan. Split the half vanilla bean lengthwise and push out the seeds with the blade of a knife. Add the vanilla pod and the seeds to the pan with the pears. Warm the pears over medium heat. When you see them begin to release their juice, stir them and cover the pan. Let the pears stew for 4 to 5 minutes, or until they are soft but still intact. They will have released quite a lot of juice; pour them into a strainer or small colander set over a bowl and capture the juice. Return the juice to the saucepan and reduce it until it thickens to the consistency of a heavy syrup. Place the pears in a bowl, pour the reduced syrup over them, and set aside.

Put the sugar and ¾ cup water in a deep saucepan on the stove over medium-high heat and stir the mixture until the sugar is completely dissolved. Bring to a low boil. When the water has evaporated, after about 10 minutes, the sugar temperature rises rapidly and caramelization begins. Watch the pot carefully at this point. When the caramel is a dark amber color but not burned, add the wine, standing away from the pot as you do so; it will sputter violently. Whisk the mixture until all the caramel is dissolved. Place the peelings of the pears in the pot. Bring the mixture to a boil and reduce it over high heat to about ⅔ cup. The sauce should be slightly viscous. Strain the sauce through a fine sieve and set it aside to cool.

Preheat the oven to 350 degrees. Whisk the yogurt so that it is very smooth and blended.

Place about 2 tablespoons of the cooked pears on the pale side of the crepes, roll them up snugly, and transfer them, seam side down, to a nonstick baking sheet. Warm the crepes in the oven for 10 to 12 minutes. Transfer them to 4 warm plates. Pour about 2 tablespoons of caramel-red wine sauce over and around the crepes. Place a dollop of yogurt to one side. Put the sugar in a small sieve and dust the tops of the crepes with it. Serve immediately.

*Serving size = 1 crepe and 2 tablespoons caramel*
*187 calories*
*0.5 gram fat*
*0.4 milligram cholesterol*
*103.1 milligrams sodium*

## CHEESE BLINTZES WITH FRESH FRUIT

Myrna Melling

*High in protein, these blintzes can be served for breakfast or brunch topped with fresh sliced peaches, figs or plums, or whole berries or stewed fruit. In short, these are good with just about any unsweetened preserves or syrup. The pancakes can be used without the cheese filling and simply tossed with preserves or fruit.*

MAKES 8 BLINTZES
SERVES 4 TO 8

**4 egg equivalent oil-free egg substitute**
**1⅛ to 1¼ cups nonfat milk**
**1 teaspoon sugar**
**½ teaspoon pure vanilla extract**
**¼ teaspoon salt**
**¾ cup all-purpose white flour**
**Vegetable oil spray**
**1 cup nonfat cottage cheese**
**1 teaspoon sugar**
**¼ teaspoon almond extract**

Stir the egg substitute, milk, sugar, vanilla, and salt together. Blend in the flour with a wire whisk. Let the mixture rest at room temperature for 10 minutes.

Spray a 10-inch nonstick frying pan with vegetable oil pan

spray and wipe away any excess with a paper towel. Pour ¼ cup batter onto the skillet and immediately tip the skillet to allow the batter to spread and fill up the bottom of the pan.

When the crepe begins to brown, the edges will separate away from the skillet. Use a long spatula to slide under the crepe and flip it over. Brown lightly on the second side, then transfer to a warm plate.

Continue with the remaining batter, wiping the skillet between each crepe with a tiny bit of oil on a paper towel. If necessary, respray the pan after 3 to 4 crepes.

Using a hand blender or food processor, blend the cottage cheese, sugar, and almond extract until smooth. Spread about 2 teaspoons of filling across the center of each pancake. Roll loosely. Arrange side by side on a warmed plate. Dust lightly with confectioners' sugar and top with fruit or preserves.

*Serving size = 2 blintzes*
*202 calories*
*2.6 grams fat*
*4.2 milligrams cholesterol*
*501.2 milligrams sodium*

## PEACH PURSES WITH RASPBERRY COULIS

Tina Salter and Christine Swett

*This is best when the peaches are at the height of the season. Surprise your guests with this elegant presentation: Flood the dessert plate with the raspberry coulis. Squeeze concentric circles of nonfat vanilla yogurt over the coulis from a plastic sauce bottle. Draw a toothpick from the center circle through the outer circles (without lifting) every 1 inch or so to create a spider web effect!*

*The dessert must be served hot from the oven, as the phyllo will become soggy very quickly if it is left to stand. Work quickly with the phyllo dough, as it dries out immediately when exposed to air. If you must let it sit for even a minute or two, cover the dough with a damp towel or plastic wrap.*

SERVES 6

- **½ cup Nonfat Yogurt Cheese (page 148)**
- **1 tablespoon plus 6 teaspoons honey**
- **1 teaspoon pure vanilla extract**
- **¼ teaspoon almond extract**
- **6 ripe peaches, peeled, halved, and pits removed**
- **6 sheets oil-free, fat-free phyllo dough**
- **Raspberry Coulis (recipe follows)**

Preheat the oven to 350 degrees.

In a small bowl, combine the yogurt cheese, 1 tablespoon honey, vanilla, and almond extract. Fill 1 peach half with a tablespoon of the yogurt mixture. Cover with the second peach half. Repeat with the remaining 5 peaches.

Fold 1 sheet of phyllo dough in half, then in half again to make 4 layers. Set a stuffed peach in the center of the phyllo dough, pull the dough up around the peach, and twist gently just above the peach to seal, creating a "purse."

Drizzle 1 teaspoon honey over the purse and place on a parchment-lined baking sheet. Repeat with the remaining 5 peaches. Bake for 10 to 12 minutes, or until golden brown. Serve immediately on a puddle of raspberry coulis.

## RASPBERRY COULIS

*This puree can be prepared and refrigerated for up to 24 hours before serving.*

MAKES 1½ CUPS

- **2 baskets raspberries**
- **¼ cup orange juice**
- **2 teaspoons honey**

In a blender or food processor, combine the raspberries, orange juice, and honey. Puree until very smooth. Strain the sauce through a fine-mesh sieve. Refrigerate until ready to serve.

*Serving size = 1 peach purse and 2 tablespoons coulis*
*178 calories*
*0.8 gram fat*
*0.7 milligram cholesterol*
*150 milligrams sodium*

## FLAN

Jean-Marc Fullsack

*This is wonderful served with a layer of blueberries or raspberries on the bottom of the baking dish. For variety, whisk in 1 teaspoon of orange, lemon, or lime zest.*

MAKES 4 CUPS
SERVES 4 TO 8

**2 cups nonfat milk**
**1 cup egg whites (approximately 8 eggs)**
**1 tablespoon pure vanilla extract**
**1 tablespoon maple syrup**
**1 teaspoon honey**

Preheat the oven to 325 degrees.

In a medium bowl, whisk together the milk, egg whites, vanilla, maple syrup, and honey. Pour the custard into a 4-cup soufflé dish, set the dish in a larger pan, pour in hot water to within 2 inches of the top of the dish, and bake for 40 to 50 minutes, or until the center is just set; do not overcook or the flan will be dry. Rest for 10 minutes before serving. Serve chilled or at room temperature.

*Serving size = ½ cup*
*52 calories*
*0.1 gram fat*
*1.1 milligrams cholesterol*
*86.6 milligrams sodium*

## APPLES AND RASPBERRIES IN APPLE-GINGER CONSOMMÉ

Hubert Keller

*You will need a juice extractor to execute this dish.*

SERVES 4

**6 Granny Smith apples**
**1 cinnamon stick**
**¼ teaspoon peeled and finely shredded fresh gingerroot**
**1 teaspoon calvados or other apple brandy**
**1 tablespoon honey**
**½ vanilla bean, halved lengthwise**
**Vegetable oil spray**
**20 large red raspberries**
**4 mint leaves**

Peel and core 4 apples. Cut them into large pieces and process them in a juice extractor. Transfer the juice into a nonreactive saucepan. Add the cinnamon stick, fresh ginger, apple brandy, honey, and vanilla bean. Bring to a boil, cover, and set aside. Meanwhile, peel and core the remaining 2 apples. Cut them into quarters and then into ¼-inch-thick slices. Heat a nonstick sauté pan over medium-high heat, spray lightly with the pan coating, and add the apple slices. Brown slowly, turning frequently to ensure uniform coloring and to prevent burning. Keep the cooked apple slices warm.

Arrange the apple slices and the fresh raspberries decoratively in individual shallow soup plates. Mince the mint leaves finely and sprinkle over the fruit. Remove the cinnamon stick and vanilla bean from the warm consommé and ladle it over the fruit.

*Serving size = ½ cup consommé and ½ cup fruit*
*122 calories*
*0.7 gram fat*
*0 milligrams cholesterol*
*0.3 milligram sodium*

## FIGS AND BLUEBERRIES IN CITRUS BROTH

Hubert Keller

*The blueberries release a very attractive reddish color into the citrus-based broth.*

SERVES 6 TO 8

- **1½ cups freshly squeezed orange juice**
- **1 cup freshly squeezed grapefruit juice**
- **3 tablespoons freshly squeezed lemon juice**
- **½ teaspoon peeled and finely shredded fresh gingerroot**
- **2 tablespoons honey**
- **1 tablespoon rum**
- **16 to 20 ripe black figs**
- **1 banana**
- **3 tablespoons blueberries**
- **8 mint leaves, for garnish**

Mix the juices together in a stainless steel or nonstick saucepan. Add the ginger, honey, and rum and bring to a boil. Meanwhile, prick each fig with a fork in a few places. Peel the banana and cut into ¼-inch-thick slices. Plunge all the fruits gently in the boiling juices. Remove from the heat, cover, and cool to room temperature. Refrigerate for 1 hour. Serve in shallow-rimmed soup plates and decorate with fresh mint leaves.

*Serving size = 6 tablespoons with fruit broth*
*152 calories*
*0.6 gram fat*
*0 milligrams cholesterol*
*2.8 milligrams sodium*

## PEACHES COOKED IN RED WINE

Donna Nicoletti

SERVES 6

**6 ripe peaches, preferably freestone**
**2 cups full-flavored red wine, such as Zinfandel**
**1 cup water**
**2 cinnamon sticks**
**2 cups sugar**
**Fresh mint leaves, for garnish**

Skin the peaches by dropping them briefly into boiling water. Cool enough to handle and slip off the skins. Cut the peaches in half and remove their pits. Cut the peaches into ½-inch slices.

Bring the wine, water, cinnamon sticks, and sugar to a full boil. Remove from the heat and add the peaches; cool to room temperature and then refrigerate overnight or for at least 4 hours.

Serve the peaches and some of the cooking liquid garnished with fresh mint leaves.

*Serving size = 1 peach and 2 tablespoons syrup*
*115 calories*
*0.1 gram fat*
*0 milligrams cholesterol*
*1.7 milligrams sodium*

## FIVE FRUIT AND BERRY COMPOTE WITH A MINT AND TEA INFUSION

Alfred Portale

SERVES 8 OR MORE

**½ cup water**
**2 tea bags**
**3 large sprigs of fresh mint**
**12 large red ripe strawberries (about 1½ cups)**

**2 cups Bing (black) cherries**
**1 cup blueberries**
**1 cup raspberries**
**1 ripe mango**
**⅔ cup sugar**
**2 vanilla beans, split in half and seeds scraped away, or 1 teaspoon pure vanilla extract**
**3¼ cups dry white wine**
**½ cup port wine**
**Fresh mint sprigs, for garnish**

Bring the water to a boil and add the tea bags and 3 large fresh mint sprigs. Stir until the mint is wilted. Remove from the heat and cover. Let stand 10 minutes or longer.

Meanwhile, trim off and discard the stems of the strawberries. Cut each strawberry in half lengthwise. Put the strawberries into a saucepan.

Pull off and discard the cherry stems. Cut each cherry in half and discard the pits. Add the cherries to the strawberries.

Rinse the blueberries and raspberries and add them to the saucepan with the other fruits.

Peel the mango. Cut the flesh into thin slices. Cut the slices into thin lengthwise strips. Add to the fruit and berries.

Put the sugar in a saucepan and add the vanilla beans or vanilla, white wine, and port. Place a sieve over the saucepan and pour the tea mixture through it into the pan. Squeeze each tea bag to release all the liquid; discard the bags. Reserve the mint sprigs. Bring the mixture to a boil, then pour it into the pan with the fruits and berries. Quickly bring to a simmer over high heat. Add the mint sprigs and remove the pan from the heat. Place in the refrigerator and chill well.

To serve the compote, remove the mint sprigs, dish into shallow soup plates, and garnish with sprigs of fresh mint.

*Serving size = ½ cup fruit and ¼ cup broth*
*159 calories*
*0.7 gram fat*
*0 milligrams cholesterol*
*6.6 milligrams sodium*

## VANILLA POACHED FRUITS

Alfred Portale

SERVES 6 TO 8

**4 dried figs**
**4 medjool dates**
**12 dried apricots**
**1 ounce dried sour cherries**
**1 ounce black raisins**
**1½ quarts white wine**
**1¼ cups sugar**
**Pinch of ground cloves**
**4 cinnamon sticks**
**2 vanilla beans, split**
**1 orange, peeled and sliced**
**1 lemon, peeled and sliced**
**2 Bosc pears, peeled**
**2 ounces dark rum**
**20 perfect raspberries**
**4 sprigs of fresh mint**

Soak the figs, dates, apricots, cherries, and raisins in warm water for 3 hours, then drain. Set aside.

Meanwhile, combine the white wine, sugar, cloves, cinnamon sticks, vanilla, and orange and lemon slices in a stainless-steel pot. Add the pears and cover with a clean white kitchen towel. Return to a simmer and poach until the pears are tender, approximately 20 minutes. Remove the pears with half the poaching liquid, cover with a towel, and chill.

Poach the figs and apricots in the remaining poaching liquid until tender, approximately 20 minutes; add the cherries, raisins, and dates. Remove from the heat, add the rum, and chill.

To serve, slice the pears in half. Arrange in 4 stemmed glasses or bowls along with the other dried fruits. Spoon a little syrup over and garnish with cinnamon sticks, raspberries, and fresh mint sprigs.

*Serving size = ¾ cup*
*127 calories*
*0.4 gram fat*
*0 milligrams cholesterol*
*3.7 milligrams sodium*

## POACHED BOSC PEAR WITH ZINFANDEL GRANITÉ

Alfred Portale

SERVES 4 TO 6

**4 cups water**
**1½ cups sugar**
**1 vanilla bean, split lengthwise**
**1 orange, cut in half**
**1 lemon, cut in half**
**4 to 6 Bosc pears, firm but ripe**
**Zinfandel Granité (recipe follows)**
**Fresh blueberries (optional)**
**Sprigs of fresh mint**

Place the water, sugar, and vanilla bean into a saucepan. Squeeze the orange and lemon halves into the water before adding them to the pan.

Peel the pears and core them from the bottom three-quarters of the way up. Leave the stems on.

Place the pears in the poaching liquid and cover with a clean towel to keep the tops of the pears moist and to keep them from discoloring.

Bring to a boil, reduce to a simmer, and cook the pears until tender. The pears are done when a fork goes in easily, but they should not get mushy.

Cool and keep the pears in their poaching liquid until ready to serve.

Spoon the granité crystals into large wineglasses or bowls, filling them about three-quarters full. Remove the pears from the poaching liquid and place one in each glass, setting it onto the granité. Arrange the blueberries around the pear and garnish with a sprig of mint.

### ZINFANDEL GRANITÉ

- **¾ cup water**
- **¾ cup sugar**
- **Juice of 3 oranges**
- **Juice of 3 lemons**
- **2 tablespoons cassis**
- **1 bottle good California Zinfandel**

Place the water and sugar in a saucepan. Bring to a boil to dissolve the sugar. Mix 1 cup of the sugar syrup, the juices, the cassis, and wine in a bowl. Pour into a shallow container and place in the freezer. Freeze overnight.

When ready to serve, use a fork to scrape the surface of the granité to form large crystals.

*Serving size = 1 pear and ½ cup granité*
*250 calories*
*0.2 gram fat*
*0 milligrams cholesterol*
*5.6 milligrams sodium*

## BAKED APPLES WITH BROWN SUGAR, CINNAMON, CURRANTS, AND APPLE CIDER YOGURT

Bradley Ogden

*This dish can be served as a main dish for breakfast or as a dessert.*

SERVES 4

- **1½ cups apple cider**
- **Juice of 1 lemon**
- **Juice of 2 oranges**
- **4 tablespoons firmly packed light brown sugar**

- ⅛ teaspoon ground cinnamon
- 1 tablespoon maple syrup
- 2 tablespoons currants
- 4 baking apples (Granny Smith or Winesap)
- Cider Yogurt (recipe follows)

Preheat the oven to 400 degrees.

In a small saucepan, combine all the ingredients except the apples and Cider Yogurt. Place on high heat and bring to a boil. Continue boiling, stirring frequently, until the liquid is reduced by half. Remove from the heat and set aside.

Core the apples, but do not cut through the bottom of each. Peel each apple one-third of the way down from the top. Place the apples in a 2-quart baking dish. Pour the cider reduction into and over the apples. Bake for 30 to 40 minutes, or until tender, basting occasionally.

To serve, place each apple in a bowl with the Cider Yogurt and top with a drizzle of the pan juices.

## APPLE CIDER YOGURT

MAKES 1 CUP

- 2 cups apple cider
- ½ tart apple, cored and cut into 1-inch chunks
- 1 tablespoon honey
- ¾ cup nonfat plain yogurt

In a stainless-steel saucepan combine the cider, apple, and honey. Bring the mixture to a boil over medium-high heat and cook, stirring occasionally, until the liquid is reduced to ⅓ cup. Cool immediately and fold into the yogurt.

*Serving size = 1 apple and ¼ cup apple cider yogurt*
*191 calories*
*0.6 gram fat*
*0.8 milligram cholesterol*
*37.6 milligrams sodium*

## PINEAPPLE AND STRAWBERRIES WITH SPICES

Alain Rondelli

SERVES 4

**1 pineapple (about 4 pounds)**
**1 tablespoon sugar**
**¼ teaspoon kosher salt**
**1 teaspoon whole black peppercorns**
**¼ teaspoon ground ginger**
**⅛ teaspoon ground cloves**
**⅛ teaspoon ground cinnamon**
**⅛ teaspoon ground allspice**
**Juice of 1 lemon**
**2 cups strawberries**

Remove the leaves from the pineapple, remove the core, and cut lengthwise into quarters; then cut away the outer peel. Cut 3 pineapple quarters into large chunks, place in a food processor, and puree. Strain the puree through a fine sieve.

Combine the pineapple puree, sugar, salt, peppercorns, spices, and lemon juice in a serving bowl. Slice the remaining pineapple quarter into ¼-inch-thick slices. Clean and stem the strawberries, and cut them in quarters. Add the strawberries to the bowl and refrigerate for at least 2 hours before serving.

*Serving size = 1 cup*
*168 calories*
*1.3 grams fat*
*0 milligrams cholesterol*
*149.4 milligrams sodium*

## POACHED APPLE WITH VANILLA SPICE GLAZE

Tracy Pikhart Ritter

SERVES 6

**3 Granny Smith apples, halved from top to bottom, peeled, and cored**
**1 quart apple juice**
**1 cup dry white wine**
**Juice of 1 orange**
**Zest of 1 orange**
**2 vanilla beans, split, or 2 tablespoons pure vanilla extract**
**2 cinnamon sticks**
**1 clove**
**3 whole allspice or ¼ teaspoon ground**
**1 whole nutmeg**
**1½ quarter-size pieces of fresh gingerroot (optional)**
**2 tablespoons honey or brown sugar**
**Frozen nonfat plain yogurt**

Place the apple halves in a shallow pan with the apple juice, wine, orange juice, and orange zest. Add water if necessary to cover the apples completely.

Tie all the remaining ingredients, except the honey or brown sugar and frozen yogurt, in a piece of cheesecloth or a handkerchief. If you are using vanilla extract instead of vanilla beans, add it to the pan. Place the cheesecloth bag with the apples and liquid.

Bring to a boil, reduce to a simmer, and poach the apples for 20 minutes, or until soft but not mushy. Carefully remove the apples and cool. Discard the spice bag.

Add the honey to the poaching liquid and reduce over medium-high heat for 20 minutes, or until reduced to ½ cup. Cool. Slice each half into 4 pieces. Fan the apple slices onto 6 individual plates. Spoon the glaze over the tops and sides. Serve with the yogurt.

*Serving size = ½ apple and ¼ cup glaze*
*69 calories*
*0.3 gram fat*
*0 milligrams cholesterol*
*1.8 milligrams sodium*

## LEMON SPEARMINT ICE WITH FRESH BERRIES

Alfred Portale

SERVES 8

**1 bunch of fresh spearmint (approximately 2 ounces)**
**1 cup sugar**
**4 cups water**
**½ cup lemon juice**
**Zest of 1 lemon**
**2 pints mixed ripe berries (strawberries, blackberries, raspberries)**

Wash the mint. Reserve 8 sprigs for garnish. Roughly chop the remaining leaves and combine in a saucepan with the sugar, water, lemon juice, and lemon zest. Bring to a boil, reduce the heat, and simmer for 2 minutes. Remove from the heat and allow to steep for 20 minutes, then strain. Pour the cooled liquid into a shallow, nonreactive pan and place in a freezer overnight.

At serving time, use the tines of a fork to scrape the surface of the ice into large crystals. Heap the crystals into chilled stemmed glasses and garnish with the berries and the reserved mint sprigs.

*Serving size = ⅓ cup "ice" and ½ cup berries*
*123 calories*
*0.3 gram fat*
*0 milligrams cholesterol*
*4.4 milligrams sodium*

## STRAWBERRIES WITH RASPBERRY SAUCE

Catherine Pantsios

*This recipe is ridiculously simple but berries at their peak deliver full flavor. Be sure to allow the time for the strawberries to macerate in the sauce—and don't serve them too cold.*

SERVES 4

**1 pint fresh strawberries**
**½ pint fresh raspberries**
**Superfine sugar to taste**

Stem the strawberries and place in a serving bowl. Puree the raspberries in a blender or food processor with only as much sugar as you need to sweeten them to taste. Strain to remove the seeds and pour over the strawberries. Set aside at room temperature for a half hour before serving.

*Serving size = ½ cup strawberries and ¼ cup raspberry sauce*
*96 calories*
*0.6 gram fat*
*0 milligrams cholesterol*
*0.9 milligram sodium*

## BANANA HEART

Jean-Marc Fullsack

*This is a very sumptuous dish and simple to execute once you master folding the edges of the parchment paper hearts.*

MAKES 4 HEARTS
SERVES 4

**¼ cup orange juice concentrate**
**1 tablespoon honey**
**4 drops pure vanilla extract**
**4 drops almond extract**

**4 drops dark rum or rum extract**
**4 large bananas, sliced**
**Parchment paper or foil**
**Fresh mint leaves, for garnish**

Preheat the oven to 425 degrees.

In a small bowl, combine the orange juice concentrate, honey, vanilla, almond extract, and rum. Set aside.

Cut 8 10-inch parchment paper hearts. Place 1 sliced banana on the center of each parchment heart. Spoon a generous tablespoon of the flavoring mixture over the banana. Place a second parchment heart directly over the banana, carefully aligning the edges. Grasp the edges of both the upper and lower parchment hearts and fold in toward the center ¼ inch 3 to 4 times to create an airtight seal around the banana.

Repeat with the remaining 3 bananas.

Transfer each heart to a baking sheet and bake for 7 to 10 minutes. If a good seal was formed, the heart will puff up during the baking.

Transfer the baked hearts to individual serving dishes. Just before serving cut a large X in the center of each heart to open. Garnish with the mint leaves and serve immediately. The banana is to be eaten out of the parchment.

*Serving size = 1 heart*
*150 calories*
*0.6 gram fat*
*0 milligrams cholesterol*
*1.9 milligrams sodium*

## BANANAS, PINEAPPLE, AND BERRIES

Jean-Marc Fullsack

SERVES 4

**1⅓ cups nonfat plain yogurt**
**4 teaspoons honey**
**½ teaspoon pure vanilla extract**

- **¼ teaspoon ground cinnamon**
- **¼ teaspoon dark rum or rum extract**
- **1⅓ cups diced fresh pineapple**
- **¼ cup pineapple juice concentrate**
- **1⅓ cups sliced bananas**
- **⅔ cup sliced fresh strawberries**
- **⅔ cup fresh raspberries**
- **4 teaspoons chiffonaded fresh mint**

In a medium-sized bowl, whisk together the yogurt, honey, vanilla, cinnamon, and rum. Cover and refrigerate until needed.

In a 2½-quart saucepan, combine the diced pineapple and the pineapple juice concentrate. Bring to a boil, reduce the heat, and simmer for 5 to 7 minutes, stirring frequently. Allow to cool.

In a large bowl, toss and combine the pineapple mixture with the bananas and berries. Serve in individual portions with the sauce spooned over. Alternatively, pour a puddle of the sauce onto each plate, then pile the fruit on it. Garnish with the mint.

*Serving size = 1 cup fruit and ⅓ cup sauce*
*169 calories*
*0.7 gram fat*
*1.4 milligrams cholesterol*
*59.6 milligrams sodium*

## STRAWBERRY RHUBARB COMPOTE

Jean-Marc Fullsack

*This is very simple to make. Try it as a "puddle" under honey-flavored Nonfat Yogurt Cheese (page 148) molded into a heart shape. This would make a nice presentation with a sprinkling of edible lavender blossoms over it. It also tastes very good all by itself.*

SERVES 4

**1 pound thin young rhubarb, sliced ½ inch thick**
**1 pound strawberries, washed and hulled**
**¼ cup honey**

In a large saucepan, combine the rhubarb, strawberries, and honey. Bring to a boil. Reduce the heat and simmer gently for 10 to 15 minutes. Cool and serve chilled or at room temperature.

*Serving size = ¾ cup*
*122 calories*
*0.6 gram fat*
*0 milligrams cholesterol*
*6.7 milligrams sodium*

## AMARETTO CUP-A-CHEESE CAKE

Michael McDermott

*This elegant dessert can be prepared and refrigerated up to 24 hours ahead of time. It has an excellent flavor and nearly duplicates a real cream cheese filling.*

SERVES 4

**1 large whole-grain muffin (approximately ¾ cup)**
**1 cup Nonfat Yogurt Cheese (page 148)**
**¼ cup all-fruit apricot jam**
**2 tablespoons Amaretto liqueur**
**½ teaspoon lime zest**
**Ground cinnamon**

Cut the muffin into ½-inch pieces and place 3 to 4 pieces in the bottom of each of 4 6-ounce ramekins or glass goblets.

In a small bowl, combine the yogurt cheese, jam, liqueur, and lime zest. Mix well. Divide the mixture over the muffin pieces. Tap the ramekin or goblet gently on the counter to smooth and settle the mixture. Cover and chill for at least 30 minutes before serving. Sprinkle with the cinnamon.

*Serving size = 1 cup*
*169 calories*
*0.4 gram fat*
*2.1 milligrams cholesterol*
*148.6 milligrams sodium*

## BLUEBERRY PANCAKES

Jean-Marc Fullsack

*Serve these with fresh fruit and yogurt; raspberries or sliced strawberries make equally delicious alternatives.*

MAKES 16 PANCAKES

- **¾ cups whole wheat pastry flour**
- **½ cup buckwheat flour**
- **½ cup wheat bran**
- **½ teaspoon baking powder**
- **½ teaspoon baking soda**
- **1 cup nonfat plain yogurt**
- **1 cup nonfat milk**
- **2 tablespoons honey**
- **1 tablespoon pure vanilla extract**
- **5 egg whites**
- **3 cups fresh blueberries**

In a large bowl, combine the pastry flour, buckwheat flour, wheat bran, baking powder, and baking soda.

In a separate bowl, combine the yogurt, milk, honey, and vanilla. Stir the yogurt mixture into the flour mixture and mix until smooth.

In a large bowl, beat the egg whites until just stiff and fold into the batter. Gently fold in the blueberries.

For each pancake, ladle ¼ cup of batter onto a hot, nonstick griddle or sauté pan. Cook over medium heat until golden brown. Flip and cook on the second side. Serve immediately.

*Serving size = 2 pancakes*
*160 calories*

*0.9 gram fat*
*1.1 milligrams cholesterol*
*128 milligrams sodium*

## PEAR RICE PUDDING WITH KIWI SAUCE

Jean-Marc Fullsack

*This delicious dessert could also be served warm for breakfast. The brown rice gives a chewy, nutty flavor that complements the fruit. For a softer texture, cook the rice for 10 to 15 minutes longer. The sauce is very tasty, but this pudding could be served without it.*

MAKES 6 CUPS
SERVES 6 TO 8

**1 cup uncooked brown rice**
**2 cups nonfat milk**
**1 large apple, peeled, cored, and cut in ½-inch dice**
**4 pears, peeled, cored, and cut in ½-inch dice**
**¼ cup water**
**4 tablespoons honey**
**1 teaspoon pure vanilla extract**
**⅛ teaspoon ground cinnamon**
**1 pound kiwis, peeled and roughly chopped**
**1 teaspoon sugar**

In a medium-sized saucepan, combine the rice and milk. Bring to a boil. Reduce the heat and simmer for 1 hour. Set aside.

Meantime, in a second medium saucepan, combine the apples, pears, water, honey, vanilla, and cinnamon. Bring to a boil, reduce the heat, and simmer for 10 minutes, or until quite tender but not mushy.

In a food processor bowl or blender, combine the kiwis and sugar. Puree until smooth. Strain to remove the seeds if desired.

Combine the rice and fruit mixtures thoroughly. Serve warm or at room temperature with the kiwi sauce.

*Serving size = ¾ cup*
*160 calories*
*0.8 gram fat*
*1.1 milligrams cholesterol*
*34.8 milligrams sodium*

## PUMPKIN "TOFU" CHEESECAKE

Jean-Marc Fullsack

*The creaminess and satisfying pumpkin flavor will delight you. This can be prepared and refrigerated up to 24 hours in advance.*

MAKES 1 10-INCH CHEESECAKE
SERVES 8 TO 10

**1 cup oat bran**
**¾ cup apple juice concentrate**
**2 cups canned pumpkin**
**1 pound soft tofu**
**1 cup egg whites (approximately 8 eggs)**
**½ cup maple syrup**
**¼ cup flour**
**1 tablespoon pure vanilla extract**
**1 teaspoon fresh lemon zest**
**½ teaspoon ground cinnamon**
**¼ teaspoon ground ginger**
**Pinch of ground cloves**

Preheat the oven to 325 degrees.

Line a 10-inch cake pan with a circle of parchment paper. In a medium-sized bowl, combine the oat bran and apple juice concentrate. Press into the base of the cake pan.

In the bowl of a food processor, combine the pumpkin, tofu, egg whites, maple syrup, flour, vanilla, lemon zest, cinnamon, ginger, and cloves. Process for 1 minute, or until thoroughly combined.

Pour the cheesecake mixture over the bran base and shake very gently to level the surface. Set the cake pan in a large pan, pour in hot water to within 2 inches of the top of the cake pan, and bake for 45 minutes, or until the center is just set. Cool to room temperature and refrigerate for at least 2 hours before serving.

*Serving size = 1/10 of cheesecake*
*164 calories*
*2.6 grams fat*
*0 milligrams cholesterol*
*56.6 milligrams sodium*

## STUFFED BAKED APPLES

Joyce Goldstein

*For a homey winter dessert nothing is better than a warm baked apple. Stuffing it with dried fruit adds a chewy contrast as the apple softens and becomes fluffy. Rome Beauty is the ideal baking apple, as it steams and becomes tender in its own skin.*

SERVES 4

**4 Rome Beauty apples**
**½ cup raisins**
**1 tablespoon grated orange zest**
**4 tablespoons brown sugar (optional)**
**2 tablespoons chopped candied ginger**
**1 teaspoon ground cinnamon**
**¼ cup honey**
**½ cup orange juice**

Preheat the oven to 375 degrees.

Core the apples. Remove an inch of peel at the top of the apple. Combine the raisins, orange zest, brown sugar, ginger, and cinnamon in the container of a food processor. Pulse to combine. Stuff this mixture into the hollowed cores of the apples, mounding a little on top. Place the apples in a baking dish and place in the oven.

Warm the honey in a small pan. When it is liquefied, add

the orange juice. Baste the apples with this mixture every 10 minutes until the apples are tender and feel soft to the touch, 40 to 60 minutes.

Serve warm with yogurt seasoned with a little honey and cinnamon, if desired.

*Serving size = 1 apple*
*179 calories*
*0.5 gram fat*
*0 milligrams cholesterol*
*7.3 milligrams sodium*

# Appendix 1: How to Read Labels

Thanks to Dr. David A. Kessler, Commissioner of the Food and Drug Administration, new labels begin appearing on foods in May 1993. These labels are designed to provide you with correct, usable nutritional information about commercially packaged foods.

This is an important step in the right direction, for accurate information is, of course, important in order to make wise food choices. Standardizing definitions of such words as *low-fat, light, healthy, low cholesterol,* and so on will help reduce some of the confusion in the supermarket.

In an attempt to help consumers understand how much fat and calories they should consume, the new labels provide a column called "% Daily Value" to give an idea of what percentage of the day's allotment of fat and calories come from this food. In the label below, for example, the food has 13 grams of fat, or 20 percent of the daily value. At the bottom of the label is a general guide for how much of each key nutrient a person should have each day based on a 2,000- or 2,500-calorie intake.

Unfortunately, these guidelines are based on a diet consisting of 30 percent of calories from fat. I am concerned that this may give many consumers the erroneous idea that a 30 percent fat diet is optimal.

Serving size ½ cup (114g)
Servings per container 4

| Amount per serving | |
|---|---|
| Calories 260 | Calories from fat 120 |
| | **% Daily Value*** |
| **Total Fat** 13g | **20%** |
| Saturated Fat 5g | **25%** |
| **Cholesterol** 30mg | **10%** |
| **Sodium** 660g | **28%** |
| **Total Carbohydrate** 31g | **11%** |
| Sugars 5g | |
| Dietary Fiber 0g | **0%** |
| **Protein** 5g | |

**Vitamin A 4% ● Vitamin C 2% ●**
**Calcium 15% ● Iron 4%**

*Percent (%) of a Daily Value are based on a 2,000 calorie diet. Your Daily Values may vary higher or lower depending on your calorie needs:

| **Nutrient** | | **2,000 Calories** | **2,500 Calories** |
|---|---|---|---|
| Total Fat | Less than | 65g | 80g |
| Sat Fat | Less than | 20g | 25g |
| Cholesterol | Less than | 300mg | 300mg |
| Sodium | Less than | 2,400mg | 2,400mg |
| Total Carbohydrate | | 300g | 375g |
| Fiber | | 25g | 30g |

**1 g Fat = 9 calories**
**1 g Carbohydrates = 4 calories**
**1 g Protein = 4 calories**

The diet I recommend is based on 10 percent of calories from fat. In this book, and in my earlier ones, I have described why a 10 percent fat diet is more healthful for most people than a 30 percent fat diet.

In any event, the new labels will make it easier for you to follow this diet, if you wish to do so. In the column labeled "% Daily Value," just *multiply* those numbers by three to determine the appropriate values on this diet. In the example shown here, the food has 13 grams of fat, or 20 percent of the "% Daily Value." On this diet, this food would provide 60 percent of your daily fat allotment—a lot—so it's probably too high in fat for you. You can apply this same procedure for the other nutrients listed, e.g., saturated fat, cholesterol, sodium, carbohydrate, and protein.

For the general guide for how much of each key nutrient you should have each day based on a 2,000- or a 2,500-calorie intake, simply *divide* these numbers by three to obtain the comparable values on this diet. For example, on a 10 percent fat, 2,000-calorie diet, you would consume less than 65 ÷ 3 = 22 grams of total fat per day. On a 2,500-calorie diet, you would consume less than 80 ÷ 3 = 27 grams of total fat per day.

# *Appendix 2: Nutrient Analysis of Common Foods*

| *Food* | *Unit* | *Weight (g)* | *Cal* | *CHO (g)* | *Prot (g)* | *Fat (g)* | *Sat Fat (g)* | *Mono Fat (g)* | *Poly Fat (g)* | *Chol (mg)* | *Na (mg)* |
|---|---|---|---|---|---|---|---|---|---|---|---|
| Almonds: dried, shelled, slivered (not packed) | 1 tbsp | 7 | 43 | 1.4 | 1.3 | 3.9 | 0.3 | 2.7 | 0.7 | 0 | tr |
| Anchovy: 1–4" flat | 1 whole | 4 | 5 | 0 | 0.8 | 0.3 | 0.1 | 0.1 | 0.1 | 5 | 32 |
| Angel food cake: see *Cake* | | | | | | | | | | | |
| Apple: raw with skin | 1 whole | 150 | 80 | 20.0 | 0.3 | 0.8 | 0 | 0 | 0.8 | 0 | 1 |
| Apple: raw, pared, ¼" slices or diced pieces | 1 cup | 110 | 59 | 15.5 | 0.2 | 0.3 | 0 | 0 | 0.3 | 0 | 1 |
| Apple butter | 1 tbsp | 18 | 33 | 8.2 | 0.1 | 0.1 | 0 | 0 | 0.1 | 0 | tr |
| Apple juice: canned or bottled | 1 cup | 248 | 117 | 29.5 | 0.2 | 0 | 0 | 0 | 0 | 0 | 2 |
| Applesauce: canned, sweetened | 1 cup | 255 | 232 | 60.7 | 0.5 | 0.3 | 0 | 0 | 0.3 | 0 | 5 |
| Apricots: raw | 3 whole | 114 | 55 | 13.7 | 1.1 | 0.2 | 0 | 0 | 0.2 | 0 | 1 |
| Apricot nectar: canned or bottled | 1 cup | 251 | 143 | 36.6 | 0.8 | 0.3 | 0 | 0 | 0.3 | 0 | tr |
| Artichoke: frozen, cooked, bud or globe | 1 whole | 300 | 52 | 11.9 | 3.4 | 0.2 | 0 | 0 | 0.2 | 0 | 36 |
| Asparagus: canned spears, ½" diameter | 4 spears | 80 | 17 | 2.7 | 1.9 | 0.3 | 0 | 0 | 0.3 | 0 | 189 |
| Asparagus: canned, cut spears, low sodium | 1 cup | 235 | 47 | 7.3 | 6.1 | 0.7 | 0 | 0 | 0.7 | 0 | 7 |
| Avocado: California, raw, 3½" diameter (unpeeled) | 1 whole | 284 | 369 | 12.9 | 4.7 | 36.7 | 7.3 | 16.5 | 4.8 | 0 | 9 |
| Avocado: California, raw, pureed, mashed, or sieved | 1 tbsp | 14 | 25 | 0.9 | 0.3 | 2.4 | 0.5 | 1.1 | 0.3 | 0 | 1 |
| Bacon: Canadian, cooked, 3⅜ × 3⁄16" | 1 oz | 28 | 78 | 0.1 | 7.7 | 5.0 | 1.7 | 1.9 | 0.4 | 25 | 726 |
| Bacon: cooked (approximately 20 slices/lb raw) | 2 slices | 15 | 86 | 0.5 | 3.8 | 7.8 | 2.7 | 3.4 | 0.8 | 11 | 153 |
| Bacon bits: with coconut oil | 1 tsp | 3 | 15 | 0.9 | 1.3 | 0.6 | 0.6 | 0 | 0 | 0 | 115 |
| Bacon bits: with soy oil | 1 tsp | 3 | 14 | 0.9 | 1.4 | 0.6 | 0.1 | 0.2 | 0.2 | 0 | 115 |

| Food | Unit | Weight (g) | Cal | CHO (g) | Prot (g) | Fat (g) | Sat Fat (g) | Mono Fat (g) | Poly Fat (g) | Chol (mg) | Na (mg) |
|---|---|---|---|---|---|---|---|---|---|---|---|
| Bagel: water | 1 whole | 73 | 212 | 41.1 | 7.9 | 1.3 | 0.2 | 0.2 | 0.3 | 0 | 120 |
| Baking powder: double acting | 1 tsp | 3 | 3 | 0.7 | 0 | 0 | 0 | 0 | 0 | 0 | 290 |
| Baking powder: low sodium | 1 tsp | 4 | 7 | 1.8 | 0 | 0 | 0 | 0 | 0 | 0 | tr |
| Baking soda | ¼ tsp | 4 | 0 | 0 | 0 | 0 | 0 | 0 | 0 | 0 | 345 |
| Banana, raw, medium | 1 whole | 175 | 101 | 26.4 | 1.3 | 0.2 | 0 | 0 | 0.2 | 0 | 1 |
| Barbecue sauce: commercial (corn oil) | 1 tbsp | 16 | 14 | 1.3 | 0.2 | 1.1 | 0.1 | 0.3 | 0.6 | 0 | 127 |
| Beans: garbanzos or chick-peas | 1 cup | 185 | 248 | 42.1 | 14.1 | 3.3 | 1.0 | 0.3 | 2.0 | 0 | 18 |
| Beans: pork and beans in tomato sauce, canned | 1 cup | 255 | 311 | 48.5 | 15.6 | 6.6 | 2.4 | 2.8 | 0.6 | 6 | 1,181 |
| Beans: kidney | 1 cup | 185 | 218 | 39.6 | 14.4 | 0.9 | 0.3 | 0.1 | 0.6 | 0 | 6 |
| Beans: lentils | 1 cup | 200 | 212 | 38.6 | 15.6 | 0 | 0 | 0 | 0 | 0 | 4 |
| Beans: lima, frozen, cooked | 1 cup | 170 | 168 | 32.5 | 10.2 | 0.2 | 0 | 0 | 0.1 | 0 | 172 |
| Beans: lima, canned | 1 cup | 170 | 163 | 31.1 | 9.2 | 0.5 | 0.2 | 0 | 0.3 | 0 | 401 |
| Beans: lima, canned, low sodium | 1 cup | 170 | 162 | 30.1 | 9.9 | 0.5 | 0.1 | 0 | 0.2 | 0 | 7 |
| Beans: pinto, calico, red Mexican | 1 cup | 185 | 218 | 39.6 | 14.4 | 0.9 | 0.3 | 0.1 | 0.6 | 0 | 6 |
| Beans: mung, sprouts, cooked and drained | 1 cup | 125 | 35 | 6.5 | 4.0 | 0.3 | 0 | 0 | 0.3 | 0 | 5 |
| Beans: mung, sprouts, uncooked | 1 cup | 105 | 37 | 6.9 | 4.0 | 0.2 | 0 | 0 | 0 | 0 | 5 |
| Beans: green, snap, fresh, frozen, cooked | 1 cup | 130 | 34 | 7.8 | 2.1 | 0.1 | 0 | 0 | 0.1 | 0 | 3 |

This information is current as of this printing. Check the manufacturer's label for updated analysis.
A dash (—) indicates that data are not available. Trace (tr) indicates that a very small amount of the constituent is present.
Abbreviations used in this table are: tbsp = tablespoon; tsp = teaspoon; oz = ounce; lb = pound; gm = gram; mg = milligrams; " = inches; Cal = calories; CHO = carbohydrate; Prot = protein; Sat Fat = saturated fat; Mono Fat = monounsaturated fat; Poly Fat = polyunsaturated fat; Chol = cholesterol; Na = Sodium.

## Nutrient Analysis of Common Foods (*continued*)

| *Food* | *Unit* | *Weight (g)* | *Cal* | *CHO (g)* | *Prot (g)* | *Fat (g)* | *Sat Fat (g)* | *Mono Fat (g)* | *Poly Fat (g)* | *Chol (mg)* | *Na (mg)* |
|---|---|---|---|---|---|---|---|---|---|---|---|
| Beans: green, snap, canned | 1 cup | 135 | 32 | 7.0 | 1.9 | 0.3 | 0 | 0 | 0 | 0 | 319 |
| Beans: green, snap, canned, low sodium | 1 cup | 135 | 30 | 6.5 | 2.0 | 0.1 | 0 | 0 | 0.1 | 0 | 3 |
| Beans: white, Great Northern, navy, cooked | 1 cup | 180 | 212 | 38.2 | 14.0 | 1.1 | 0.3 | 0.1 | 0.7 | 0 | 13 |
| Beans: yellow or wax, frozen, cooked | 1 cup | 125 | 28 | 5.8 | 1.8 | 0.3 | 0 | 0 | 0.3 | 0 | 4 |
| Beans: yellow or wax, canned | 1 cup | 135 | 32 | 7.0 | 1.9 | 0.4 | 0 | 0 | 0.4 | 0 | 319 |
| Beans: yellow or wax, canned, low sodium | 1 cup | 135 | 28 | 6.3 | 1.6 | 0.1 | 0 | 0 | 0.1 | 0 | |
| Beef: dried, chipped, uncooked | 1 oz | 28 | 58 | 0 | 9.7 | 1.8 | 0.8 | 0.8 | 0 | 26 | 1,219 |
| Beef: < 6% fat; flank, round (lean only) | 1 oz | 28 | 53 | 0 | 8.9 | 1.7 | 0.9 | 0.8 | 0.1 | 26 | 19 |
| Beef: 10% fat; chuck, filet mignon, New York strip, porterhouse, T-bone, tenderloin, ground round, choice grade (lean only) | 1 oz | 28 | 61 | 0 | 8.5 | 2.7 | 1.3 | 1.1 | 0.1 | 26 | 19 |
| Beef: 15% fat; club, rib eye roast (lean only) | 1 oz | 28 | 74 | 0 | 8.1 | 4.4 | 2.2 | 2.0 | 0.2 | 27 | 18 |
| Beef: 20% fat; ground chuck | 1 oz | 28 | 82 | 0 | 7.7 | 5.5 | 2.9 | 2.6 | 0.2 | 27 | 16 |
| Beef: 25% fat; ground beef (hamburger), chuck, steak, pot roast (lean and fat) | 1 oz | 28 | 93 | 0 | 7.4 | 6.8 | 3.4 | 3.1 | 0.3 | 27 | 16 |
| Beef: >30% fat; brisket, rib eye steak, standing rib roast, spareribs (lean and fat) | 1 oz | 28 | 110 | 0 | 6.5 | 9.1 | 4.8 | 4.4 | 0.3 | 27 | 15 |
| Beef: corned | 1 oz | 28 | 110 | 0 | 6.5 | 9.1 | 4.8 | 4.4 | 0.3 | 27 | 264 |
| Beef tongue: medium-fat, cooked, 3 × 2 × ⅛" | 1 slice | 20 | 49 | 0.1 | 4.3 | 3.3 | 1.8 | 2.0 | 0.1 | 18 | 12 |
| Beef: kidney, cooked, ½ × ½ × ¼" | 1 oz | 140 | 353 | 1.1 | 46.2 | 16.8 | 6.6 | 2.5 | 2.7 | 1,126 | 354 |
| Beef: liver | 1 oz | 28 | 40 | 1.5 | 5.7 | 1.1 | 0.4 | 0.2 | 0.2 | 86 | 39 |

| Food | Unit | Weight (g) | Cal | CHO (g) | Prot (g) | Fat (g) | Sat Fat (g) | Mono Fat (g) | Poly Fat (g) | Chol (mg) | Na (mg) |
|---|---|---|---|---|---|---|---|---|---|---|---|
| Beef tallow: suet | 1 tbsp | 14 | 120 | 0 | 0.2 | 13.2 | 6.8 | 5.9 | 0.6 | 11 | 0 |
| Beer: regular | 12 oz | 360 | 151 | 13.7 | 1.1 | 0 | 0 | 0 | 0 | 0 | 25 |
| Beets: red, canned, diced, sliced, or whole | 1 cup | 170 | 63 | 15.0 | 1.7 | 0.2 | 0 | 0 | 0.2 | 0 | 401 |
| Beets: red, canned, diced, sliced, or whole, low sodium | 1 cup | 170 | 63 | 14.8 | 1.5 | 0.2 | 0 | 0 | 0.2 | 0 | 78 |
| Biscuit: made with shortening | 1 whole | 28 | 103 | 12.8 | 2.1 | 4.8 | — | — | — | — | 175 |
| Blackberries: raw (also boysenberries, dewberries) | 1 cup | 144 | 84 | 18.6 | 1.7 | 1.3 | 0.3 | 0.3 | 0.7 | 0 | 1 |
| Bologna: 1 slice | 1 oz | 28 | 86 | 0.3 | 3.4 | 8.3 | 3.4 | 4.0 | 0.3 | 52 | 287 |
| Bouillon cube: all kinds (1 tsp instant bouillon) | 1 cube | 4 | 5 | 0.2 | 0.8 | 0.1 | 0.1 | 0 | 0 | 0 | 960 |
| Braunschweiger (liver sausage) | 1 oz | 28 | 90 | 0.7 | 4.2 | 9.2 | 3.1 | 4.4 | 1.2 | — | 287 |
| Bread: cracked wheat | 1 slice | 25 | 66 | 13.0 | 2.2 | 0.6 | 0.1 | 0.2 | 0.2 | 0 | 132 |
| Bread: English muffin | 1 whole | 57 | 133 | 25.5 | 4.4 | 1.4 | 0.4 | 0.6 | 0.4 | 0 | 263 |
| Bread: French, enriched, 2½ × 2 × ½" | 1 slice | 15 | 44 | 8.3 | 1.4 | 0.5 | 0.1 | 0.2 | 0.1 | 0 | 87 |
| Bread: pita, pocket | 1 large | 52 | 145 | 30.0 | 5.0 | 1.0 | 0.3 | 0.4 | 0.2 | 0 | 86 |
| Bread: pumpernickel (dark rye) | 1 slice | 32 | 79 | 17.0 | 2.9 | 0.4 | 0.1 | 0.2 | 0.1 | 0 | 182 |
| Bread: raisin | 1 slice | 25 | 66 | 13.4 | 1.7 | 0.7 | 0.1 | 0.3 | 0.2 | 0 | 91 |
| Bread: rye (light) | 1 slice | 25 | 61 | 13.0 | 2.3 | 0.3 | 0.1 | 0.2 | 0.1 | 0 | 139 |
| Bread: white, enriched | 1 slice | 25 | 68 | 12.6 | 2.2 | 0.8 | 0.2 | 0.4 | 0.2 | 0 | 127 |
| Bread: whole wheat, firm crumb | 1 slice | 25 | 61 | 11.9 | 2.6 | 0.8 | 0.1 | 0.3 | 0.2 | 0 | 132 |
| Bread: white, low sodium | 1 slice | 28 | 76 | 14.1 | 2.4 | 0.9 | 0.2 | 0.4 | 0.2 | 0 | 3 |
| Broccoli: medium stalk, fresh, cooked, and drained | 1 stalk | 180 | 47 | 8.1 | 5.6 | 0.5 | 0 | 0 | 0.5 | 0 | 18 |

## Nutrient Analysis of Common Foods (*continued*)

| *Food* | *Unit* | *Weight (g)* | *Cal* | *CHO (g)* | *Prot (g)* | *Fat (g)* | *Sat Fat (g)* | *Mono Fat (g)* | *Poly Fat (g)* | *Chol (mg)* | *Na (mg)* |
|---|---|---|---|---|---|---|---|---|---|---|---|
| Brussels sprouts: frozen, cooked, and drained | 1 cup | 155 | 51 | 10.1 | 5.0 | 0.3 | 0 | 0 | 0.3 | 0 | 22 |
| Butter: 1 pat | 1 tsp | 5 | 36 | 0 | 0 | 4.1 | 2.5 | 1.2 | 0.2 | 12 | 49 |
| Buttermilk: made from skim milk | 1 cup | 245 | 88 | 12.5 | 8.8 | 0.2 | 0.1 | 0.1 | 0 | 2 | 319 |
| Buttermilk: made from low-fat milk | 1 cup | 245 | 99 | 11.7 | 8.1 | 2.2 | 1.3 | 0.6 | 0.1 | 9 | 257 |
| Cabbage: common or Chinese; shredded, cooked, and drained | 1 cup | 145 | 29 | 6.2 | 1.6 | 0.3 | 0 | 0 | 0.3 | 0 | 20 |
| Cabbage: common or Chinese varieties, raw, shredded | 1 cup | 90 | 22 | 4.9 | 1.2 | 0.2 | 0 | 0 | 0.2 | 0 | 18 |
| Cake: angel food, 1/12 of 10" tube cake | 1 slice | 60 | 161 | 36.1 | 4.3 | 0.1 | 0.1 | 0 | 0.1 | 0 | 170 |
| Cake: coffee cake (mix), 2⅝ × 2¾ × 1¼" | 1 slice | 72 | 232 | 37.7 | 4.5 | 6.9 | 2.0 | 3.2 | 1.3 | 35 | 310 |
| Cake: cream cheese, without crust or topping | 1 slice | 85 | 368 | 25.7 | 7.6 | 26.8 | 6.0 | 6.0 | 1.0 | 163 | 173 |
| Cake: devil's food (frozen), ⅛ of 7½" cake | 1 slice | 85 | 323 | 47.3 | 3.7 | 15.0 | 7.7 | 5.4 | 0.7 | 37 | 357 |
| Cake: devil's food cupcake with icing (mix), 2½" diameter | 1 whole | 35 | 119 | 20.4 | 1.5 | 4.3 | 1.8 | 2.1 | 0.4 | 17 | 92 |
| Cake: gingerbread (mix), 2¾ × 2¾ × 1⅜" | 1 slice | 63 | 174 | 32.2 | 2.0 | 4.3 | 1.1 | 2.1 | 1.0 | 0.6 | 192 |
| Cake: marble with white icing (mix), 1/12 of layer cake | 1 slice | 87 | 288 | 53.9 | 3.8 | 7.6 | 4.8 | 2.1 | 0.7 | 40 | 225 |
| Cake: yellow with chocolate icing (mix), 1/12 of layer cake | 1 slice | 92 | 310 | 53.0 | 3.8 | 10.4 | 4.6 | 5.5 | 0.9 | 44 | 209 |
| Candy: candy corn, approximately 72 pieces | ¼ cup | 50 | 182 | 44.8 | 0 | 1.0 | 0.3 | 0.5 | 0.2 | 0 | 106 |
| Candy*: chocolate, bittersweet | 1 oz | 28 | 135 | 13.3 | 2.2 | 11.3 | 6.3 | 4.2 | 0.2 | 5 | 1 |
| Candy*: chocolate, sweet | 1 oz | 28 | 150 | 16.4 | 1.2 | 10.0 | 5.6 | 3.7 | 0.2 | 5 | 9 |

| Food | Unit | Weight (g) | Cal | CHO (g) | Prot (g) | Fat (g) | Sat Fat (g) | Mono Fat (g) | Poly Fat (g) | Chol (mg) | Na (mg) |
|---|---|---|---|---|---|---|---|---|---|---|---|
| Candy: chocolate covered mint, 1⅜ × ⅜" | 1 small | 11 | 45 | 8.9 | 0.2 | 1.2 | 0.4 | 0.7 | 0.1 | 0.6 | 20 |
| Candy: chocolate covered raisins | 1 cup | 190 | 808 | 134.0 | 10.3 | 32.5 | 18.1 | 11.8 | 0.7 | 19 | 122 |
| Candy: chocolate covered vanilla cream | 1 piece | 13 | 56 | 9.1 | 0.5 | 2.2 | 0.8 | 1.0 | 0.1 | 2 | 24 |
| Candy: fudge, plain, 1 cubic inch | 1 piece | 21 | 84 | 15.8 | 0.6 | 2.6 | 0.9 | 1.2 | 0.4 | 1 | 44 |
| Candy: gum drops, 1 large or 8 small | 1 large | 10 | 34 | 8.7 | 0 | 0.1 | 0 | 0 | 0.1 | 0 | 4 |
| Candy: jellybeans | 10 pieces | 28 | 104 | 26.4 | 0 | 0.1 | 0 | 0 | 0.5 | 0 | 3 |
| Candy: M&M's® type | ¼ cup | 49 | 230 | 35.8 | 2.6 | 9.7 | 5.4 | 3.5 | 0.2 | 3 | 36 |
| Candy: peanut brittle, 2½ × 2½ × ⅓" piece | 1 oz | 28 | 119 | 23.0 | 1.6 | 2.9 | 0.6 | 1.3 | 0.9 | 0 | 9 |
| Candy: chocolate-flavored roll (Tootsie Roll®) 1 × ½" | 1 piece | 7 | 28 | 5.8 | 0.2 | 0.6 | 0.2 | 0.3 | 0.1 | 1 | 14 |
| Candy bar*: chocolate coated almonds, or peanut bar (Mr. Goodbar®) | 1 oz | 28 | 161 | 11.2 | 3.5 | 12.4 | 2.1 | 8.2 | 1.6 | — | 17 |
| Candy bar*: chocolate coated with coconut center (Mound®) | 1 oz | 28 | 124 | 20.4 | 0.8 | 5.0 | 2.9 | 1.9 | 0 | 3 | 56 |
| Candy bar*: fudge, peanut, caramel (Oh! Henry®, Snickers®, Rally®, Baby Ruth®) | 1 oz | 28 | 130 | 16.6 | 2.7 | 6.5 | 1.8 | 3.5 | 1.0 | 3 | 36 |
| Candy bar*: Hershey Krackel® or Nestlé Crunch® | 1 oz | 28 | 144 | 15.0 | 2.3 | 8.3 | 4.4 | 3.1 | 0.6 | 3 | 35 |
| Candy bar*: milk chocolate bar or 7 chocolate kisses | 1 oz | 28 | 147 | 16.1 | 2.2 | 9.2 | 5.1 | 3.3 | 0.2 | 5 | 27 |
| Cantaloupe: 5" diameter | 1 whole | 91 | 159 | 39.8 | 3.7 | 0.5 | 0 | 0 | 0.5 | 0 | 64 |

*The weight of candy bars often changes. The analysis here is given for 1 ounce and can be calculated for the total unit (1 piece of candy).

## Nutrient Analysis of Common Foods (*continued*)

| *Food* | *Unit* | *Weight (g)* | *Cal* | *CHO (g)* | *Prot (g)* | *Fat (g)* | *Sat Fat (g)* | *Mono Fat (g)* | *Poly Fat (g)* | *Chol (mg)* | *Na (mg)* |
|---|---|---|---|---|---|---|---|---|---|---|---|
| Cantaloupe: cubed or diced, approximately 20/cup | 1 cup | 160 | 48 | 12.0 | 1.1 | 0.2 | 0 | 0 | 0.2 | 0 | 19 |
| Carbonated beverage: Coca-Cola® | 12 oz | 369 | 144 | 37.2 | 0 | 0 | 0 | 0 | 0 | 0 | 30 |
| Carbonated beverage: ginger ale | 12 oz | 366 | 108 | 28.8 | 0 | 0 | 0 | 0 | 0 | 0 | — |
| Carbonated beverage: Sprite® | 12 oz | 366 | 143 | 36.0 | 0 | 0 | 0 | 0 | 0 | 0 | 63 |
| Carbonated beverage: Sprite® without sugar | 12 oz | 366 | 5 | 0 | 0 | 0 | 0 | 0 | 0 | 0 | 63 |
| Carbonated beverage: Fresca® | 12 oz | 366 | 3 | 0 | 0 | 0 | 0 | 0 | 0 | 0 | 86 |
| Carbonated beverage: Tab® | 12 oz | 366 | 1 | 0.1 | 0 | 0 | 0 | 0 | 0 | 0 | 45 |
| Carrot: raw, approximately 1⅛ × 7½" | 1 whole | 81 | 30 | 7.0 | 0.8 | 0.1 | 0 | 0 | 0.1 | 0 | 34 |
| Carrots: fresh, cooked, sliced | 1 cup | 155 | 48 | 11.0 | 1.4 | 0.3 | 0 | 0 | 0.3 | 0 | 51 |
| Carrots: canned solids, sliced | 1 cup | 155 | 47 | 10.4 | 1.2 | 0.5 | 0 | 0 | 0.5 | 0 | 366 |
| Carrots: canned solids, sliced, low sodium | 1 cup | 155 | 39 | 8.7 | 1.2 | 0.2 | 0 | 0 | 0.2 | 0 | 60 |
| Cashew: roasted in oil, unsalted (14 large, 18 medium, or 26 small) | 1 oz | 28 | 159 | 8.3 | 4.9 | 12.8 | 2.6 | 7.3 | 2.1 | 0 | 4 |
| Catfish: freshwater, raw | 1 oz | 28 | 29 | 0 | 5.0 | 1.0 | 0.2 | 0.3 | 0.3 | — | 17 |
| Cauliflower: frozen, cooked, approximately 7 florets | 1 cup | 180 | 32 | 5.9 | 3.4 | 0.4 | 0 | 0 | 0.4 | 0 | 18 |
| Caviar: sturgeon, granular | 1 tbsp | 16 | 42 | 0.5 | 4.3 | 2.4 | 0.6 | 0.7 | 1.0 | 48 | 352 |
| Celery: green, raw, 8 × 1½" stalk | 1 stalk | 40 | 7 | 1.6 | 0.4 | 0 | 0 | 0 | 0 | 0 | 50 |
| Cereal: bran, unprocessed, 1.17 cup | 1 oz | 28 | 91 | 12.3 | 3.9 | 0.4 | 0.2 | 0.2 | 0.7 | 0 | 2 |
| Cereal: bran buds | 1 cup | 60 | 144 | 44.6 | 7.6 | 1.8 | 0.3 | 0.3 | 1.1 | 0 | 493 |
| Cereal: 40% bran flakes | 1 cup | 35 | 106 | 28.2 | 3.6 | 0.6 | 0.1 | 0.1 | 0.3 | 0 | 207 |

| Food | Unit | Weight (g) | Cal | CHO (g) | Prot (g) | Fat (g) | Sat Fat (g) | Mono Fat (g) | Poly Fat (g) | Chol (mg) | Na (mg) |
|---|---|---|---|---|---|---|---|---|---|---|---|
| Cereal: Cheerios® or puffed oats | 1 cup | 25 | 99 | 18.8 | 3.0 | 1.4 | 0.3 | 0.5 | 0.6 | 0 | 317 |
| Cereal: corn flakes | 1 cup | 25 | 97 | 21.3 | 2.0 | 0.1 | 0 | 0 | 0.1 | 0 | 251 |
| Cereal: corn grits, enriched, cooked without salt | 1 cup | 245 | 125 | 27.0 | 2.9 | 0.2 | 0 | 0 | 0.1 | 0 | 2 |
| Cereal: cream of rice, cooked without salt | 1 cup | 245 | 123 | 27.4 | 2.0 | 0 | 0 | 0 | 0 | 0 | 2 |
| Cereal: cream of wheat, cooked without salt | 1 cup | 240 | 180 | 40.6 | 5.3 | 1.0 | 0.2 | 0.1 | 0.5 | 0 | 2 |
| Cereal: farina, enriched, regular, cooked without salt | 1 cup | 245 | 103 | 21.3 | 3.2 | 0.5 | 0.1 | 0 | 0.2 | 0 | 4 |
| Cereal: farina, enriched, quick-cooking, cooked with salt | 1 cup | 245 | 105 | 21.8 | 3.2 | 0.5 | 0.1 | 0 | 0.2 | 0 | 466 |
| Cereal: farina, enriched, instant-cooking, cooked without salt | 1 cup | 245 | 135 | 27.9 | 4.2 | 0.5 | 0.1 | 0 | 0.2 | 0 | 13 |
| Cereal: granola, without coconut or other saturated fat | ¼ cup | 28 | 139 | 16.9 | 2.9 | 6.7 | 5.1 | 0 | 0.6 | 0 | 30 |
| Cereal: granola, cooked (¼ cup dry = ½ cup cooked) | ½ cup | 120 | 100 | 21.0 | 3.0 | 1.0 | 0.2 | 0.4 | 0.4 | 0 | 30 |
| Cereal: Grape-Nuts® | 1 cup | 110 | 430 | 92.8 | 11.0 | 0.7 | 0 | 0 | 0.7 | 0 | 814 |
| Cereal: oatmeal, cooked without salt | 1 cup | 240 | 132 | 23.3 | 4.8 | 2.4 | 0.4 | 0.8 | 1.0 | 0 | 2 |
| Cereal: puffed rice | 1 cup | 15 | 60 | 13.4 | 0.9 | 0.1 | 0 | 0 | 0.1 | 0 | 0 |
| Cereal: puffed wheat | 1 cup | 15 | 54 | 11.8 | 2.3 | 0.2 | 0 | 0 | 0.2 | 0 | 1 |
| Cereal: raisin bran | 1 cup | 50 | 144 | 39.7 | 4.2 | 0.7 | 0.1 | 0.1 | 0.4 | 0 | 212 |
| Cereal: Rice Krispies® | 1 cup | 30 | 117 | 26.3 | 1.8 | 0.1 | 0 | 0 | 0.1 | 0 | 283 |
| Cereal: Spoon Size Shredded Wheat®, approximately 50 biscuits per cup | 1 cup | 50 | 180 | 40.0 | 5.0 | 1.3 | 0.2 | 0.2 | 0.7 | 0 | 2 |

## Nutrient Analysis of Common Foods (*continued*)

| *Food* | *Unit* | *Weight (g)* | *Cal* | *CHO (g)* | *Prot (g)* | *Fat (g)* | *Sat Fat (g)* | *Mono Fat (g)* | *Poly Fat (g)* | *Chol (mg)* | *Na (mg)* |
|---|---|---|---|---|---|---|---|---|---|---|---|
| Cereal: Shredded Wheat® biscuit, 3¾ × 2¼ × 1" | 1 whole | 25 | 90 | 20.0 | 2.5 | 0.6 | 0.1 | 0.1 | 0.3 | 0 | 1 |
| Cereal: sugar-coated corn flakes | 1 cup | 40 | 154 | 36.5 | 1.8 | 0.1 | 0 | 0 | 0.1 | 0 | 267 |
| Cereal: Wheat Chex® | ⅓ cup | 28 | 110 | 23.0 | 2.0 | 1.0 | 0.9 | 0.1 | 0 | 0 | 198 |
| Cereal: wheat germ | 1 tbsp | 6 | 23 | 3.0 | 1.8 | 0.7 | 0.1 | 0.1 | 0.4 | 0 | 1 |
| Cereal: Wheaties® or Total® | 1 cup | 30 | 104 | 24.2 | 3.1 | 0.7 | 0.1 | 0.1 | 0.4 | 0 | 310 |
| Cheese: American | 1 oz | 28 | 106 | 0.5 | 6.3 | 8.9 | 5.6 | 2.5 | 0.3 | 27 | 406 |
| Cheese: blue | 1 oz | 28 | 100 | 0.7 | 6.1 | 8.2 | 5.3 | 2.2 | 0.2 | 21 | 396 |
| Cheese: brick | 1 oz | 28 | 105 | 0.8 | 6.6 | 8.4 | 5.3 | 2.4 | 0.2 | 27 | 159 |
| Cheese: brie | 1 oz | 28 | 95 | 0.1 | 5.9 | 7.9 | — | — | — | 28 | 178 |
| Cheese: camembert | 1 oz | 28 | 85 | 0.1 | 5.6 | 6.9 | 4.3 | 2.0 | 0.2 | 20 | 239 |
| Cheese: cheddar | 1 oz | 28 | 114 | 0.4 | 7.1 | 9.4 | 6.0 | 2.7 | 0.3 | 30 | 176 |
| Cheese: colby | 1 oz | 28 | 112 | 0.4 | 6.7 | 9.1 | 5.7 | 2.6 | 0.3 | 27 | 171 |
| Cheese: cottage, creamed (4% fat) | ¼ cup | 53 | 54 | 1.4 | 6.6 | 2.4 | 1.5 | 0.7 | 0.1 | 8 | 212 |
| Cheese: cottage, low-fat (2% fat) | ¼ cup | 57 | 51 | 2.1 | 7.8 | 1.1 | 0.7 | 0.3 | 0 | 5 | 230 |
| Cheese: cottage, dry curd | ¼ cup | 36 | 31 | 0.7 | 6.3 | 0.2 | 0.1 | 0 | 0 | 3 | 5 |
| Cheese: cream cheese, 2 tbsp | 1 oz | 28 | 99 | 0.8 | 2.1 | 9.9 | 6.2 | 2.8 | 0.4 | 31 | 84 |
| Cheese: edam | 1 oz | 28 | 101 | 0.4 | 7.1 | 7.9 | 5.0 | 2.3 | 0.2 | 25 | 274 |
| Cheese: feta | 1 oz | 28 | 75 | 1.2 | 4.0 | 6.0 | 4.2 | 1.3 | 0.2 | 25 | 316 |
| Cheese: gouda | 1 oz | 28 | 101 | 0.6 | 7.1 | 7.8 | 5.0 | 2.2 | 0.2 | 32 | 232 |
| Cheese: gruyère | 1 oz | 28 | 117 | 0.1 | 8.5 | 9.2 | 5.4 | 2.9 | 0.5 | 31 | 95 |
| Cheese: monterey | 1 oz | 28 | 106 | 0.2 | 6.9 | 8.6 | — | — | — | — | 152 |

| Food | Unit | Weight (g) | Cal | CHO (g) | Prot (g) | Fat (g) | Sat Fat (g) | Mono Fat (g) | Poly Fat (g) | Chol (mg) | Na (mg) |
|---|---|---|---|---|---|---|---|---|---|---|---|
| Cheese: mozzarella, part-skim, low-moisture | 1 oz | 28 | 79 | 0.9 | 7.8 | 4.9 | 3.1 | 1.4 | 0.1 | 15 | 150 |
| Cheese: mozzarella, whole milk | 1 oz | 28 | 80 | 0.6 | 5.5 | 6.1 | 3.7 | 1.9 | 0.2 | 22 | 106 |
| Cheese: muenster | 1 oz | 28 | 104 | 0.3 | 6.6 | 8.5 | 5.4 | 2.5 | 0.2 | 27 | 178 |
| Cheese: neufchatel | 1 oz | 28 | 74 | 0.8 | 2.8 | 6.6 | 4.2 | 1.9 | 0.2 | 22 | 113 |
| Cheese: parmesan, grated | 1 tbsp | 5 | 23 | 0.2 | 2.1 | 1.5 | 1.0 | 0.4 | 0 | 4 | 93 |
| Cheese: provolone | 1 oz | 28 | 100 | 0.6 | 7.3 | 7.6 | 4.8 | 2.1 | 0.2 | 20 | 248 |
| Cheese: ricotta, whole milk (13% fat) | ¼ cup | 62 | 108 | 1.9 | 7.0 | 8.1 | 5.2 | 2.3 | 0.2 | 32 | 52 |
| Cheese: ricotta, part skim milk (8% fat) | ¼ cup | 62 | 86 | 3.2 | 7.1 | 4.9 | 3.1 | 1.4 | 0.2 | 19 | 77 |
| Cheese: romano | 1 oz | 28 | 110 | 1.0 | 9.0 | 7.6 | — | — | — | 29 | 340 |
| Cheese: roquefort | 1 oz | 28 | 105 | 0.6 | 6.1 | 8.7 | 5.5 | 2.4 | 0.4 | 26 | 513 |
| Cheese: Swiss | 1 oz | 28 | 95 | 0.6 | 7.0 | 7.1 | 4.6 | 2.0 | 0.2 | 24 | 388 |
| Cheese: Velveeta® (cheese spread) | 1 oz | 28 | 82 | 2.5 | 4.7 | 6.0 | 3.8 | 1.8 | 0.2 | 16 | 381 |
| Cheese: 1% butterfat (Countdown®) | 1 oz | 28 | 40 | 3.6 | 6.6 | 0.3 | 0.2 | 0.1 | 0 | 1 | 409 |
| Cheese: 4–8% butterfat, processed (Breeze®, Chef's Delight®, Country Club®, Mellow Age®, Tasty®, Lite-Line®, low-fat DI-ET®) | 1 oz | 28 | 50 | 2.8 | 5.8 | 1.7 | 1.1 | 0.5 | 0 | 10 | 428 |
| Cheese: 5% butterfat, natural (St. Otho) | 1 oz | 28 | 49 | 3.1 | 9.1 | 1.1 | 0.8 | 0.3 | 0 | 10 | — |
| Cheese: 19–32% polyunsaturated fat (Golden®, Image®, Cheez-ola®, Dorman®, Nutrend®, Scandic®, Unique®) | 1 oz | 28 | 98 | 1.1 | 6.2 | 7.5 | 1.5 | 1.4 | 4.1 | 4 | 330 |
| Cheese: 23% polyunsaturated fat, low sodium (Cheez-ola®) | 1 oz | 28 | 90 | 0.6 | 6.8 | 6.3 | 0.8 | 1.5 | 3.6 | 1 | 156 |

## Nutrient Analysis of Common Foods (*continued*)

| *Food* | *Unit* | *Weight (g)* | *Cal* | *CHO (g)* | *Prot (g)* | *Fat (g)* | *Sat Fat (g)* | *Mono Fat (g)* | *Poly Fat (g)* | *Chol (mg)* | *Na (mg)* |
|---|---|---|---|---|---|---|---|---|---|---|---|
| Cherries: raw, sweet, unpitted | 10 whole | 75 | 47 | 11.7 | 0.9 | 0.2 | 0 | 0 | 0.2 | 0 | 1 |
| Cherries: canned, sweet, syrup-packed, pitted | 1 cup | 257 | 208 | 52.7 | 2.3 | 0.5 | 0 | 0 | 0.5 | 0 | 3 |
| Chicken: gizzard, all classes, cooked, chopped | 1 cup | 145 | 215 | 1.0 | 39.2 | 4.8 | 1.4 | 1.8 | 1.2 | 283 | 83 |
| Chicken: light meat, no skin | 1 oz | 28 | 51 | 0 | 9.2 | 1.4 | 0.4 | 0.7 | 0.3 | 22 | 18 |
| Chicken: dark meat, no skin | 1 oz | 28 | 52 | 0 | 8.3 | 1.8 | 0.5 | 0.6 | 0.4 | 26 | 24 |
| Chicken: dark and light meat, with skin | 1 oz | 28 | 70 | 0 | 7.7 | 4.2 | 1.2 | 1.4 | 1.0 | 25 | — |
| Chicken fat | 1 tbsp | 14 | 126 | 0 | 0 | 14.0 | 4.6 | 6.4 | 2.5 | 9 | 0 |
| Chicken liver: cooked, whole, 2 × 2 × ⅝" | 1 liver | 25 | 41 | 0.2 | 6.6 | 1.1 | 0.4 | 0.3 | 0.2 | 158 | 13 |
| Chick-peas: see *Beans* | | | | | | | | | | | |
| Chocolate: bitter or baking | 1 oz | 28 | 143 | 8.2 | 3.0 | 15.0 | 8.4 | 5.6 | 0.3 | 0 | 1 |
| Chocolate syrup (or topping): fudge type | 2 tbsp | 38 | 124 | 20.3 | 1.9 | 5.1 | 2.6 | 1.9 | 0.2 | 0 | 33 |
| Clams: canned solids (chopped or minced) | 1 cup | 160 | 143 | 3.0 | 25.3 | 2.4 | 0.7 | 0.4 | 0.9 | 101 | 192 |
| Cocoa: dry powder, medium fat, plain | 1 tbsp | 5 | 14 | 2.8 | 0.9 | 1.0 | 0.6 | 0.4 | 0 | 0 | tr |
| Cocoa mix: 1 oz package | 1 pkg | 28 | 102 | 20.1 | 5.3 | 0.8 | 0.6 | 0.3 | 0 | 2 | 149 |
| Coconut: shredded, fresh, meat only | 1 cup | 80 | 277 | 7.5 | 2.8 | 28.2 | 25.0 | 1.7 | 0.5 | 0 | 18 |
| Cookie: commercial, chocolate chip, 2¼ × ⅜" | 1 cookie | 11 | 50 | 7.3 | 0.6 | 2.2 | 0.7 | 0.8 | 0.5 | 5 | 42 |
| Cookie: commercial, fig bar, 1⅝ × 1⅝" | 1 cookie | 14 | 50 | 10.6 | 0.6 | 0.8 | 0.2 | 0.4 | 0.2 | 0 | 35 |
| Cookie: commercial, gingersnap, 2 × ¼" | 1 cookie | 7 | 29 | 5.6 | 0.4 | 0.6 | 0.2 | 0.3 | 0.1 | 0 | 40 |
| Cookie: commercial, macaroon, 2¾ × ¼" | 1 cookie | 19 | 91 | 12.5 | 1.0 | 4.4 | 1.9 | 0.2 | 0.1 | 0 | 7 |
| Cookie: commercial, marshmallow, chocolate-coated, 1¾ × ¾" | 1 cookie | 13 | 53 | 9.4 | 0.5 | 1.7 | 0.9 | 0.9 | 0 | 4 | 27 |

| Food | Unit | Weight (g) | Cal | CHO (g) | Prot (g) | Fat (g) | Sat Fat (g) | Mono Fat (g) | Poly Fat (g) | Chol (mg) | Na (mg) |
|---|---|---|---|---|---|---|---|---|---|---|---|
| Cookie: commercial, oatmeal with raisins, 2⅝ × ¼" | 1 cookie | 13 | 59 | 9.6 | 0.8 | 2.0 | 0.5 | 1.0 | 0.5 | 4 | 21 |
| Cookie: commercial, peanut butter sandwich, 1¾ × ½" | 1 cookie | 12 | 58 | 8.2 | 1.2 | 2.4 | 0.6 | 1.2 | 0.6 | 5 | 21 |
| Cookie: commercial, sandwich, round, 1¾ × ⅜" | 1 cookie | 10 | 50 | 6.9 | 0.5 | 2.3 | 0.6 | 1.1 | 0.5 | 5 | 48 |
| Cookie: commercial, vanilla wafer, 1¾ × ¼" | 1 wafer | 4 | 19 | 2.9 | 0.2 | 0.6 | 0.2 | 0.3 | 0.2 | 1 | 10 |
| Cookie: prepared mix, brownies, 1¾ × 1¾ × ⅞" | 1 piece | 20 | 86 | 12.6 | 1.0 | 4.0 | 0.8 | 1.5 | 1.3 | 17 | 33 |
| Cordial: apricot brandy, benedictine, anisette, crème de menthe, or curaçao | 4 tsp | 20 | 66 | 6.3 | 0 | 0 | 0 | 0 | 0 | 0 | 0 |
| Corn: canned, whole kernel | 1 cup | 165 | 139 | 32.7 | 4.3 | 1.3 | 0.4 | 0.1 | 0.7 | 0 | 389 |
| Corn: canned, whole kernel, low sodium | 1 cup | 165 | 152 | 29.7 | 4.1 | 1.2 | 0.4 | 0.1 | 0.7 | 0 | 3 |
| Corn: canned, cream style, low sodium | 1 cup | 256 | 210 | 47.4 | 6.7 | 2.8 | 0.8 | 0.3 | 1.7 | 0 | 5 |
| Corn chips: 1½ oz package = 1¼ cups or 60 chips | 1¼ cup | 43 | 239 | 22.7 | 2.9 | 15.8 | 3.8 | 7.9 | 3.8 | 0 | 240 |
| Cornmeal: white and yellow, enriched, degermed | 1 cup | 138 | 502 | 108.2 | 10.9 | 1.7 | 0.5 | 0.2 | 1.0 | 0 | 1 |
| Corned beef: see *Beef* | | | | | | | | | | | |
| Cornstarch: not packed | 1 tbsp | 8 | 29 | 7.0 | 0 | 0 | 0 | 0 | 0 | 0 | tr |
| Cottage cheese: see *Cheese* | | | | | | | | | | | |
| Crab: fresh, cooked, not packed | 1 cup | 125 | 106 | 0.6 | 21.6 | 1.3 | 0.2 | 0.2 | 0.4 | 125 | 263 |
| Crab: canned solids, packed | 1 cup | 160 | 149 | 1.8 | 27.8 | 2.6 | 0.4 | 0.5 | 0.9 | 162 | 1,600 |
| Crackers: animal | 10 whole | 26 | 112 | 20.8 | 1.7 | 2.4 | 0.6 | 1.2 | 0.5 | 16 | 79 |

# Nutrient Analysis of Common Foods (*continued*)

| *Food* | *Unit* | *Weight (g)* | *Cal* | *CHO (g)* | *Prot (g)* | *Fat (g)* | *Sat Fat (g)* | *Mono Fat (g)* | *Poly Fat (g)* | *Chol (mg)* | *Na (mg)* |
|---|---|---|---|---|---|---|---|---|---|---|---|
| Cracker: graham, chocolate-coated, 2½ × 2 × ¼" | 1 whole | 13 | 62 | 8.8 | 0.7 | 3.1 | 0.9 | 1.9 | 0.2 | 7 | 53 |
| Crackers: graham, sugar honey, 2 squares, 2½" each | 2 whole | 14 | 58 | 10.8 | 1.0 | 1.6 | 0.4 | 0.8 | 0.4 | 1 | 72 |
| Cracker: matzo | 1 whole | 30 | 118 | 26.1 | 3.2 | 0.3 | 0 | 0 | 0.1 | 0 | 10 |
| Crackers: melba toast | 3 whole | 12 | 60 | 9.0 | 2.0 | 2.0 | 0.8 | 0.9 | 0.2 | 0.6 | 2 |
| Crackers: melba toast, low sodium | 3 whole | 12 | 60 | 9.0 | 2.0 | 2.0 | 0.8 | 0.9 | 0.2 | 0.6 | 1 |
| Crackers: saltines, single crackers | 4 whole | 11 | 48 | 8.0 | 1.0 | 1.3 | 0.3 | 0.6 | 0.3 | 1 | 123 |
| Crackers: sandwich, cheese and peanut butter (1 oz pack) | 4 whole | 28 | 139 | 15.9 | 4.3 | 6.8 | 1.8 | 3.1 | 1.6 | 6 | 281 |
| Crackers: Triscuit® | 1 whole | 4 | 21 | 3.0 | 0.4 | 0.8 | 0.4 | 0.4 | 0.1 | 0 | 20 |
| Cranberries: raw, chopped | 1 cup | 110 | 51 | 11.9 | 0.4 | 0.8 | 0 | 0 | 0.8 | 0 | 2 |
| Cranberry juice: cocktail, sweetened | 1 cup | 253 | 164 | 41.7 | 0.3 | 0.3 | 0 | 0 | 0.3 | 0 | 3 |
| Cranberry sauce: sweetened, canned | 1 cup | 277 | 404 | 103.9 | 0.3 | 0.6 | 0 | 0 | 0.6 | 0 | 3 |
| Cream: fluid, half and half (11.7% fat) | 1 tbsp | 15 | 20 | 0.7 | 0.5 | 1.7 | 1.1 | 0.5 | 0.1 | 6 | 6 |
| Cream: fluid, light (20.6% fat) | 1 tbsp | 15 | 29 | 0.6 | 0.4 | 2.9 | 1.8 | 0.8 | 0.1 | 10 | 6 |
| Cream: fluid, light, whipping (31.3% fat), approximately 2 cups whipped | 1 cup | 239 | 699 | 7.1 | 5.2 | 73.9 | 46.2 | 21.7 | 2.1 | 265 | 82 |
| Cream: fluid, heavy or whipping (37.6% fat), approximately 2 cups whipped | 1 cup | 238 | 821 | 6.6 | 4.9 | 88.1 | 54.8 | 25.4 | 3.3 | 326 | 89 |
| Cream: sour | 1 tbsp | 14 | 31 | 0.6 | 0.5 | 3.0 | 1.9 | 0.9 | 0.1 | 6 | 8 |
| Cream: sour, imitation (IMO®, Wonder®) | 1 tbsp | 15 | 26 | 0.7 | 0.5 | 2.4 | 2.0 | 0.3 | 0.1 | 1 | 7 |

| Food | Unit | Weight (g) | Cal | CHO (g) | Prot (g) | Fat (g) | Sat Fat (g) | Mono Fat (g) | Poly Fat (g) | Chol (mg) | Na (mg) |
|---|---|---|---|---|---|---|---|---|---|---|---|
| Creamer: nondairy, powder, containing saturated fat (Cremora® and Coffee-mate®) | 1 tbsp | 6 | 33 | 3.3 | 0.3 | 2.1 | 2.1 | 0 | 0 | 0 | 12 |
| Creamer: nondairy, liquid, containing saturated fat (Coffee Rich®) | 1 tbsp | 15 | 20 | 1.7 | 0.2 | 1.5 | 1.4 | 0 | 0 | 0 | 12 |
| Creamer: nondairy, liquid, containing polyunsaturated fat (Poly Perx® and Mocha Mix®) | 1 tbsp | 15 | 20 | 1.8 | 0.1 | 1.5 | 0.2 | 0.7 | 0.6 | 0 | 1 |
| Cucumbers: raw, pared, whole, 2⅛ × 8¼" | 1 whole | 280 | 39 | 9.0 | 1.7 | 0.3 | 0 | 0 | 0.3 | 0 | 17 |
| Dates: hydrated, without pits | 10 whole | 80 | 219 | 58.3 | 1.8 | 0.4 | 0 | 0 | 0.4 | 0 | 1 |
| Dessert topping: frozen, semisolid (Cool Whip®) | 1 tbsp | 4 | 13 | 0.9 | 0.1 | 1.0 | 0.9 | 0.1 | 0 | 0 | 1 |
| Dessert topping: nondairy, pressurized | 1 tbsp | 4 | 11 | 0.6 | 0 | 0.9 | 0.8 | 0.1 | 0 | 0 | 2 |
| Doughnut: cake type, plain, 1½ × ¾" | 1 whole | 14 | 55 | 7.2 | 0.6 | 2.6 | 0.7 | 1.3 | 0.5 | 7 | 70 |
| Doughnut: yeast leavened, plain, 3¾ × 1¼" | 1 whole | 42 | 176 | 16.0 | 2.7 | 11.3 | 2.8 | 5.6 | 2.5 | 12 | 99 |
| Duck: flesh only, raw, domesticated | 1 oz | 28 | 47 | 0 | 6.1 | 2.3 | 0.5 | 1.1 | 0.3 | — | 21 |
| Duck: flesh and skin, raw, domesticated | 1 oz | 28 | 92 | 0 | 4.5 | 8.1 | 1.9 | 4.1 | 0.9 | — | 21 |
| Eclair: custard filling with chocolate, 5 × 2 × 1¾" | 1 whole | 100 | 239 | 23.2 | 6.2 | 13.6 | 4.4 | 6.2 | 2.1 | 145 | 82 |
| Egg: chicken, fresh, medium | 1 whole | 50 | 79 | 0.6 | 6.1 | 5.6 | 1.7 | 2.2 | 0.7 | 274 | 69 |
| Egg: chicken, white, fresh | 1 white | 33 | 16 | 0.4 | 3.4 | tr | 0 | 0 | 0 | 0 | 50 |
| Egg: chicken, yolk, fresh | 1 yolk | 17 | 63 | 0 | 2.8 | 5.6 | 1.7 | 2.2 | 0.7 | 272 | 8 |
| Eggnog: commercial | 1 cup | 254 | 342 | 34.4 | 9.7 | 19.0 | 11.3 | 5.7 | 0.9 | 149 | 138 |

## Nutrient Analysis of Common Foods (*continued*)

| *Food* | *Unit* | *Weight (g)* | *Cal* | *CHO (g)* | *Prot (g)* | *Fat (g)* | *Sat Fat (g)* | *Mono Fat (g)* | *Poly Fat (g)* | *Chol (mg)* | *Na (mg)* |
|---|---|---|---|---|---|---|---|---|---|---|---|
| Egg substitute: Egg Beaters®, 1 egg equivalent | ¼ cup | 60 | 40 | 3.0 | 7.0 | 0 | 0 | 0 | 0 | 0 | 130 |
| Egg substitute: Second Nature®, 1 egg equivalent | 3 tbsp | 47 | 35 | 0.5 | 4.7 | 1.6 | 0.3 | 0.6 | 0.8 | 0 | 79 |
| Egg substitute: Lucern®, 1 egg equivalent | ¼ cup | 60 | 50 | 2.0 | 6.0 | 2.0 | — | — | — | tr | — |
| Eggplant: cooked, diced | 1 cup | 200 | 38 | 8.2 | 2.0 | 0.4 | 0 | 0 | 0.4 | 0 | 2 |
| English muffin: see *Bread* | | | | | | | | | | | |
| Fig: raw, whole, 1½" diameter | 1 small | 40 | 32 | 8.1 | 0.5 | 0.1 | 0 | 0 | 0.1 | 0 | 1 |
| Fish: see *Catfish, Haddock, Halibut, Herring, Snapper, Flounder, Sole* | | | | | | | | | | | |
| Fish sticks: breaded, cooked, frozen, 4 × 1 × ½" | 1 oz | 28 | 50 | 1.0 | 4.7 | 2.5 | 0.7 | 1.0 | 0.7 | 17 | 20 |
| Flounder: raw | 1 oz | 28 | 22 | 0 | 4.7 | 0.2 | 0 | 0 | 0.1 | 14 | 22 |
| Flour: white, all purpose, enriched, unsifted | 1 cup | 125 | 455 | 95.1 | 13.1 | 1.3 | 0.3 | 0.1 | 0.8 | 0 | 3 |
| Flour: white, self-rising, enriched, unsifted | 1 cup | 125 | 440 | 92.8 | 11.6 | 1.3 | 0.4 | 0.1 | 0.8 | 0 | 1,349 |
| Flour: whole wheat | 1 cup | 120 | 400 | 85.2 | 16.0 | 2.4 | 0.7 | 0.2 | 1.4 | 0 | 4 |
| Frankfurter: 5 × ¾" | 1 whole | 45 | 139 | 0.8 | 5.6 | 12.4 | 4.7 | 5.9 | 0.8 | 27 | 495 |
| Frosting mix: prepared | 1 tbsp | 15 | 61 | 13.2 | 0.3 | 1.5 | 0.4 | 0.8 | 0.1 | 0 | 9 |
| Frosting: ready to spread (with animal or vegetable shortening) | 1 tbsp | 15 | 55 | 10.8 | 0.1 | 1.6 | 0.5 | 0.9 | 0.2 | 0 | 9 |
| Fruit cocktail: canned, solids and liquid, water-packed | 1 cup | 245 | 91 | 23.8 | 1.0 | 0.2 | 0 | 0 | 0.2 | 0 | 12 |

| Food | Unit | Weight (g) | Cal | CHO (g) | Prot (g) | Fat (g) | Sat Fat (g) | Mono Fat (g) | Poly Fat (g) | Chol (mg) | Na (mg) |
|---|---|---|---|---|---|---|---|---|---|---|---|
| Garbanzos: see *Beans* | | | | | | | | | | | |
| Gelatin: dry, unflavored, 1 envelope | 1 pkg | 7 | 23 | 0 | 6.0 | 0 | 0 | 0 | 0 | 0 | 0 |
| Gelatin: sweetened dessert powder (Jell-O®), prepared with water, plain | ½ cup | 120 | 71 | 16.9 | 1.8 | 0 | 0 | 0 | 0 | 0 | 61 |
| Gelatin: low calorie, prepared with water | ½ cup | 120 | 8 | 0 | 2.0 | 0 | 0 | 0 | 0 | 0 | 8 |
| Gin: see *Liquor* | | | | | | | | | | | |
| Gizzard: chicken, all classes, cooked, chopped | ¼ cup | 36 | 54 | 0.3 | 9.8 | 1.2 | 0.4 | 0.5 | 0.3 | 71 | 21 |
| Goose: flesh only, raw | 1 oz | 28 | 45 | 0 | 6.3 | 2.0 | 0.5 | 0.9 | 0.2 | — | 24 |
| Grapes: raw, seedless (Thompson) | 10 grapes | 50 | 34 | 8.7 | 0.3 | 0.2 | 0 | 0 | 0.2 | 0 | 2 |
| Grape juice: frozen concentrate, sweetened, diluted | 1 cup | 250 | 133 | 33.3 | 0.5 | 0 | 0 | 0 | 0 | 0 | 3 |
| Grapefruit: all varieties | 1 whole | 400 | 80 | 20.8 | 1.0 | 0.2 | 0 | 0 | 0.2 | 0 | 2 |
| Grapefruit juice: unsweetened, frozen concentrate, diluted | 1 cup | 247 | 101 | 24.2 | 1.2 | 0.2 | 0 | 0 | 0.2 | 0 | 2 |
| Greens, collard: frozen, cooked | 1 cup | 170 | 51 | 9.5 | 4.9 | 0.7 | 0 | 0 | 0.7 | 0 | 27 |
| Haddock: raw | 1 oz | 28 | 29 | 0 | 6.6 | 0.1 | 0 | 0 | 0.1 | 17 | 17 |
| Halibut: Atlantic or Pacific, broiled | 1oz | 28 | 28 | 0 | 5.9 | 0.3 | 0.1 | 0 | 0.1 | 14 | 15 |
| Ham: see *Pork* | | | | | | | | | | | |
| Hamburger: see *Beef* | | | | | | | | | | | |
| Herring: canned, solids and liquid, plain | 1 oz | 28 | 59 | 0 | 5.6 | 3.1 | 0.7 | 1.6 | 0.5 | 24 | — |
| Honey: strained | 1 tbsp | 21 | 64 | 17.3 | 0.1 | 0 | 0 | 0 | 0 | 0 | 1 |
| Honeydew: 7 × 2" wedge, 1/10 of melon | 1 slice | 226 | 49 | 11.5 | 1.2 | 0.4 | 0 | 0 | 0.4 | 0 | 18 |
| Horseradish: prepared | 1 tbsp | 15 | 6 | 1.4 | 0.2 | 0 | 0 | 0 | 0 | 0 | 14 |

## Nutrient Analysis of Common Foods (*continued*)

| *Food* | *Unit* | *Weight (g)* | *Cal* | *CHO (g)* | *Prot (g)* | *Fat (g)* | *Sat Fat (g)* | *Mono Fat (g)* | *Poly Fat (g)* | *Chol (mg)* | *Na (mg)* |
|---|---|---|---|---|---|---|---|---|---|---|---|
| Ice cream: rich, approximately 16% fat, hardened | 1 cup | 148 | 349 | 32.0 | 4.1 | 23.7 | 14.7 | 6.8 | 0.9 | 88 | 108 |
| Ice cream: regular, approximately 10% fat, hardened | 1cup | 133 | 269 | 31.7 | 4.8 | 14.3 | 8.9 | 4.1 | 0.5 | 59 | 116 |
| Ice cream bar: chocolate-covered (Eskimo Pie) | 1 bar | 85 | 270 | 22.0 | 2.9 | 19.1 | 14.7 | 2.8 | 0.5 | 35 | — |
| Ice cream sandwich: 3 oz size | 1 whole | 85 | 238 | 35.8 | 4.3 | 8.5 | 4.0 | 2.2 | 0.4 | 34 | — |
| Ice cream cone | 1 cone | 3 | 11 | 2.3 | 0.3 | 0.1 | 0 | 0.1 | 0 | 0 | 1 |
| Ice milk: 5.1% fat, soft serve | 1 cup | 175 | 223 | 38.4 | 8.0 | 4.6 | 2.9 | 1.3 | 0.2 | 13 | 163 |
| Ice milk: 5.1% fat, hardened | 1 cup | 131 | 184 | 29.0 | 5.2 | 5.6 | 3.5 | 1.6 | 0.2 | 18 | 105 |
| Instant breakfast: dry powder, all flavors except eggnog | 1¼ oz | 36 | 130 | 23.4 | 7.2 | 0.9 | 0.5 | 0.3 | 0.1 | 4 | tr |
| Jelly: sweetened | 1 tbsp | 18 | 49 | 12.7 | 0 | 0 | 0 | 0 | 0 | 0 | 3 |
| Knockwurst link: 4 × 1⅛" | 1 link | 68 | 165 | 1.5 | 9.6 | 18.5 | 6.8 | 8.8 | 1.8 | 42 | 748 |
| Ladyfingers | 1 whole | 11 | 40 | 7.1 | 0.9 | 0.9 | 0.3 | 0.4 | 0.1 | 39 | 8 |
| Lamb: < 7% fat, chop, leg, roast, sirloin chop (lean only) | 1 oz | 28 | 53 | 0 | 8.2 | 2.0 | 0.9 | 0.8 | 0.1 | 28 | 15 |
| Lamb: 10% fat, shank, shoulder (lean only) | 1 oz | 28 | 58 | 0 | 7.6 | 2.8 | 1.4 | 1.2 | 0.2 | 28 | 15 |
| Lamb: 20% fat, leg, roast, sirloin chop (lean and fat) | 1 oz | 28 | 79 | 0 | 7.2 | 5.4 | 2.8 | 2.4 | 0.4 | 28 | 14 |
| Lamb: 30% fat, breast, chop, rib (lean and fat) | 1 oz | 28 | 96 | 0 | 6.2 | 7.7 | 3.6 | 3.1 | 0.4 | 28 | 14 |
| Lard | 1 tbsp | 13 | 117 | 0 | 0 | 12.8 | 5.1 | 5.7 | 1.5 | 12 | 0 |
| Lemon: raw, 1 wedge (⅛ of 2⅛" lemon) | 1 slice | 18 | 3 | 1.0 | 0.1 | 0 | 0 | 0 | 0 | 0 | 0 |

| *Food* | *Unit* | *Weight (g)* | *Cal* | *CHO (g)* | *Prot (g)* | *Fat (g)* | *Sat Fat (g)* | *Mono Fat (g)* | *Poly Fat (g)* | *Chol (mg)* | *Na (mg)* |
|---|---|---|---|---|---|---|---|---|---|---|---|
| Lemon juice: canned, unsweetened | 1 tbsp | 15 | 4 | 1.2 | 0.1 | tr | 0 | 0 | tr | 0 | tr |
| Lemonade: concentrate, frozen, diluted | 1 cup | 248 | 88 | 22.9 | 0.2 | 0 | 0 | 0 | 0 | 0 | 0 |
| Lentils: see *Beans* | | | | | | | | | | | |
| Lettuce: raw, crisp head varieties, chopped or shredded | 1 cup | 55 | 7 | 1.6 | 0.5 | 0.1 | 0 | 0 | 0.1 | 0 | 5 |
| Liquor: gin, rum, vodka, whiskey | 1 oz | 28 | 70 | 0 | 0 | 0 | 0 | 0 | 0 | 0 | 0 |
| Liver: see *Beef* or *Chicken* | | | | | | | | | | | |
| Lobster: northern, cooked, ½" cubes | 1 cup | 145 | 138 | 0.4 | 27.1 | 1.5 | 0.2 | 0.2 | 0.5 | 123 | 305 |
| Luncheon meat: see *Salami, Bologna, Braunschweiger, Sausage, Turkey* | | | | | | | | | | | |
| Macadamia nuts: 15 whole nuts | 1 oz | 28 | 196 | 4.5 | 2.2 | 20.3 | 3.1 | 16.3 | 0.6 | 0 | — |
| Macaroni: enriched, cooked, hot | 1 cup | 140 | 155 | 32.2 | 4.8 | 0.6 | 0 | 0.3 | 0.3 | 0 | 1 |
| Mackerel: canned, solids and liquids | ¼ cup | 35 | 64 | 0 | 7.5 | 3.5 | 0.9 | 1.3 | 0.8 | 33 | 148 |
| Mango: raw | 1 whole | 300 | 152 | 38.8 | 1.6 | 0.9 | 0 | 0 | 0.9 | 0 | 16 |
| Margarine: P/S > 3.1 (Promise® soft, Parkay® soft safflower, Hains® soft, Saffola® soft) | 1 tbsp | 14 | 102 | 0.1 | 0.1 | 11.5 | 1.5 | 3.5 | 6.3 | 0 | 140 |
| Margarine: P/S 2.6 to 3.0 (Mrs. Filbert's® soft corn oil, Promise® stick, Parkay® liquid squeeze) | 1 tbsp | 14 | 102 | 0.1 | 0.1 | 11.5 | 1.7 | 4.6 | 4.9 | 0 | 140 |
| Margarine: P/S 2.0 to 2.5 (Fleischmann's® soft, Chiffon® soft, Parkay® corn oil soft) | 1 tbsp | 14 | 102 | 0.1 | 0.1 | 11.5 | 2.1 | 4.1 | 5.0 | 0 | 110 |
| Margarine: P/S 1.6 to 1.9 (Fleischmann's® stick, Chiffon® stick, Meadow Gold® stick) | 1 tbsp | 14 | 102 | 0.1 | 0.1 | 11.5 | 2.1 | 5.0 | 3.6 | 0 | 110 |

## Nutrient Analysis of Common Foods (*continued*)

| *Food* | *Unit* | *Weight (g)* | *Cal* | *CHO (g)* | *Prot (g)* | *Fat (g)* | *Sat Fat (g)* | *Mono Fat (g)* | *Poly Fat (g)* | *Chol (mg)* | *Na (mg)* |
|---|---|---|---|---|---|---|---|---|---|---|---|
| Margarine: P/S 1.0 to 1.5 (Mazola® stick, Parkay® corn oil stick, Imperial® stick) | 1 tbsp | 14 | 100 | 0.1 | 0.1 | 11.3 | 2.0 | 5.1 | 4.0 | 0 | 115 |
| Margarine: low sodium, P/S 1.7 (Fleischmann's®, Mazola®) | 1 tbsp | 14 | 100 | 0.1 | 0.1 | 11.2 | 2.1 | 5.0 | 3.6 | 0 | tr |
| Margarine: P/S < 0.5, all vegetable fat (Kraft® all purpose stick, Swift® all purpose stick) | 1 tbsp | 14 | 102 | 0.1 | 0.1 | 11.5 | 2.2 | 7.5 | 1.5 | 0 | 140 |
| Margarine: P/S < 0.5, vegetable and animal or all animal (Gaylord® stick, Meadowlake® stick) | 1 tbsp | 14 | 102 | 0.1 | 0.1 | 11.5 | 4.7 | 5.6 | 1.0 | 0 | 140 |
| Margarine: P/S 2.4, (diet tub Fleischmann's® soft, Imperial® soft) | 1 tbsp | 14 | 50 | 0.1 | 0 | 5.6 | 1.0 | 2.1 | 2.4 | 0 | 135 |
| Mellorine | 1 cup | 131 | 244 | 30.8 | 5.9 | 11.1 | 9.5 | 0.6 | 0.2 | 18 | 105 |
| Milk: skim (less than 1% fat) | 1 cup | 245 | 86 | 11.9 | 8.4 | 0.4 | 0.3 | 0.1 | 0 | 4 | 126 |
| Milk: low fat (1% to 2% fat) | 1 cup | 244 | 102 | 11.7 | 8.0 | 2.6 | 1.6 | 0.8 | 0.1 | 10 | 123 |
| Milk: whole (3.3% fat) | 1 cup | 244 | 150 | 11.4 | 8.0 | 8.2 | 5.1 | 2.4 | 0.3 | 33 | 120 |
| Milk: canned, evaporated, whole | 1 cup | 252 | 338 | 25.3 | 17.2 | 19.1 | 11.6 | 5.9 | 0.6 | 74 | 267 |
| Milk: canned, evaporated, skim | 1 cup | 256 | 200 | 29.0 | 19.4 | 0.6 | 0.4 | 0.2 | 0 | 10 | 294 |
| Milk: nonfat, dry powder, approximately 1 cup reconstituted | ⅓ cup | 23 | 81 | 11.8 | 8.0 | 0.2 | 0.1 | 0 | 0 | 4 | 124 |
| Milk: canned, condensed, sweetened | 1 cup | 306 | 982 | 166.2 | 24.2 | 26.6 | 16.8 | 7.4 | 1.0 | 104 | 389 |
| Milk: chocolate drink, fluid, commercial, made with whole milk | 1 cup | 250 | 213 | 27.5 | 8.5 | 8.5 | 5.3 | 2.5 | 0.3 | 30 | 118 |

| Food | Unit | Weight (g) | Cal | CHO (g) | Prot (g) | Fat (g) | Sat Fat (g) | Mono Fat (g) | Poly Fat (g) | Chol (mg) | Na (mg) |
|---|---|---|---|---|---|---|---|---|---|---|---|
| Milk: low sodium (whole) | 1 cup | 244 | 149 | 10.9 | 7.6 | 8.4 | 5.3 | 2.4 | 0.3 | 33 | 6 |
| Milkshake: chocolate | 11 oz | 311 | 369 | 65.9 | 9.5 | 8.4 | 5.2 | 2.4 | 0.3 | 33 | 346 |
| Milkshake: vanilla | 11 oz | 313 | 350 | 55.6 | 12.1 | 9.5 | 5.9 | 2.7 | 0.4 | 37 | 299 |
| Molasses: light | 1 tbsp | 21 | 52 | 13.3 | 0 | 0 | 0 | 0 | 0 | 0 | 3 |
| Mushrooms: raw, sliced, chopped, or diced | 1 cup | 70 | 20 | 3.1 | 1.9 | 0.2 | 0 | 0 | 0.2 | 0 | 11 |
| Mustard: prepared, yellow | 1 tsp | 5 | 4 | 0.3 | 0.2 | 0.2 | 0 | 0 | 0.2 | 0 | 63 |
| Nectarine: raw, 2½" diameter | 1 whole | 150 | 88 | 23.6 | 0.8 | 0 | 0 | 0 | 0 | 0 | 8 |
| Noodles: egg, enriched, cooked | 1 cup | 160 | 200 | 37.3 | 6.6 | 2.4 | 0.8 | 1.1 | 0.2 | 50 | 3 |
| Noodles: chow mein, canned | 1 cup | 45 | 220 | 26.1 | 5.9 | 10.6 | 2.8 | 4.3 | 2.9 | 5 | — |
| Oil: coconut | 1 tbsp | 14 | 120 | 0 | 0 | 13.6 | 11.7 | 0.8 | 0.2 | 0 | 0 |
| Oil: cod liver | 1 tbsp | 14 | 120 | 0 | 0 | 13.6 | 2.4 | 7.0 | 3.5 | — | 0 |
| Oil: corn | 1 tbsp | 14 | 120 | 0 | 0 | 13.6 | 1.7 | 3.4 | 7.9 | 0 | 0 |
| Oil: cottonseed | 1 tbsp | 14 | 120 | 0 | 0 | 13.6 | 3.6 | 2.6 | 6.9 | 0 | 0 |
| Oil: olive | 1 tbsp | 14 | 119 | 0 | 0 | 13.5 | 1.9 | 9.8 | 1.2 | 0 | 0 |
| Oil: palm kernel | 1 tbsp | 14 | 120 | 0 | 0 | 13.6 | 11.1 | 1.6 | 0.2 | 0 | 0 |
| Oil: peanut | 1 tbsp | 14 | 119 | 0 | 0 | 13.5 | 2.6 | 6.2 | 4.1 | 0 | 0 |
| Oil: safflower | 1 tbsp | 14 | 120 | 0 | 0 | 13.6 | 1.3 | 1.7 | 10.0 | 0 | 0 |
| Oil: soybean | 1 tbsp | 14 | 120 | 0 | 0 | 13.6 | 2.0 | 3.1 | 7.8 | 0 | 0 |
| Oil: soybean-cottonseed blend | 1 tbsp | 14 | 120 | 0 | 0 | 13.6 | 2.2 | 3.1 | 7.7 | 0 | 0 |
| Oil: sunflower | 1 tbsp | 14 | 120 | 0 | 0 | 13.6 | 1.4 | 2.8 | 8.7 | 0 | 0 |
| Okra: frozen, cooked, cuts | 1 cup | 185 | 70 | 16.3 | 4.1 | 0.2 | 0 | 0 | 0.2 | 0 | 4 |
| Olives: ripe, whole, extra large | 10 whole | 55 | 61 | 1.2 | 0.5 | 6.5 | 0.7 | 5.0 | 0.5 | 0 | 385 |
| Olives: green, whole, large | 10 whole | 46 | 45 | 0.5 | 0.5 | 4.9 | 0.5 | 3.7 | 0.3 | 0 | 926 |
| Onions: green, raw, 4⅛ × ⅝" | 2 med | 30 | 14 | 3.2 | 0.3 | 0.1 | 0 | 0 | 0.1 | 0 | 2 |
| Onions: mature, raw, chopped | 1 cup | 170 | 65 | 14.8 | 2.6 | 0.2 | 0 | 0 | 0.2 | 0 | 17 |

## Nutrient Analysis of Common Foods (*continued*)

| *Food* | *Unit* | *Weight (g)* | *Cal* | *CHO (g)* | *Prot (g)* | *Fat (g)* | *Sat Fat (g)* | *Mono Fat (g)* | *Poly Fat (g)* | *Chol (mg)* | *Na (mg)* |
|---|---|---|---|---|---|---|---|---|---|---|---|
| Onions: mature, cooked, whole or sliced | 1 cup | 210 | 61 | 13.7 | 2.5 | 0.2 | 0 | 0 | 0.2 | 0 | 15 |
| Orange: Florida, medium, 2 11⁄16" diameter | 1 whole | 204 | 71 | 18.1 | 1.1 | 0.3 | 0 | 0 | 0.3 | 0 | 2 |
| Orange juice: concentrate, frozen, unsweetened, diluted | 1 cup | 249 | 122 | 28.9 | 1.7 | 0.2 | 0 | 0 | 0.2 | 0 | 2 |
| Oysters: canned, 18 to 27 medium or 27 to 44 small | 12 oz | 340 | 224 | 11.6 | 28.6 | 6.1 | 1.8 | 0.7 | 2.0 | 170 | 248 |
| Oysters: raw, 13 to 19 medium or 19 to 31 small | 1 cup | 240 | 158 | 8.2 | 20.2 | 4.3 | 1.2 | 0.5 | 1.4 | 120 | 175 |
| Pancake: made from mix, 6 × ½" | 1 cake | 73 | 164 | 23.7 | 5.3 | 5.3 | — | — | — | — | 412 |
| Peach: raw, pared, 2¾" diameter, approximately 2½ per lb | 1 whole | 175 | 51 | 12.9 | 0.8 | 0.1 | 0 | 0 | 0.1 | 0 | 1 |
| Peaches: canned, syrup packed, halves, slices, or chunks | 1 cup | 256 | 200 | 51.5 | 1.0 | 0.3 | 0 | 0 | 0.3 | 0 | 5 |
| Peanut butter | 1 cup | 258 | 1,520 | 48.5 | 65.0 | 130.5 | 27.1 | 60.7 | 39.0 | 0 | 1,561 |
| Peanuts: roasted, salted, 10 Virginia, 20 Spanish, or 1 tbsp, chopped | 10 nuts | 9 | 53 | 1.7 | 2.3 | 4.5 | 0.8 | 2.1 | 1.3 | 0 | 38 |
| Pear: raw, Bartletts, 2½ × 3½" | 1 whole | 180 | 100 | 25.1 | 1.1 | 0.7 | 0 | 0 | 0.7 | 0 | 3 |
| Pear: canned, syrup-packed, with 1⅔ tbsp liquid | 1 half | 76 | 58 | 14.9 | 0.2 | 0.2 | 0 | 0 | 0.2 | 0 | 1 |
| Pear nectar: canned | 1 cup | 250 | 130 | 33.0 | 0.8 | 0.5 | 0 | 0 | 0.5 | 0 | 3 |
| Peas: cow or black-eyed, canned, cooked | 1 cup | 255 | 179 | 31.6 | 12.8 | 0.8 | 0.2 | 0 | 0.3 | 0 | 602 |
| Peas: green, immature, canned solids | 1 cup | 170 | 150 | 28.6 | 8.0 | 0.7 | 0 | 0.4 | 0.7 | 0 | 401 |

| Food | Unit | Weight (g) | Cal | CHO (g) | Prot (g) | Fat (g) | Sat Fat (g) | Mono Fat (g) | Poly Fat (g) | Chol (mg) | Na (mg) |
|---|---|---|---|---|---|---|---|---|---|---|---|
| Peas: green, immature, canned solids, low sodium | 1 cup | 170 | 122 | 22.1 | 7.5 | 0.7 | 0 | 0.4 | 0.7 | 0 | 5 |
| Pecans: chopped or pieces | 1 tbsp | 7 | 51 | 1.1 | 0.7 | 5.2 | 0.5 | 3.1 | 1.3 | 0 | tr |
| Pepper: immature, green, raw, 3¾ × 3" | 1 whole | 200 | 36 | 7.9 | 2.0 | 0.3 | 0 | 0 | 0.3 | 0 | 21 |
| Pepper: jalapeño, canned | 1 whole | 18 | 5 | 1.1 | 0.2 | 0 | 0 | 0 | 0 | 0 | 72 |
| Pepper: jalapeño, fresh | 1 whole | 18 | 7 | 1.6 | 0.2 | 0 | 0 | 0 | 0 | 0 | 5 |
| Pheasant: flesh only, raw | 1 oz | 28 | 46 | 0 | 6.7 | 1.9 | 0.5 | 0.8 | 0.2 | — | — |
| Pickle: dill or sour, large, 4 × 1¾" | 1 whole | 135 | 15 | 3.0 | 0.9 | 0.3 | 0 | 0 | 0.3 | 0 | 1,928 |
| Pickle: dill or sour, 3¾ × 1¼", low sodium | 1 whole | 65 | 7 | 1.4 | 0.5 | 0.1 | 0 | 0 | 0.1 | 0 | 4 |
| Pickles: fresh, sweetened (bread and butter), 1½ × ¼" | 2 slices | 15 | 11 | 2.7 | 0.1 | 0 | 0 | 0 | 0 | 0 | 101 |
| Pickle: sweet, gherkins, large, 3 × 1" | 1 whole | 35 | 51 | 12.8 | 0.2 | 0.1 | 0 | 0 | 0.1 | 0 | 500 |
| Pickle relish: finely chopped, sweet | 1 tbsp | 15 | 21 | 5.1 | 0.1 | 0.1 | 0 | 0 | 0.1 | 0 | 107 |
| Pie: frozen, baked, apple, 8" diameter | 1 pie | 550 | 1,386 | 219.0 | 10.6 | 54.8 | 13.6 | 27.3 | 12.2 | 0 | 1,168 |
| Pie: frozen, baked, cherry, 8" diameter | 1 pie | 580 | 1,690 | 257.4 | 12.5 | 70.0 | 17.4 | 34.8 | 15,6 | 0 | 1,333 |
| Pie: mix, baked, coconut custard (eggs and milk), 8" diameter | 1 pie | 797 | 1,618 | 231.9 | 34.3 | 63.0 | 27.1 | 31.1 | 8.0 | 837 | 1,873 |
| Pineapple: raw, diced pieces | 1 cup | 155 | 81 | 21.2 | 0.6 | 0.3 | 0 | 0 | 0.3 | 0 | 2 |
| Pineapple: canned, syrup-packed, chunk, tidbit, or crushed | 1 cup | 255 | 189 | 49.5 | 0.8 | 0.3 | 0 | 0 | 0.3 | 0 | 3 |
| Pineapple: canned, water-packed, tidbits | 1 cup | 246 | 96 | 25.1 | 0.7 | 0.2 | 0 | 0 | 0.2 | 0 | 2 |
| Pineapple: in its own juice (no sugar added), 4 slices with juice or 1 cup with juice | 1 cup | 227 | 140 | 35.0 | 1.0 | 1.0 | 0 | 0 | 1.0 | 0 | 2 |
| Pineapple juice: canned, unsweetened | 1 cup | 250 | 138 | 33.8 | 1.0 | 0.3 | 0 | 0 | 0.3 | 0 | 3 |

## Nutrient Analysis of Common Foods (*continued*)

| *Food* | *Unit* | *Weight (g)* | *Cal* | *CHO (g)* | *Prot (g)* | *Fat (g)* | *Sat Fat (g)* | *Mono Fat (g)* | *Poly Fat (g)* | *Chol (mg)* | *Na (mg)* |
|---|---|---|---|---|---|---|---|---|---|---|---|
| Plum: hybrid, fresh, 2⅛" diameter | 1 whole | 70 | 32 | 8.1 | 0.3 | 0.1 | 0 | 0 | 0.1 | 0 | 1 |
| Plums: canned, served with 2¾ tbsp syrup | 3 whole | 140 | 110 | 28.7 | 0.5 | 0.1 | 0 | 0 | 0.1 | 0 | 1 |
| Popcorn: no salt or fat added to popped corn | 1 cup | 6 | 23 | 4.6 | 0.8 | 0.3 | 0 | 0.1 | 0.2 | 0 | tr |
| Pork: fresh, 10% fat, ham or picnic ham (lean only) | 1 oz | 28 | 61 | 0 | 8.4 | 2.8 | 0.9 | 1.2 | 0.3 | 25 | 18 |
| Pork: fresh, 13–20% fat, Boston butt roast, chop, loin, shoulder (lean only) | 1 oz | 28 | 71 | 0 | 8.0 | 3.9 | 1.6 | 2.1 | 0.5 | 25 | 20 |
| Pork: fresh, 23–30% fat, Boston butt, ground pork, ham, loin picnic, shoulder (lean and fat) | 1 oz | 28 | 103 | 0 | 6.6 | 8.3 | 2.9 | 3.8 | 0.9 | 25 | 16 |
| Pork: spareribs, 37% fat (lean and fat) | 1 oz | 28 | 125 | 0 | 5.9 | 11.0 | 3.8 | 5.1 | 1.2 | 25 | 10 |
| Pork: cured, 7–10% fat, ham or picnic ham (lean only) | 1 oz | 28 | 56 | 0 | 7.6 | 2.7 | 0.9 | 1.1 | 0.2 | 25 | 273 |
| Pork: cured, 13–20% fat, Boston butt, shoulder (lean only) | 1 oz | 28 | 75 | 0 | 6.9 | 5.1 | 1.8 | 2.4 | 0.6 | 25 | 247 |
| Pork: cured, 23–30% fat, ham, picnic, shoulder (lean and fat) | 1 oz | 28 | 93 | 0 | 6.4 | 7.2 | 2.5 | 3.4 | 0.8 | 25 | 230 |
| Pork: deviled ham, canned | ¼ cup | 56 | 198 | 0 | 7.8 | 18.2 | 6.4 | 8.5 | 2.0 | 35 | 703 |
| Potato chips | 10 chips | 20 | 114 | 10.0 | 1.1 | 8.0 | 2.0 | 1.7 | 4.0 | 0 | 200 |
| Potatoes: fresh, boiled, diced, or sliced | 1 cup | 155 | 101 | 22.5 | 2.9 | 0.2 | 0 | 0 | 0.2 | 0 | 3 |
| Potato: fresh, baked in skin, 2⅓ × 4¾" | 1 whole | 202 | 145 | 32.8 | 4.0 | 0.2 | 0 | 0 | 0.2 | 0 | 6 |
| Potato: frozen, French fried, 4" strips (oven-heated) | 10 strips | 78 | 172 | 26.3 | 2.8 | 6.6 | 1.6 | 1.4 | 3.3 | 0 | 3 |

| Food | Unit | Weight (g) | Cal | CHO (g) | Prot (g) | Fat (g) | Sat Fat (g) | Mono Fat (g) | Poly Fat (g) | Chol (mg) | Na (mg) |
|---|---|---|---|---|---|---|---|---|---|---|---|
| Potato, sweet: fresh, baked, 5 × 2" | 1 whole | 146 | 161 | 37.0 | 2.4 | 0.6 | 0 | 0 | 0.6 | 0 | 14 |
| Potatoes, sweet: pieces, canned in syrup | 1 cup | 200 | 216 | 49.8 | 4.0 | 0.4 | 0 | 0 | 0.4 | 0 | 96 |
| Pretzels: extruded type, rods, 7½ × ½" | 1 whole | 14 | 55 | 10.6 | 1.4 | 0.6 | 0.2 | 0.4 | 0.1 | 0 | 235 |
| Pretzels: twisted type, rings (3), 1⅞ × 1¾ × ¼" | 10 whole | 30 | 117 | 22.8 | 2.9 | 1.4 | 0.3 | 0.8 | 0.2 | 0 | 504 |
| Prunes: dried, uncooked, without pits | 10 whole | 102 | 260 | 68.7 | 2.1 | 0.6 | 0 | 0 | 0.6 | 0 | 8 |
| Prunes: dried, cooked, no added sugar | 1 cup | 250 | 253 | 66.7 | 2.1 | 0.6 | 0 | 0 | 0.6 | 0 | 9 |
| Prune juice: canned or bottled | 1 cup | 256 | 197 | 48.6 | 1.0 | 0.3 | 0 | 0 | 0.3 | 0 | 5 |
| Pudding mix: chocolate, regular, prepared with whole milk | 1 cup | 260 | 322 | 59.3 | 8.8 | 7.8 | 4.3 | 2.6 | 0.2 | 36 | 335 |
| Pudding mix: chocolate, instant, prepared with whole milk | 1 cup | 260 | 325 | 63.4 | 7.8 | 6.5 | 3.6 | 2.2 | 0.3 | 36 | 322 |
| Pudding mix: low calorie, dry form, 1 package (all kinds) | 4 oz | 128 | 100 | 24.0 | 0 | 0 | 0 | 0 | 0 | 0 | 280 |
| Pumpkin: canned | 1 cup | 245 | 81 | 19.4 | 2.5 | 0.7 | 0 | 0 | 0.7 | 0 | 5 |
| Quail: flesh and skin, raw | 1 oz | 28 | 48 | 0 | 7.2 | 2.0 | 0.5 | 0.9 | 0.5 | — | 11 |
| Raisins: natural, seedless, uncooked, whole, not packed | 1 tbsp | 9 | 26 | 7.0 | 0.2 | tr | 0 | 0 | tr | 0 | 2 |
| Raspberries: raw, red | 1 cup | 123 | 70 | 16.7 | 1.5 | 0.6 | 0 | 0 | 0.6 | 0 | 1 |
| Rhubarb: frozen, sweetened | 1 cup | 270 | 381 | 97.2 | 1.4 | 0.3 | 0 | 0 | 0.3 | 0 | 5 |
| Rice: brown, cooked without salt | 1 cup | 195 | 232 | 49.7 | 4.9 | 1.2 | 0.3 | 0.3 | 0.6 | 0 | 5 |
| Rice: white, enriched, cooked without salt | 1 cup | 205 | 221 | 49.6 | 4.1 | 0.4 | 0.1 | 0.1 | 0.1 | 0 | 5 |
| Roll: hard, enriched | 1 roll | 25 | 78 | 14.9 | 2.5 | 0.8 | 0.2 | 0.4 | 0.2 | 0 | 157 |
| Roll: soft, enriched, brown and serve, or Parker House | 1 roll | 28 | 83 | 14.8 | 2.3 | 1.6 | 0.4 | 0.7 | 0.4 | 0 | 142 |

| Food | Unit | Weight (g) | Cal | CHO (g) | Prot (g) | Fat (g) | Sat Fat (g) | Mono Fat (g) | Poly Fat (g) | Chol (mg) | Na (mg) |
|---|---|---|---|---|---|---|---|---|---|---|---|
| Roll: enriched, hotdog (6 × 2") or hamburger (3½ × 1½") | 1 whole | 40 | 119 | 21.2 | 3.3 | 2.2 | 0.5 | 1.1 | 0.5 | 0 | 202 |
| Rum: see *Liquor* | | | | | | | | | | | |
| Salad dressing: blue or roquefort | 1 tbsp | 15 | 76 | 1.1 | 0.7 | 8.0 | 1.6 | 1.8 | 3.8 | 10 | 164 |
| Salad dressing: blue or roquefort, low calorie | 1 tbsp | 16 | 12 | 0.7 | 0.5 | 0.9 | 0.5 | 0.3 | 0 | 1 | 177 |
| Salad dressing: French | 1 tbsp | 16 | 66 | 2.8 | 0.1 | 6.2 | 1.1 | 1.3 | 3.2 | 0 | 219 |
| Salad dressing: French, low calorie | 1 tbsp | 16 | 15 | 2.5 | 0.1 | 0.7 | 0.1 | 0.1 | 0.4 | 0 | 126 |
| Salad dressing: Italian | 1 tbsp | 15 | 83 | 1.0 | tr | 9.0 | 1.5 | 1.9 | 4.6 | 0 | 314 |
| Salad dressing: Italian, low calorie | 1 tbsp | 15 | 8 | 0.4 | tr | 0.7 | 0.1 | 0.2 | 0.4 | 0 | 118 |
| Salad dressing: mayonnaise | 1 tbsp | 15 | 101 | 0.3 | 0.2 | 11.2 | 2.0 | 2.4 | 5.5 | 9 | 84 |
| Salad dressing: mayonnaise, low sodium | 1 tbsp | 14 | 99 | 0.3 | 0.2 | 11.0 | 2.0 | 2.4 | 5.5 | 9 | 2 |
| Salad dressing: mayonnaise type (Miracle Whip®) | 1 tbsp | 15 | 65 | 2.2 | 0.2 | 6.3 | 1.1 | 1.4 | 3.1 | 7 | 88 |
| Salad dressing: mayonnaise type, low calorie | 1 tbsp | 16 | 22 | 0.8 | 0.2 | 2.0 | 0.4 | 0.4 | 1.0 | 0 | 19 |
| Salad dressing: Russian | 1 tbsp | 15 | 74 | 1.6 | 0.2 | 7.6 | 1.4 | 1.7 | 3.9 | 7 | 130 |
| Salad dressing: Thousand Island | 1 tbsp | 16 | 80 | 2.5 | 0.1 | 8.0 | 1.4 | 1.7 | 3.9 | 7 | 112 |
| Salad dressing: Thousand Island, low calorie | 1 tbsp | 15 | 27 | 2.3 | 0.1 | 2.1 | 0.4 | 0.5 | 1.1 | 0 | 105 |
| Salami: cooked, 4½" diameter slice | 1 oz | 28 | 73 | 0.4 | 5.0 | 5.8 | 2.1 | 2.7 | 0.6 | 15 | 297 |
| Salmon: fresh, broiled or baked, no added fat | 1 oz | 28 | 48 | 0 | 7.7 | 1.6 | 0.5 | 0.8 | 0.1 | 10 | 33 |
| Salmon: canned, drained, pink | 1 oz | 28 | 49 | 0 | 5.7 | 1.9 | 0.2 | 0.3 | 1.0 | 10 | 135 |
| Salmon: smoked (Lox) | 1 oz | 28 | 50 | 0 | 6.1 | 2.6 | 0.5 | 0.8 | 0.1 | 10 | 135 |
| Salt: table | 1 tsp | 6 | 0 | 0 | 0 | 0 | 0 | 0 | 0 | 0 | 2,196 |

| Food | Unit | Weight (g) | Cal | CHO (g) | Prot (g) | Fat (g) | Sat Fat (g) | Mono Fat (g) | Poly Fat (g) | Chol (mg) | Na (mg) |
|---|---|---|---|---|---|---|---|---|---|---|---|
| Salt pork | 1 oz | 28 | 219 | 0 | 1.1 | 24.0 | 8.5 | 11.3 | 2.7 | 20 | 340 |
| Sandwich spread: with chopped pickle | 1 tbsp | 15 | 58 | 2.4 | 0.1 | 5.5 | 1.1 | 1.4 | 3.1 | 8 | 96 |
| Sandwich spread: low calorie | 1 tbsp | 15 | 17 | 1.2 | 0.2 | 1.4 | 0.3 | 0.3 | 0.8 | 0 | 94 |
| Sardine: canned in oil, 3 × 1 × ½" | 1 whole | 12 | 24 | 0 | 2.9 | 1.3 | 0.4 | 0.4 | 0.4 | 17 | 99 |
| Sauerkraut: canned, solids and liquid | 1 cup | 235 | 42 | 9.4 | 2.4 | 0.5 | 0 | 0 | 0.5 | 0 | 1,755 |
| Sausage, Polish: 5⅝ × 1" | 1 link | 76 | 231 | 0.9 | 11.9 | 19.6 | 6.9 | 9.1 | 1.7 | 47 | 836 |
| Sausage, pork: 4 × ⅞" (uncooked) | 1 link | 13 | 49 | 0 | 2.4 | 4.2 | 1.5 | 2.0 | 0.5 | 8 | 125 |
| Sausage, Vienna: canned, 2 × ⅞" diameter | 1 whole | 16 | 56 | 0 | 2.2 | 5.2 | 1.8 | 2.5 | 0.6 | 10 | 157 |
| Scallops: fresh, cooked, steamed | 1 oz | 28 | 32 | — | 6.6 | 0.3 | 0 | 0 | 0.1 | 15 | 75 |
| Sesame seeds: dry, hulled | 1 tbsp | 8 | 47 | 1.4 | 1.5 | 4.4 | 0.6 | 1.6 | 1.8 | 0 | — |
| Sherbet: orange | 1 cup | 193 | 270 | 58.7 | 2.2 | 3.8 | 2.4 | 1.1 | 0.1 | 14 | 88 |
| Shortening: animal | 1 tbsp | 13 | 111 | 0 | 0 | 12.5 | 6.3 | 5.5 | 0.8 | 10 | 0 |
| Shortening: animal-vegetable | 1 tbsp | 13 | 111 | 0 | 0 | 12.5 | 5.6 | 5.5 | 1.1 | 6 | 0 |
| Shortening: vegetable | 1 tbsp | 13 | 111 | 0 | 0 | 12.5 | 3.3 | 5.8 | 3.5 | 0 | 0 |
| Shrimp: 4½ oz can drained | 1 cup | 128 | 148 | 0.8 | 31.0 | 1.5 | 0.2 | 0.2 | 0.6 | 192 | — |
| Shrimp: canned, approximately 2" long (small) | 10 whole | 17 | 20 | 0.1 | 4.1 | 0.2 | 0 | 0 | 0.1 | 26 | — |
| Shrimp: fresh, cooked, 8 shrimp, each 3¼" long | 2 oz | 58 | 67 | 0.4 | 14.0 | 0.7 | 0.1 | 0.1 | 0.3 | 87 | 81 |
| Snapper: red or gray, raw | 1 oz | 28 | 26 | 0 | 5.6 | 0.3 | 0.1 | 0.1 | 0.1 | — | 19 |
| Sole: raw | 1 oz | 28 | 22 | 0 | 4.7 | 0.2 | 0 | 0 | 0.1 | — | 22 |
| Soup: canned, bean with pork, prepared with equal volume of water | 1 cup | 250 | 170 | 21.8 | 8.0 | 6.0 | 1.5 | 2.2 | 1.8 | 4 | 1,008 |
| Soup: canned, beef broth, prepared with equal volume of water | 1 cup | 240 | 31 | 2.6 | 5.0 | 0 | 0 | 0 | 0 | 0 | 782 |

## Nutrient Analysis of Common Foods (*continued*)

| *Food* | *Unit* | *Weight (g)* | *Cal* | *CHO (g)* | *Prot (g)* | *Fat (g)* | *Sat Fat (g)* | *Mono Fat (g)* | *Poly Fat (g)* | *Chol (mg)* | *Na (mg)* |
|---|---|---|---|---|---|---|---|---|---|---|---|
| Soup: canned, cream of celery, prepared with equal volume of water | 1 cup | 240 | 86 | 8.9 | 1.7 | 5.5 | 1.4 | 1.2 | 2.4 | 7 | 955 |
| Soup: canned, cream of chicken, prepared with equal volume of water | 1 cup | 240 | 94 | 7.9 | 2.9 | 5.8 | 2.0 | 3.2 | 1.4 | 8 | 970 |
| Soup: canned, cream of mushroom, prepared with equal volume of water | 1 cup | 240 | 132 | 10.1 | 2.4 | 9.4 | 2.5 | 1.8 | 4.4 | 6 | 955 |
| Soup: canned, chicken noodle, prepared with equal volume of water | 1 cup | 240 | 67 | 7.9 | 3.4 | 2.4 | 0.6 | 1.0 | 0.5 | 6 | 979 |
| Soup: canned, clam chowder, Manhattan style, prepared with equal volume of water | 1 cup | 245 | 78 | 12.3 | 2.2 | 2.2 | 0.4 | 0.4 | 1.3 | 6 | 938 |
| Soup: canned, minestrone, prepared with equal volume of water | 1 cup | 245 | 105 | 14.2 | 4.9 | 2.7 | 0.6 | 0.7 | 1.2 | 2 | 995 |
| Soup: canned, onion, prepared with equal volume of water | 1 cup | 240 | 65 | 5.3 | 5.3 | 2.4 | 0.8 | 1.0 | 0.6 | 6 | 1,051 |
| Soup: canned, split pea, prepared with equal volume of water | 1 cup | 245 | 145 | 20.6 | 8.6 | 3.2 | 1.0 | 1.5 | 0.3 | 6 | 941 |
| Soup: canned, tomato, prepared with equal volume of water | 1 cup | 245 | 88 | 15.7 | 2.0 | 2.0 | 0.4 | 0.4 | 0.9 | 2 | 970 |
| Soup: canned, vegetable beef, prepared with equal volume of water | 1 cup | 245 | 89 | 9.6 | 5.3 | 3.4 | 0.8 | 0.9 | 1.6 | 6 | 1,046 |
| Soup: canned, vegetarian vegetable, prepared with equal volume of water | 1 cup | 245 | 80 | 13.2 | 2.2 | 2.2 | 0.5 | 0.6 | 0.9 | 2 | 838 |
| Soup: dehydrated, onion, 1 package | 1½ oz | 43 | 150 | 23.2 | 6.0 | 4.6 | 1.0 | 2.0 | 1.0 | 0 | 2,871 |

| Food | Unit | Weight (g) | Cal | CHO (g) | Prot (g) | Fat (g) | Sat Fat (g) | Mono Fat (g) | Poly Fat (g) | Chol (mg) | Na (mg) |
|---|---|---|---|---|---|---|---|---|---|---|---|
| Sour cream: see *Cream* | | | | | | | | | | | |
| Soy sauce | 1 tbsp | 18 | 12 | 1.7 | 1.0 | 0.2 | 0 | 0 | 0.2 | 0 | 1,319 |
| Soybeans: mature seeds, cooked | 1 cup | 180 | 234 | 19.4 | 19.8 | 10.3 | 1.5 | 2.1 | 5.3 | 0 | 4 |
| Soybean curd (tofu): 2½ × 2¾ × 1" | 1 piece | 120 | 86 | 2.9 | 9.4 | 5.0 | 0.8 | 1.0 | 2.6 | 0 | 8 |
| Soybean seeds: sprouted, raw | 1 cup | 105 | 48 | 5.6 | 6.5 | 1.5 | 0.5 | 0.1 | 0.9 | 0 | — |
| Soybean seeds: sprouted, cooked | 1 cup | 125 | 48 | 4.6 | 6.6 | 1.8 | 0.5 | 0.2 | 1.1 | 0 | — |
| Spaghetti: enriched, cooked without salt | 1 cup | 140 | 155 | 32.2 | 4.8 | 0.6 | 0 | 0 | 0.6 | 0 | 1 |
| Spaghetti with meat balls and tomato sauce: canned, rings | 1 cup | 250 | 258 | 28.5 | 12.3 | 10.3 | 2.2 | 3.3 | 3.9 | 39 | 1,220 |
| Spinach: frozen, cooked | 1 cup | 205 | 47 | 7.6 | 6.2 | 0.6 | 0 | 0 | 0.6 | 0 | 107 |
| Spinach: canned, low sodium | 1 cup | 205 | 53 | 8.2 | 6.6 | 1.0 | 0.3 | 0.1 | 0.6 | 0 | 66 |
| Squash, summer: fresh, cooked, sliced | 1 cup | 180 | 25 | 5.6 | 1.6 | 0.2 | 0 | 0 | 0.2 | 0 | 2 |
| Squash, winter: frozen, cooked | 1 cup | 240 | 91 | 22.1 | 2.9 | 0.7 | 0 | 0 | 0.7 | 0 | 2 |
| Steak: see *Beef* | | | | | | | | | | | |
| Stew: beef and vegetable, canned | 1 cup | 245 | 194 | 17.4 | 14.2 | 7.6 | 3.2 | 3.1 | 0.2 | 36 | 1,007 |
| Strawberries: fresh, whole | 1 cup | 149 | 55 | 12.5 | 1.0 | 0.7 | 0 | 0 | 0.7 | 0 | 1 |
| Sugar: brown, packed | 1 cup | 220 | 821 | 212.1 | 0 | 0 | 0 | 0 | 0 | 0 | 66 |
| Sugar: granulated | 1 tbsp | 12 | 46 | 11.9 | 0 | 0 | 0 | 0 | 0 | 0 | tr |
| Sugar: powdered (confectioners'), unsifted | 1 tbsp | 8 | 31 | 8.0 | 0 | 0 | 0 | 0 | 0 | 0 | tr |
| Sunflower seed kernels: dry, hulled | 1 tbsp | 9 | 51 | 1.8 | 2.2 | 4.3 | 0.5 | 0.9 | 2.7 | 0 | 3 |
| Sweet roll: Danish pastry, without nuts or fruit, 4½ × 1" | 1 whole | 65 | 274 | 29.6 | 4.8 | 15.3 | 4.5 | 7.1 | 2.8 | 17 | 238 |
| Sweetbreads (thymus), beef | 1 oz | 28 | 90 | 0 | 7.3 | 6.6 | — | — | — | 132 | 99 |
| Syrup: cane and maple | 1 tbsp | 20 | 50 | 12.8 | 0 | 0 | 0 | 0 | 0 | 0 | tr |

## Nutrient Analysis of Common Foods (*continued*)

| Food | Unit | Weight (g) | Cal | CHO (g) | Prot (g) | Fat (g) | Sat Fat (g) | Mono Fat (g) | Poly Fat (g) | Chol (mg) | Na (mg) |
|---|---|---|---|---|---|---|---|---|---|---|---|
| Taco shell: fried tortilla | 1 whole | 30 | 146 | 19.7 | 2.6 | 5.6 | 1.5 | 2.3 | 1.5 | 0 | tr |
| Tangerine: large, 2½" diameter | 1 whole | 136 | 46 | 11.7 | 0.8 | 0.2 | 0 | 0 | 0.2 | 0 | 2 |
| Tapioca: dry | 1 tbsp | 10 | 33 | 8.2 | 0.1 | tr | 0 | 0 | tr | 0 | tr |
| Tartar sauce | 1 tbsp | 14 | 76 | 0.6 | 0.2 | 8.3 | 1.0 | 2.1 | 4.1 | 7 | 102 |
| Tofu: see *Soybean curd* | | | | | | | | | | | |
| Tomatoes: canned, solids and liquid | 1 cup | 241 | 51 | 10.4 | 2.4 | 0.5 | 0 | 0 | 0.5 | 0 | 313 |
| Tomatoes: fresh, raw, 3 × 2⅛" high (tomato = 6 slices) | 1 whole | 200 | 40 | 8.6 | 2.0 | 0.4 | 0 | 0 | 0.4 | 0 | 5 |
| Tomatoes: fresh, cooked | 1 cup | 241 | 63 | 13.3 | 3.1 | 0.5 | 0 | 0 | 0.5 | 0 | 10 |
| Tomatoes: canned, solids and liquid, low sodium | 1 cup | 241 | 48 | 10.1 | 2.4 | 0.5 | 0 | 0 | 0.5 | 0 | 7 |
| Tomato chili sauce: bottled | 1 cup | 273 | 284 | 67.7 | 6.8 | 0.8 | 0 | 0 | 0.8 | 0 | 3,653 |
| Tomato juice: canned or bottled | 1 cup | 243 | 46 | 10.4 | 2.2 | 0.2 | 0 | 0 | 0.2 | 0 | 486 |
| Tomato juice: canned or bottled, low sodium | 1 cup | 242 | 46 | 10.4 | 1.9 | 0.2 | 0 | 0 | 0.2 | 0 | 7 |
| Tomato ketchup: canned or bottled | 1 cup | 273 | 289 | 69.3 | 5.5 | 1.1 | 0 | 0 | 1.1 | 0 | 2,845 |
| Tomato paste: canned | 1 cup | 262 | 215 | 48.7 | 8.9 | 1.0 | 0.3 | 0.1 | 0.6 | 0 | 100 |
| Tomato paste: low sodium | 1 cup | 262 | 215 | 48.7 | 8.9 | 1.0 | 0.3 | 0.1 | 0.6 | 0 | 40 |
| Tomato sauce | 1 cup | 240 | 80 | 18.0 | 3.0 | 0 | 0 | 0 | 0 | 0 | 882 |
| Tomato sauce: low sodium | 1 cup | 240 | 80 | 18.0 | 3.0 | 0 | 0 | 0 | 0 | 0 | 13 |
| Tortilla: corn, 6" diameter | 1 whole | 30 | 70 | 13.4 | 1.6 | 0.6 | 0 | 0 | 0 | 0 | tr |
| Tortilla: flour | 1 whole | 30 | 108 | 22.4 | 2.9 | 1.2 | 0.6 | 0.8 | 0.3 | 0 | 120 |
| Tuna: water-packed, canned, chunk style, solids and liquid, low sodium | 6½ oz | 184 | 234 | 0 | 51.5 | 1.5 | 0.4 | 0.3 | 0.4 | 115 | 75 |

| Food | Unit | Weight (g) | Cal | CHO (g) | Prot (g) | Fat (g) | Sat Fat (g) | Mono Fat (g) | Poly Fat (g) | Chol (mg) | Na (mg) |
|---|---|---|---|---|---|---|---|---|---|---|---|
| Tuna: oil-packed, canned (drained), 1 cup | 4½ oz | 127 | 295 | 0 | 46.1 | 10.9 | 3.6 | 2.8 | 2.9 | 104 | 1,280 |
| Turkey: light meat, without skin | 1 oz | 28 | 45 | 0 | 9.3 | 0.7 | 0.2 | 0.2 | 0.2 | 22 | 23 |
| Turkey: dark meat, without skin | 1 oz | 28 | 48 | 0 | 8.5 | 1.5 | 0.4 | 0.4 | 0.4 | 29 | 28 |
| Turkey: light and dark with skin | 1 oz | 28 | 63 | 0 | 9.0 | 2.9 | 0.8 | 1.0 | 0.8 | 30 | — |
| Turkey bologna or franks | 1 oz | 28 | 71 | 2.1 | 3.5 | 5.4 | 2.4 | 2.1 | 0.9 | 37 | 336 |
| Turkey ham | 1 oz | 28 | 40 | 0.5 | 5.5 | 1.5 | 0.4 | 0.4 | 0.4 | 28 | 280 |
| Turkey pastrami | 1 oz | 28 | 34 | 0.8 | 5.2 | 1.6 | 0.4 | 0.4 | 0.4 | 29 | 525 |
| Turkey salami: with skin | 1 oz | 28 | 50 | 0.5 | 4.6 | 3.6 | 0.8 | 1.0 | 0.8 | 26 | 454 |
| Turnip greens: frozen, chopped, cooked | 1 cup | 165 | 38 | 6.4 | 4.1 | 0.5 | 0 | 0 | 0.5 | 0 | 28 |
| Turnips: fresh, cooked, cubes | 1 cup | 155 | 36 | 7.6 | 1.2 | 0.3 | 0 | 0 | 0.3 | 0 | 53 |
| Veal: <6% fat, breast riblet, cutlet, leg, loin, rump, shank, shoulder steak (lean only) | 1 oz | 28 | 40 | 0 | 5.7 | 1.7 | 0.9 | 0.8 | 0.1 | 28 | 16 |
| Veal: 10% fat, cutlet, leg, rump, shank, shoulder, steak (lean and fat) | 1 oz | 28 | 61 | 0 | 8.2 | 3.0 | 1.4 | 1.3 | 0.2 | 28 | 13 |
| Veal: 15% fat, loin (lean and fat) | 1 oz | 28 | 67 | 0 | 7.5 | 3.8 | 1.8 | 1.6 | 0.2 | 29 | 13 |
| Veal: 20% fat, rib (lean and fat) | 1 oz | 28 | 86 | 0 | 7.4 | 6.0 | 3.2 | 2.9 | 0.3 | 29 | 14 |
| Veal: 25% fat, breast riblet (lean and fat) | 1 oz | 28 | 89 | 0 | 4.7 | 7.7 | 3.6 | 3.1 | 0.4 | 29 | 14 |
| Vodka: see *Liquor* | | | | | | | | | | | |
| Vinegar: cider | 1 cup | 240 | 34 | 14.2 | 0 | 0 | 0 | 0 | 0 | 0 | 2 |
| Waffle: made from mix, 7 × ⅝" | 1 waffle | 75 | 206 | 27.2 | 6.6 | 8.0 | — | — | — | — | 515 |
| Walnuts: English, chopped pieces | 1 tbsp | 8 | 49 | 1.2 | 1.1 | 4.8 | 0.5 | 0.7 | 3.1 | 0 | tr |
| Water chestnuts | 4 nuts | 25 | 20 | 4.8 | 0.4 | 0.1 | 0 | 0 | 0.1 | 0 | 5 |
| Watermelon: diced pieces | 1 cup | 160 | 42 | 10.2 | 0.8 | 0.3 | 0 | 0 | 0.3 | 0 | 2 |

| *Food* | *Unit* | *Weight (g)* | *Cal* | *CHO (g)* | *Prot (g)* | *Fat (g)* | *Sat Fat (g)* | *Mono Fat (g)* | *Poly Fat (g)* | *Chol (mg)* | *Na (mg)* |
|---|---|---|---|---|---|---|---|---|---|---|---|
| Watermelon: 10 × 1" wedge, or 4" arc × 8" radius | 1 slice | 926 | 111 | 27.3 | 2.1 | 0.9 | 0 | 0 | 0.9 | 0 | 4 |
| Whiskey: see *Liquor* | | | | | | | | | | | |
| Weiner: 5 × ¾" | 1 whole | 45 | 139 | 0.8 | 5.6 | 12.4 | 4.7 | 5.9 | 0.8 | 27 | 495 |
| Wine: dessert (port, madeira, sweet sherry) | 1 oz | 30 | 41 | 2.3 | 0 | 0 | 0 | 0 | 0 | 0 | 1 |
| Wine: table (burgundy, rosé, white, dry sherry) | 1 oz | 29 | 25 | 1.2 | 0 | 0 | 0 | 0 | 0 | 0 | 1 |
| Worcestershire sauce | 1 tbsp | 15 | 6 | 1.4 | 0.1 | 0 | 0 | 0 | 0 | 0 | 267 |
| Yeast: bakers, dry package, scant tbsp | ¼ oz | 7 | 20 | 2.7 | 2.6 | 0.1 | 0 | 0 | 0.1 | 0 | 4 |
| Yogurt: skim, home recipe | 1 cup | 227 | 127 | 17.4 | 13.0 | 0.4 | 0.3 | 0.1 | 0 | 4 | 174 |
| Yogurt: plain, low fat | 1 cup | 227 | 144 | 16.0 | 11.9 | 3.5 | 2.3 | 1.0 | 0.1 | 14 | 159 |
| Yogurt: whole milk | 1 cup | 227 | 139 | 10.6 | 7.9 | 7.4 | 4.8 | 2.0 | 0.2 | 29 | 105 |
| Yogurt: with fruit (1–2% fat) | 1 cup | 227 | 225 | 42.3 | 9.0 | 2.6 | 1.7 | 0.7 | 0.1 | 10 | 121 |
| Yogurt: frozen (2% fat) | 1 cup | 227 | 244 | 48.0 | 6.0 | 3.0 | 1.9 | 0.7 | 0.1 | 10 | 121 |

# *List of Contributors*

**Paul Bertolli** has been head chef at Chez Panisse in Berkeley, California, since 1982. Prior to Chez Panisse, he worked in restaurants in Florence, Italy. He is the author of *Chez Panisse Cooking* (Random House) with Alice Waters.

**David Boulud** has been executive chef at Le Cirque in New York City. He recently opened a new restaurant, Daniel, in New York. He is author of a cookbook published in the fall of 1993 by Random House.

**Judith Ets-Hokin** is the director of the Judith Ets-Hokin's Homechef Cooking School in San Francisco. She is the author of *The San Francisco Dinner Party Cookbook* (Houghton Mifflin) and *The Home Chef: Fine Cooking Made Simple* (Celestial Arts).

**Susan Feniger and Mary Sue Milliken** are co-chefs and co-proprietors of Los Angeles's City Restaurant and Border Grill. They are the authors of *City Cuisine* (Morrow).

**Jean-Marc Fullsack** was born in Strasbourg, France, where he graduated from the Culinary School in 1972. For the past eleven years, he has been the chef for Dr. Ornish's Lifestyle Heart Trial. Prior to that, he was a chef at L'Ermitage in Beverly Hills and Lutèce in New York City, and an instructor at the California Culinary Academy in San Francisco.

**Joyce Goldstein** is the chef and proprietor of Square One restaurant in San Francisco. She has been a columnist for *Rolling Stone* and *Bon Appétit* and writes a monthly food column for the *San Francisco Chronicle.* She is the author of *The Mediterranean Kitchen* (Morrow) and *Back to Square One* (Morrow).

**Hubert Keller** is chef and co-owner of Fleur de Lys restaurant in San Francisco, voted the best restaurant in the United States by *Esquire* magazine. He was selected one of the top ten chefs in America in 1988 by *Food & Wine* magazine.

**Michael Lomonaco** is the executive chef of the famed "21" Club in New York City.

**Sharon Luce** is a California realtor and part-time aerobics teacher with a taste for healthy low-fat cuisine.

**Deborah Madison** is author of *The Greens Cookbook* and *The Savory Way* (Bantam). A co-founder of Greens restaurant on San Francisco Bay, she is currently chef and proprietor of Cafe Escalera in Santa Fe, New Mexico.

**Margaret Malone** is a chef at Milly's in San Rafael, California.

**Michael McDermott** is the creator and host of *The Food Show* and author of *The Healthful Gourmet.*

**Donna Nicoletti** is chef and co-owner of the Undici restaurant in San Francisco, where she re-creates dishes of her southern Italian heritage.

**Jill O'Connor,** former pastry chef at the Golden Door Fitness Spa, is author of *Sweet Nothings* (Chronicle Books).

**Bradley Ogden** is co-owner and executive chef of the Lark Creek Inn in Larkspur, California, and One Market Street in San Francisco. He is the author of *Bradley Ogden's Breakfast, Lunch & Dinner* (Random House).

**Natalie Ornish** is the mother of Dean Ornish and three others. She has composed and produced music, books, plays, and films for children. She currently lectures and writes about early Texas history.

**Catherine Pantsios** was chef and co-owner of Zola's restaurant in San Francisco. She has contributed to the *Open Hand* cookbook and several other publications.

**Alfred Portale** is executive chef at the Gotham Bar & Grill in New York City. He graduated first in his class from the Culinary Institute of America in 1981 and won the 1990 Ivy award.

**Wolfgang Puck** is chef and co-owner of several restaurants, including Spago and Eureka in Los Angeles, Chinois on Main in Santa Monica, Granita in Malibu, and Postrio in San Francisco. He is the author of several books, including *The Wolfgang Puck Cookbook* and *Adventures in the Kitchen* (Random House).

**Tracy Pikhart Ritter** is the former executive chef at the Golden Door Fitness Spa. She is the owner of Stamina Cuisine in San Diego.

**Alain Rondelli** was chef for French president Valéry Giscard d'Estaing at the Palais de l'Eysée. He is currently the executive chef at Ernie's in San Francisco.

**Tina Salter and Christine Swett** contributed to the California Culinary Academy's book *Cooking A–Z.* They also act as cooking consultants to major department stores and cookware manufacturers.

**Martha Rose Shulman** is the author of several books, including *The Vegetarian Feast, Fast Vegetarian Feasts, Mediterranean Light,* and *Entertaining Light* (Bantam). She developed the recipes for Dr. Ornish's first book, *Stress, Diet & Your Heart,* and is a frequent contributor to *Eating Well* magazine.

**Barbara Tropp** is a China scholar turned Chinese cook. She is the chef and owner of China Moon restaurant in San Francisco, and the author of *The Modern Art of Chinese Cooking* (Morrow) and the *China Moon Cookbook* (Workman).

Recipes were also provided by participants and staff of the Lifestyle Heart Trial, including: John and Phyllis Cardozo, Joe and Anita Cecena, Hank and Phyllis Ginsberg, Victor and Lydia Karpenko, Conrad and Marsha Knudsen, Myrna Melling, Paul Paulsen, and Don Vaupel.

# Notes

**PAGE** **CHAPTER 1**

4 "Over the years": G. Kolata, "Vindication for a Leading Proponent of Theory, 'People Are Born to Be Fat,' " *The New York Times,* 2/25/88, sec. B, p. 5; and J. Hirsch, and R. L. Leibel, "New light on obesity" [editorial], *New England Journal of Medicine,* 1988, 318:509–10.

5 "At least half of obese people": Jane E. Brody, "Research Lifts Blame from Many of the Obese," *The New York Times,* 3/24/87, sec. C, p. 1.

5 "There is not one single": Sandy Rovner, "Diets Don't Work, Obesity Experts Are Told," *The Washington Post,* 6/25/86, Health section, p. 10.

5 "I can see": Ibid.

5 "A growing number of women": Molly O'Neil, *The New York Times,* 4/12/92.

6 Over one-third of children were overweight: Nanci Hellmich, "Today's Kids Weigh In Heavier," *USA Today,* 9/25/92.

6 One out of three girls: Larry Thompson, "Young Girls Diet to Please Mother," *The Washington Post,* 5/10/88, p. Z5.

15 Your weight is partially determined: T. I. Sorensen, C. Holst, A. J. Stunkard, and L. T. Skovgaard, "Correlations

of body mass index of adult adoptees and their biological and adoptive relatives," *International Journal of Obesity,* 1992, 16(3):227–36; and A. J. Stunkard, T. T. Foch, and Z. Hrubec, "A twin study of human obesity," *Journal of the American Medical Association,* 1986, 256(1):51–4.

15 "you have to have the environment": Gina Kolata, "The Burdens of Being Overweight," *The New York Times,* 11/22/92, sec. 1, p. 18.

15 overweight parents tend: Rovner, "Diets Don't Work," quoting Dr. William Dietz; and W. H. Dietz, Jr., "Prevention of childhood obesity," *Pediatric Clinics of North America,* 1986, 33(4):823–33.

**CHAPTER 3**

25 Only about 1 percent of dietary protein: Jane Brody, "Research Lifts Blame from Many of the Obese," *The New York Times,* 3/24/87, sec. C, p. 1.

29 rats who lost and regained weight: K. D. Brownell, M. R. Greenwood, E. Stellar, and E. E. Shrager, "The effects of repeated cycles of weight loss and regain in rats," *Physiology and Behavior,* 1986, 38(4):459–64.

29 changes in metabolism of wrestlers: S. N. Steen, R. A. Oppliger, and K. D. Brownell, "Metabolic effects of repeated weight loss and regain in adolescent wrestlers," *Journal of the American Medical Association,* 1988, 260(1):47–50.

30 the more your weight fluctuates: L. Lissner, P. M. Odell, R. B. D'Agostino, J. Stokes, 3d, B. E. Kreger, A. J. Belanger, and K. D. Brownell, "Variability of body weight and health outcomes in the Framingham population," *New England Journal of Medicine,* 1991, 324(26):1839–44.

30 Dr. Olaf Mickelsen: Cited in Marian Burros, "Carbohydrates Are a Dieter's Best Friend," *The New York Times,* 3/6/91, sec. C, p. 1.

31 "These results demonstrate": A. Kendall, D. A. Levitsky, B. J. Strupp, and L. Lissner, "Weight loss on a low-fat diet: consequence of the imprecision of the control of food

intake in humans," *American Journal of Clinical Nutrition,* 1991, 53(5):1124–9.

31 "Maybe the body can't detect": Quoted by Marian Burros in "Eating Well," *The New York Times,* 5/22/91, sec. C, p. 3.

32 thyroid hormone: R. A. Mathieson, J. L. Walberg, F. C. Gwazdauskas, et al., "The effect of varying carbohydrate content of a very-low-caloric diet on resting metabolic rate and thyroid hormones," *Metabolism,* 1986, 35:394–8; E. Danforth, Jr., E. S. Horton, M. O'Connell, E. A. Sims, A. G. Burger, S. H. Ingbar, L. Braverman, and A. G. Vagenakis, "Dietary-induced alterations in thyroid hormone metabolism during overnutrition," *Journal of Clinical Investigation,* 1979, 64(5):1336–47; and S. W. Spaulding, I. J. Chopra, R. S. Sherwin, and S. S. Lyall, "Effect of caloric restriction and dietary composition of serum T3 and reverse T3 in man," *Journal of Clinical Endocrinology and Metabolism,* 1976, 42(1):197–200.

32 grazing is good for you: J. A. Jenkins-David, Thomas Wolever, Vladimir Vuksan, Furio Brighenti, Stephen C. Cunnane, A. Venketshwer Rao, Alexandra L. Jenkins, Gloria Buckley, Robert Patten, William Singer, Paul Corey, and Robert G. Josse, "Nibbling versus gorging: metabolic advantages of increased meal frequency," *New England Journal of Medicine,* 1989, 321 (14):929–34.

33 increases the uptake of fat: P. A. Kern, J. M. Ong, B. Saffari, and J. Carty, "The effects of weight loss on the activity and expression of adipose-tissue lipoprotein lipase in very obese humans," *New England Journal of Medicine,* 1990, 322(15):1053–9.

33 When your insulin levels rise: J. M. Dietschy and M. S. Brown, "Effect of alterations of the specific activity of the intracellular acetyl CoA pool on apparent rates of hepatic cholesterogenesis," *Journal of Lipid Research,* 1974, 15: 508–16.

33 insulin enhances the growth: R. W. Stout, "Insulin-stimulated lipogenesis in arterial tissue in relation to diabetes and atheroma," *Lancet,* 1968, 2:702–3; and Y. Sato, S. Shiraishi, Y. Oshida, T. Ishiguro, and N. Sakamoto,

"Experimental atherosclerosis-like lesions induced by hyperinsulinism in Wistar rats," *Diabetes,* 1989, 38:91–6.

34 people with high insulin levels: P. Fabry and J. Tepperman, "Meal frequency—a possible factor in human pathology," *American Journal of Clinical Nutrition,* 1970, 23:1059–68.

34 people with high blood pressure: P. Singer, W. Godicke, S. Voigt, I. Hajdu, and M. Weiss, "Postprandial hyperinsulinemia in patients with mild essential hypertension," *Hypertension,* 1985, 7(2):182–6.

34 increased risk of breast cancer: D. V. Schapira, N. B. Kumar, G. H. Lyman, D. Cavanagh, W. S. Roberts, and J. LaPolla, "Upper-body fat distribution and endometrial cancer risk," *Journal of the American Medical Association,* 1991, 266(13):1808–11.

34 LDL ("bad") cholesterol: R. R. Wing, K. A. Matthews, L. H. Kuller, E. N. Meilahn, and P. Plantinga, "Waist to hip ratio in middle-aged women. Associations with behavioral and psychosocial factors and with changes in cardiovascular risk factors," *Arteriosclerosis and Thrombosis,* 1991, 11(5):1250–7.

36 Nonvegetarian women: B. R. Goldin, H. Adlercreutz, J. T. Dwyer, L. Swenson, J. H. Warram, and S. L. Gorbach, "Effect of diet on excretion of estrogens in pre- and postmenopausal women," *Cancer Research,* 1981, 41(9 Pt. 2):3771–3; and B. R. Goldin, H. Adlercreutz, S. L. Gorbach, J. H. Warram, J. T. Dwyer, L. Swenson and M. N. Woods, "Estrogen excretion patterns and plasma levels in vegetarian and omnivorous women," *New England Journal of Medicine,* 1982, 307(25):1542–7.

36 shown to retard aging: E. J. Masoro, I. Shimokawa, and B. P. Yu, "Retardation of the aging processes in rats by food restriction," *Annals of the New York Academy of Sciences,* 1991, 621:337–52.

36 "Clearly, although energy intake": C. Kubo, B. C. Johnson, A. Gajjar, and R. A. Good, "Crucial dietary factors in maximizing life span and longevity in autoimmune-prone mice," *Journal of Nutrition,* 1987, 117(6):1129–35.

36 restricting calories "typically and strongly lowers": R. Weindruch, (National Institute on Aging, Biomedical Research and Clinical Medicine Program, Bethesda, MD 20892), "Dietary restriction, tumors, and aging in rodents," *Journal of Gerontology,* 1989, 44(6):67–71.

36 "Restriction of dietary energy": E. J. Masoro, "Aging and proliferative homeostasis: modulation by food restriction in rodents," *Laboratory Animal Science,* 1992, 42(2):132–7.

36 "In experimental animals": M. T. Tacconi, L. Lligona, M. Salmona, N. Pitsikas, and S. Algeri, "Aging and food restriction: effect on lipids of cerebral cortex," *Neurobiology of Aging,* 1991, 12(1):55–9.

36 Eating fewer calories: C. Pieri, "Food restriction slows down age-related changes in cell membrane parameters," *Annals of the New York Academy of Sciences,* 1991, 621:353–62.

37 "Restricting the food intake of rodents": E. J. Masoro, "Assessment of nutritional components in prolongation of life and health by diet," *Proceedings of the Society for Experimental Biology and Medicine,* 1990, 193(1):31–4.

37 iron is a potent risk factor: J. T. Salonen, K. Nyyssonen, H. Korpela, J. Tuomilehto, R. Seppanen, and R. Salonen, "High stored iron levels are associated with excess risk of myocardial infarction in eastern Finnish men," *Circulation,* 1992, 86(3):803–11; and J. L. Sullivan, "Iron and the sex difference in heart disease risk," *Lancet,* 1981, 1(8233):1293–4.

## CHAPTER 4

40 In 1910, Americans: Marion Burros, "Carbohydrates Are a Dieter's Best Friend," *The New York Times,* 3/6/91, sec. C, p. 1.

41 A study at Stanford: D. M. Dreon, B. Frey-Hewlett, N. Ellsworth, et al., "Dietary fat: carbohydrate ratio and obesity in middle-aged men," *American Journal of Clinical Nutrition,* 1988, 47:995–1000.

41 a comprehensive study of more than 6,500 Chinese: J. Chen, T. C. Campbell, J. Li, and R. Peto, *Diet, Lifestyle, and Mortality in China: A Study of the Characteristics of 65 Chinese Counties* (Oxford: Oxford University Press, 1990).

42 In 1991, 408 fat-free products: L. Miller, "Pizza Joins Ranks of Fat-free Foods," *USA Today,* 10/13/92, sec. D, p. 6.

44 Many others have recognized: R. Berry, *Famous Vegetarians & Their Favorite Recipes* (Los Angeles: Panjandrum Books, 1989).

45 "If you can't *be* a vegetarian": G. C. Griffin and W. P. Castelli, *Good Fat, Bad Fat* (Tucson: Fisher Books, 1989).

46 "Plant Products" table: *Agriculture Handbook No. 8, Revised, Composition of Foods, Raw, Processed, Prepared,* sections 8-1 through 8-20, U.S. Department of Agriculture, Washington, D.C.

48 "How do actresses": *McCall's* Tells All, *McCall's,* November 1992, p. 159.

48 "Madonna works out": *Mirabella,* December 1992.

49 adding complex carbohydrates to food: L. Lissner, D. Levitsky, B. J. Strupp, et al., "Dietary fat and the regulation of energy intake in human subjects," *American Journal of Clinical Nutrition,* 1987, 46(6):886–92.

50 three ounces of alcohol: P. M. Suter, Y. Schutz, and E. Jequier, "The effect of ethanol on fat storage in healthy subjects," *New England Journal of Medicine,* 1992, 326(15):983–7.

51 caffeine may increase your metabolism: A. G. Dulloo, C. A. Geissler, T. Horton, A. Collins, and D. S. Miller, "Normal caffeine consumption: influence on thermogenesis and daily energy expenditure in lean and postobese human volunteers," *American Journal of Clinical Nutrition,* 1989, 49(1):44–50.

59 "gut hungry": J. P. Foreyt and G. K. Goodrick, *Living Without Dieting* (Houston: Harrison Publishing, 1992).

59 moderately overweight women who regularly skipped breakfast: D. G. Schlundt, J. O. Hill, T. Sbrocco, J. Pope-Cordle, and T. Sharp, "The role of breakfast in the treatment of obesity: a randomized clinical trial," *American Journal of Clinical Nutrition,* 1992, 55(3)645–51.

**CHAPTER 5**

60 self-described couch potatoes: E. M. Bennett (Center for Disease Control, 1987), quoted in *The Los Angeles Times,* 8/4/89, part 1, p. 2.

61 Moderate exercise gives you most: S. N. Blair, H. W. Kohl, 3d, R. S. Paffenbarger, Jr., D. G. Clark, K. H. Cooper, and L. W. Gibbons, "Physical fitness and all-cause mortality. A prospective study of healthy men and women," *Journal of the American Medical Association,* 1989, 262(17):2395–401; R. S. Paffenbarger, Jr., R. T. Hyde, A. L. Wing, and C. C. Hsieh, "Physical activity, all-cause mortality, and longevity of college alumni," *New England Journal of Medicine,* 1986, 314(10):605–13; and A. S. Leon, J. Connett, D. R. Jacobs, Jr., and R. Rauramaa, "Leisure-time physical activity levels and risk of coronary heart disease and death. The Multiple Risk Factor Intervention Trial," *Journal of the American Medical Association,* 1987, 258(17):2388–95.

61 strollers lost more weight: J. J. Duncan, N. F. Gordon, and C. B. Scott, "Women walking for health and fitness. How much is enough?" *Journal of the American Medical Association,* 1991, 266(23):3295–9.

61 regular, moderate exercise: C. M. Grilo, K. D. Brownell, and A. J. Stunkard, "The metabolic and psychological importance of exercise in weight control," in A. J. Stunkard and T. A. Wadden eds. *Obesity: Theory and Therapy* (New York: Raven Press, 1992).

62 When you exercise intensely: J. Rodin, *Body Traps* (New York: William Morrow, 1992).

62 Moderate exercise may also improve: H. Northoff and A. Berg, "Immunologic mediators as parameters of the

reaction to strenuous exercise," *International Journal of Sports Medicine,* 1991, 12:S9–S15.

62 excessive exercise may depress: L. Fitzgerald, "Overtraining increases the susceptibility to infection," *International Journal of Sports Medicine,* 1991, 12:S5–S8.

62 A study of 2,300 marathon runners: D. C. Neiman, "Exercise: How Much Is Enough?" *Women's Sports and Fitness,* June 1989.

62 low to moderate levels of exercise: R. K. Dishman, "Medical psychology in exercise and sports," *Medical Clinics of North America,* 1985, 69:123–43.

62 high-intensity exercise: J. Rodin and T. G. Plante, "The psychological effects of exercise," in R. S. William and A. Wallace eds., *Biological Effects of Physical Activity* (Champaign, Ill: Human Kinetics Books, 1989); and A. Luger, P. A. Deuster, S. B. Kyle, et al., "Acute hypothalamic-pituitary-adrenal responses to the stress of treadmill exercise. Physiologic adaptations to physical training," *New England Journal of Medicine,* 1987, 316(21):1309–15.

62 "For some exercise-dependent people": J. Rodin, *Body Traps* (New York: William Morrow, 1992).

63 they had a higher percentage of body fat: J. S. Stern and E. A. Applegate, "Exercise termination effects on food intake, plasma insulin, and adipose tissue lipoprotein lipase activity in the Osborne-Mendel rat," *Metabolism,* 1987, 36:709–14.

63 Even athletes who start and stop: K. D. Brownell, S. N. Steen, and J. M. Wilmore, "Weight regulation practices in athletes," *Medicine and Science in Sports and Exercise,* 1987, 19:552–60.

64 "Most of the decline": W. Evans and I. Rosenberg, *Biomarkers* (New York: Simon & Schuster, 1991).

64 "The findings that moderate levels": C. M. Grillo, D. E. Wilfley, and K. D. Brownell, "Physical activity and weight control: why is the link so strong?" *Weight Control Digest,* 1992, 2:153–68.

## CHAPTER 6

68 major international scientific meeting: "Symposium I: Prevention: From Children to the Elderly," The Second International Symposium on Multiple Risk Factors in Cardiovascular Disease, October 5–8, 1992, Osaka, Japan, sponsored by the National Heart, Lung, and Blood Institute, NIH, and the Giovanni Lorenzini Medical Foundation.

68 Cholesterol levels in Japanese boys: R. J. Deckelbaum, ibid.

73 heart disease improves, and so on: D. Ornish and S. E. Brown, "Treatment and screening for hyperlipidemia," *New England Journal of Medicine,* 1993, 329(15):1124–25.

79 *People who feel socially isolated:* J. S. House, K. R. Landis, and D. Umberson, "Social relationships and health," *Science,* 1988, 241(4865):540–45.

79 studied three groups of women: S. Kayman, W. Bruvold and J. S. Stern, "Maintenance and relapse after weight loss in women: behavioral aspects," *American Journal of Clinical Nutrition,* 1990, 52(5):800–7.

80 one of the most recent and well-designed prospective studies: L. Berkman, presented to the International Society of Behavioral Medicine, Hamburg, Germany; also, Lisa Berkman, Linda Leo-Summers, and Ralph Horwitz, *Annals of Internal Medicine, 1992,* 1992, 117(12):1003–9.

86 a very overweight millionaire: C. S. Rand and A. M. MacGregor, "Successful weight loss following obesity surgery and the perceived liability of morbid obesity," *International Journal of Obesity,* 1991, 15(9):577–79.

86 "The problem is": G. Leonard, *Mastery* (New York: Dutton, 1991), p. 110.

## CHAPTER 7

93 carbohydrates may increase the levels: J. D. Fernstrom, "Dietary effects on brain serotonin synthesis: relationship to appetite regulation," *American Journal of Clinical Nutrition,* 1985, 42(5 Suppl):1072–82.

93 a diet rich in complex carbohydrates: J. J. Wurtman, "Carbohydrate craving. Relationship between carbohydrate intake and disorders of mood," *Drugs,* 1990, 39 (Suppl. 3):49–52.

93 alpha-amylase activity: D. R. Morse, G. R. Schacterle, L. Furst, M. Zaydenberg, and R. L. Pollack, "Oral digestion of a complex-carbohydrate cereal: effects of stress and relaxation on physiological and salivary measures," *American Journal of Clinical Nutrition,* 1989, 49(1):97–105.

96 The state of relaxation: H. Benson, "Systemic hypertension and the relaxation response," *New England Journal of Medicine,* 1977, 296:1152–56.

100 Learning communication skills: D. Ornish, *Dr. Dean Ornish's Program for Reversing Heart Disease* (New York: Ballantine Books, 1992).

103 "All of my life I thought": P. Farrell, "Diets and Other Decisions: Admitting Weight Is a Problem—But Not *the* Problem," *The Washington Post,* 2/28/89, Health section, p. Z17.

105 "Self is everywhere": Mundaka Upanishad, in S. Mitchell, *The Enlightened Heart: An Anthology of Sacred Poetry* (New York: Harper & Row, 1989).

# For Further Reading

There are many excellent books on the various topics discussed in this book. Here are only a few:

BARNARD, NEAL D. *A Physician's Slimming Guide for Permanent Weight Control.* Summertown, TN: The Book Publishing Company, 1992.

BASKIN, ROSEMARY. *How Many Calories? How Much Fat?* Yonkers, NY: Consumer Reports Books, 1991.

BELLERSON, KAREN J. *The Complete & Up-to-Date Fat Book.* Garden City Park, NY: Avery Publishing Group, 1991.

BENSON, HERBERT. *Beyond the Relaxation Response.* New York: Times Books, 1984.

BORYSENKO, JOAN. *Minding the Body, Mending the Mind.* New York: Bantam Books, 1988.

DAVID, MARC. *Nourishing Wisdom.* New York: Bell Tower Books, 1991.

FERGUSON, TOM. *The No-Nag, No-Guilt, Do-It-Your-Own-Way Guide to Quitting Smoking.* New York: Ballantine Books, 1989.

FOREYT, JOHN P., and GOODRICK, G. KEN. *Living Without Dieting.* Houston: Harrison Publishing, 1992.

GOLEMAN, DANIEL. *The Meditative Mind.* Los Angeles: Jeremy Tarcher, 1988.

GOOR, RON, and GOOR, NANCY. *The Choose to Lose Diet.* Boston: Houghton Mifflin Company, 1990.

KABAT-ZINN, JON. *Full Catastrophe Living: A Practical Guide to Mindfulness, Meditation, and Healing.* New York: Delacorte Press, 1990.

LANGER, ELLEN J. *Mindfulness.* New York: Addison-Wesley, 1989.

LEONARD, GEORGE. *Mastery.* New York: Dutton, 1991.

MATELJAN, GEORGE. *Cooking Without Fat.* Irwindale, CA: Health Valley Foods, 1992.

MCDOUGALL, JOHN. *McDougall's Medicine.* Clinton, NJ: New Win Publishing, 1985.

MITCHELL, STEPHEN. *The Enlightened Heart.* New York: Harper & Row, 1989.

———. *The Enlightened Mind.* New York: HarperCollins, 1991.

MORAN, VICTORIA. *The Love-Powered Diet.* San Rafael, CA: New World Library, 1992.

MURPHY, MICHAEL. *The Future of the Body.* Los Angeles: Jeremy Tarcher, 1992.

ORNISH, DEAN. *Dr. Dean Ornish's Program for Reversing Heart Disease.* New York: Ballantine Books, 1992.

———. "Changing Life Habits." In Moyers, Bill. *Healing and the Mind.* New York: Doubleday, 1993.

PRABHAVANANDA, SWAMI, and ISHERWOOD, CHRISTOPHER. *How to Know God.* Hollywood: Vedanta Press, 1953.

PRITIKIN, NATHAN, and MCGRADY, PATRICK. *Pritikin Program for Diet & Exercise.* New York: Grosset & Dunlap, 1979.

ROBBINS, JOHN. *May All Be Fed.* New York: William Morrow, 1992.

RODIN, JUDITH. *Body Traps: Breaking the Binds That Keep You from Feeling Good About Your Body.* New York: William Morrow, 1992.

ROSSMAN, MARTIN. *Healing Yourself.* New York: Pocket Books, 1987.

ROTH, GENEEN. *When Food Is Love: Exploring the Relationship Between Eating and Intimacy.* New York: Plume Books, 1992.

SATCHIDANANDA, SWAMI. *Beyond Words.* New York: Holt, Rinehart & Winston, 1977.

———. *The Golden Present.* Yogaville, VA: Integral Yoga Publications, 1987.

———. *Integral Yoga Hatha.* New York: Holt, Rinehart & Winston, 1970.

SIEGEL, BERNARD. *Peace, Love, and Healing.* New York: HarperCollins, 1989.

WOLF, NAOMI. *The Beauty Myth.* New York: Anchor Books/Doubleday, 1992.

# *General Index*

# *Recipe Index*

The Preventive Medicine Research Institute (PMRI) is a non-profit public institute dedicated to research, education, and service. My colleagues and I at PMRI and at other organizations offer a variety of resources and educational opportunities.

Please call (415) 332-2525 or write to the address below if you want to be put on our mailing list for information on our various activities, including hospital programs, foods, educational materials, training programs, and residential retreats.

We are also on the World Wide Web at *www.Ornish.com* or at *www.ivillage.com.*

I am very interested in learning of your experience with this book or with my program, and I welcome and would be grateful for any comments and suggestions. Due to the volume of correspondence, I am sorry that I am not able to reply personally or to answer medical questions. Please write to me at:

Preventive Medicine Research Institute
1001 Bridgeway, Box 305
Sausalito, CA 94965
USA

Thank you very much for your interest.

—Dean Ornish, M.D.